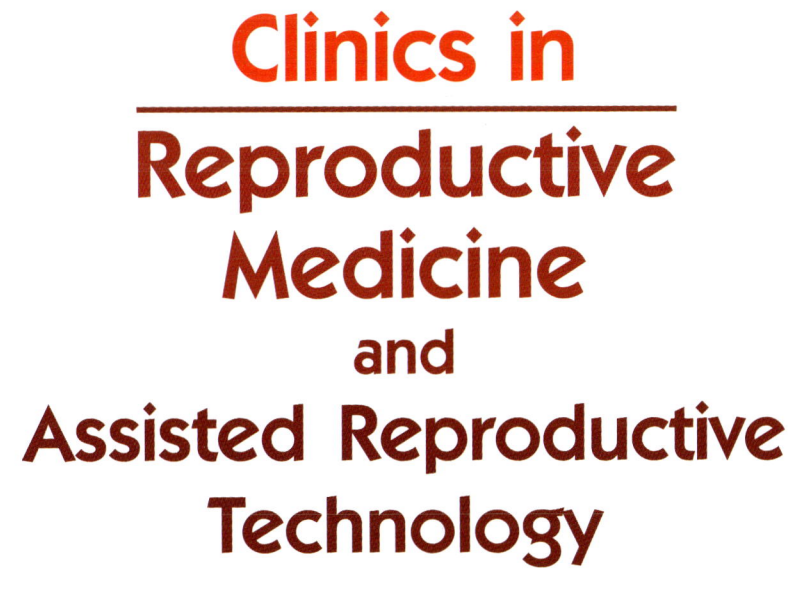

Clinics in
Reproductive
Medicine
and
Assisted Reproductive
Technology

Volume 1

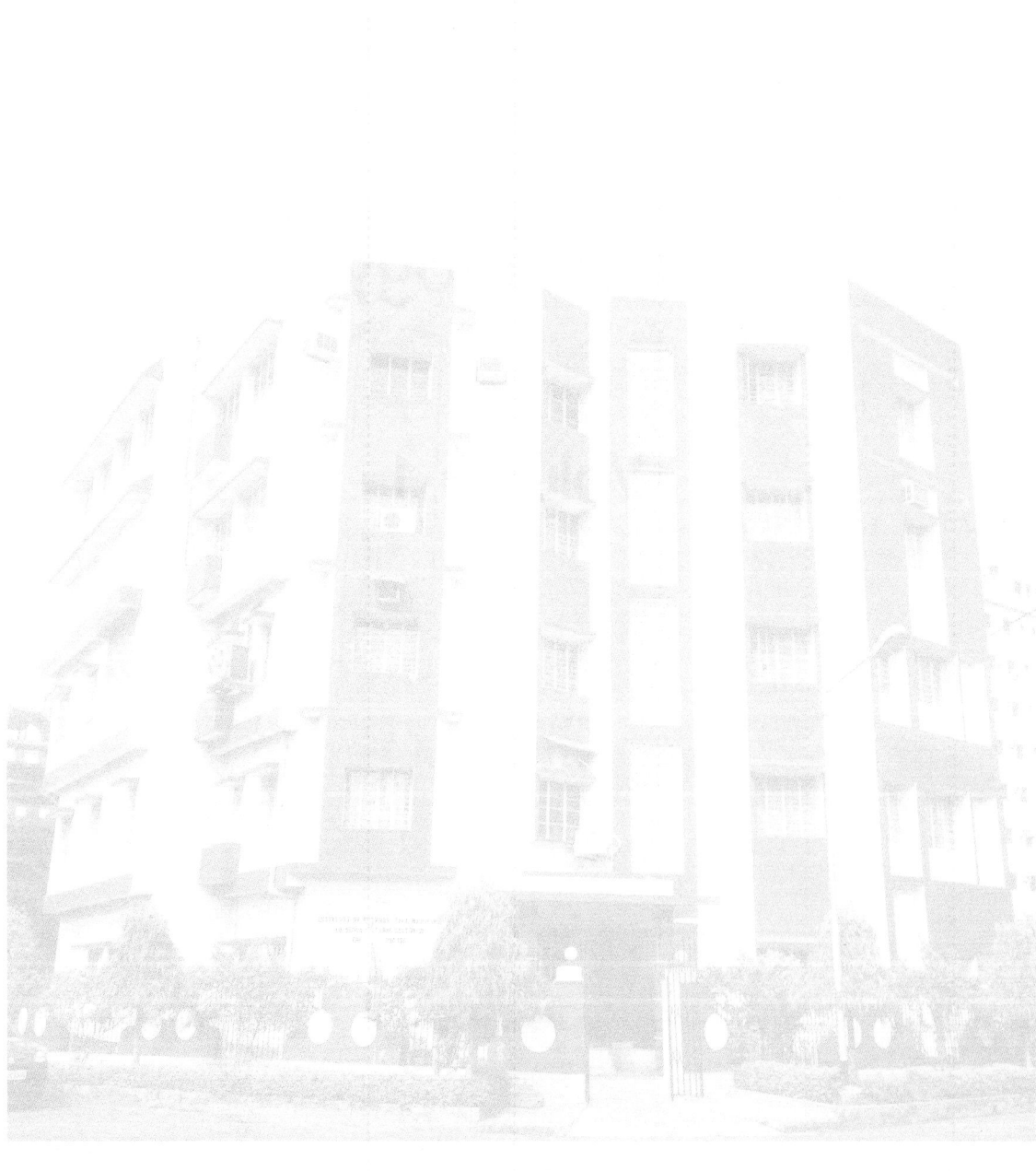

Clinics in
Reproductive
Medicine
and
Assisted Reproductive
Technology

Volume 1

BN Chakravarty
MO (Cal), FRCOG (Lond), DSc (hon)

Director
Institute of Reproductive Medicine
Kolkata, WB
India

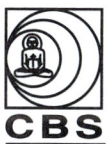

CBS

CBS Publishers & Distributors Pvt Ltd

New Delhi • Bengaluru • Chennai • Kochi • Kolkata • Mumbai
Bhopal • Bhubaneswar • Hyderabad • Jharkhand • Nagpur • Patna • Pune
Uttarakhand • Dhaka (Bangladesh)

Clinics in
Reproductive Medicine and
Assisted Reproductive Technology
Volume 1

ISBN: 978-81-239-2645-2

Copyright © Author and Publisher

First Edition: 2015

Reprint: 2019

Published by Satish Kumar Jain and Produced by Varun Jain for

CBS Publishers & Distributors Pvt Ltd
4819/XI Prahlad Street, 24 Ansari Road, Daryaganj, New Delhi 110 002, India.
Ph: 23289259, 23266861, 23266867   Fax: 011-23243014   Website: www.cbspd.com
                                                                 e-mail: delhi@cbspd.com; cbspubs@airtelmail.in.
Corporate Office: 204 FIE, Industrial Area, Patparganj, Delhi 110 092
Ph: 4934 4934   Fax: 4934 4935   e-mail: publishing@cbspd.com; publicity@cbspd.com

Branches

- **Bengaluru:** Seema House 2975, 17th Cross, K.R. Road, Banasankari 2nd Stage, Bengaluru 560 070, Karnataka
  Ph: +91-80-26771678/79   Fax: +91-80-26771680   e-mail: bangalore@cbspd.com
- **Chennai:** 7, Subbaraya Street, Shenoy Nagar, Chennai 600 030, Tamil Nadu
  Ph: +91-44-26680620, 26681266   Fax: +91-44-42032115   e-mail: chennai@cbspd.com
- **Kochi:** 42/1325, 1326, Power House Road, Opp. KSEB Power House Ernakulam 682 018, Kochi, Kerala
  Ph: +91-484-4059061-65   Fax: +91-484-4059065   e-mail: kochi@cbspd.com
- **Kolkata:** 6/B, Ground Floor, Rameswar Shaw Road, Kolkata-700 014, West Bengal
  Ph: +91-33-22891126, 22891127, 22891128   e-mail: kolkata@cbspd.com
- **Mumbai:** 83-C, Dr E Moses Road, Worli, Mumbai-400018, Maharashtra
  Ph: +91-22-24902340/41   Fax: +91-22-24902342   e-mail: mumbai@cbspd.com

Representatives

• Bhopal	0-8319310552	• Bhubaneswar	0-9911037372	• Hyderabad	0-9885175004	• Jharkhand	0-9811541605
• Nagpur	0-9021734563	• Patna	0-9334159340	• Pune	0-9623451994	• Uttarakhand	0-9716462459
• Dhaka (Bangladesh)	01912-003485						

Printed at Nutech Print Services, Faridabad, India

to

---

the students
whom I have taught
and the patients
whom I have treated

Preface

Around 1950s, soon after the Second World War, there were numerous innovations in the vast field of medical science. As a consequence, several superspecialties were identified for the purpose of specialised training and treatment. Most of them have already been recognised for postdoctoral training and specialisation. Examples include cardiology, ophthalmology, otolaryngology, paediatrics, radiology and oncology. On the other hand, recognition of reproductive medicine, a newborn superspecialty in medical curriculum, was relatively late. This discipline, as a superspecialty, was well-established following the advent of assisted reproductive technology (ART). Though science of embryology was documented as early as 1875 by Oscar Hertwig in Germany, it was a difficult subject to study in humans. At that time most knowledge of human reproduction was achieved through animal experiments. Scope of observation and research directly in humans has only been possible following the introduction of assisted reproductive technology in the treatment of infertility. The process of gametogenesis, their maturation, sperm egg interaction, fertilisation and implantation are a few of the major information which have been derived through clinical application of assisted reproduction.

Endocrine background of human reproduction was realised much earlier from late 1920s. Fertility enhancing drugs like gonadotropin, clomiphene and bromocriptine, in addition to fertility preventing drugs like oral contraceptives were discovered and introduced for clinical use around the early 1960s. Knowledge and expertise for clinical use of these hormones expanded further with introduction of gadgets and technologies like ultrasound, laparoscope, RIA and EIA. These technologies have opened up avenues for better understanding of physiology at molecular level of folliculogenesis and ovulation, pathophysiology of PCOS, precocious puberty, premature menopause and many others.

ART has brought about an unprecedented revolution in the treatment of human infertility. The procedure has not only provided help to relieve the distress of childless couples but also has opened up avenues of potential research. One of them is stem cell research which is heading towards another medical discovery through tissue engineering and has already established the foundation stone of a new superspecialty—regenerative medicine. Apart from stem cell research, ART has also provided novel protocols for fertility preservation during and preceding oncotherapy in young cancer victims, both boys and girls.

In 1990s, there has been a breakthrough in the treatment of male infertility through introduction of intracytoplasmic sperm injection (ICSI) procedure. However, till now we do not know the exact treatment of male infertility because in ICSI gametes are treated, but not the individual. Andrology and spermatology are expanding fast and it is expected that many obscure areas in male reproduction will be explored in the near future. Expansion of genetic and immunological knowledge has widened our views on amenorrhoea, recurrent miscarriage and sexual ambiguity.

In spite of all these advances in science and technology, ART still has practical limitations, primarily in four areas which have become a source of concern for the clinician. These are

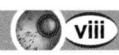

(*a*) cost, (*b*) complexities of treatment, (*c*) complications and (*d*) results, at least the prediction of outcome. Clinicians and researchers alike have joined hands to overcome these problems.

Enormous volumes of publications have accumulated over the years discussing ways and procedures for solving these persistent deficiencies of ART through development of good quality embryos, generating effective endometrial receptivity and finding ways for performing smooth and atraumatic embryo replacement. Though to some extent some of the objectives have been achieved, yet many more remained elusive.

Recent publications emphasise more on optimising stimulation protocol, redirecting approaches for mild ovarian stimulation, a move towards single embryo transfer, reducing embryo stress by introducing metabolomics in culture system, time-lapse embryoscope, and attempting to predict endometrial receptivity through non-invasive markers like uterine fluid, follicular fluid components and many others.

From the academic point of view, it is apparent that comprehensive knowledge in reproductive medicine demands a sound background of different branches of basic science and their intelligent application in clinical medicine. Unfortunately, in our medical postgraduate teaching and examinations, these two aspects of the same superspecialty have been segregated. For example, in MD (Obs and Gynae) examination, the emphasis is more on clinical aspect, whereas the PhD course syllabus and training has been oriented more on the basic aspect rather than its clinical application. There is an urgent need for bridging the gap between the two.

However, as far as I am concerned, during my professional career which covers nearly a period of five decades, I had the privilege of being continuously associated with medical teaching, both undergraduate and postgraduate. This uninterrupted commitment has helped me immensely in keeping myself updated with contemporary advances, both basic and clinical aspects of my respective discipline.

I have been teaching reproductive medicine in fellowship and PhD course for the last 20 years. Over the years I have updated and upgraded my teaching slides with contemporary information and novel experiences that I had gathered during my clinical practice. This has provided some opportunities for me to unify both basic and clinical aspects together which I learnt during the last decade of my teaching career. The incentive for writing a book came from my students whom I taught and from my colleagues with whom I have worked from the beginning of my career. Nevertheless, one of my ambitions was not fulfilled owing to my busy schedule during my working years. I could hardly get some time to concentrate and write a book, which I felt was a difficult task for me. The chapters of this book have been written in the way in which I teach my students—meaning thereby that each topic has been discussed from different angles. For example, the topic of PCOS has been covered in 5 different lectures:

  a. Adolescent PCOS—current management strategy
  b. Pubertal metabolic and endocrine changes—their relevance to adolescent PCOS
  c. Overview and management of PCOS
  d. Optimising ovarian stimulation of PCOS patients
  e. Changing concept in PCOS.

Each of these lecture notes has been converted into an individual chapter. To accommodate all these lecture notes, it was not possible to include them in a single publication. Therefore, it has been decided to publish the book in three or four different volumes.

My primary interest in infertility and subsequently in the discipline of reproductve medicine was created by my renowned colleague late Prof Subhas Mukherjee MBBS, DGO, PhD (Edin) who had pioneered the delivery of first 'test-tube baby' in India in 1978 and the second in

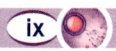

the world. My initial experience in ART was gathered through a small team of doctors (all my students) organised by me following the tragic death of Dr Mukherjee in 1981. The team primarily consisted of Dr Sudarshan Ghosh Dastidar, Dr Siddhartha Chatterjee, Dr Arup Kumar Majhi, Dr Sourendra Kanta Goswami, Dr Bani Kumar Mitra, Dr Sanghamitra Ghosh and Dr Ratna Chattopadhyay.

For writing this book I got continuous encouragement from Prof Dr Gita Ganguly Mukherjee MD, FICOG, FRCOG; Prof BB Hore MBBS DA, MS (Cal); Prof Subir Kumar Dutta MBBS, DCP, MD (Cal); Prof BB Sarkar MBBS, DGO, MO (Cal); Dr Biman Kumar Ghosh MBBS, DGO (Cal), DRCOG, EPA, FRCOG; Prof Hiralal Konar MD, DNB, FRCOG, FICOG; Dr Arup Kumar Majhi MBBS; DGO, MD (Cal); and all my students, present and past.

I express my deep appreciation to Dr Ratna Chattopadhyay, Dr Sourendra Kanta Goswami, Dr Sanghamitra Ghosh, Dr Radhika Kandula, Dr Rita Modi, Dr Geetha Rani BS, and Dr Anwesha Ghosh for their meticulous care and painstaking effort and for their assistance in repeated corrections, criticism and revision of my manuscript. I acknowledge and sincerely thank Dr Ratna Chattopadhyay and Dr Pratip Chakraborty for their individual contribution of two chapters on 'Nutraceutical in Male Infertility' and 'Insulin Resistance' respectively in this publication. I also thank and appreciate the efforts and devotion of my computer assistants Mr Ashis Shit, Mr Arup Ranjan Sarker and Ms Ria Chakraborty who have worked continuously and retyped the corrected manuscripts time and again.

Lastly, I have no words to appreciate the silent help offered by my wife Dr Manjusree Chakravarty, who has spared me from my domestic commitments and has continuously encouraged me to express my ideas through writing a book which might help the future generation.

I will be only too happy if the contents of the current and future volumes of this book are of benefit, both for information and for practice of the students and practitioners in reproductive medicine, for whom the book has been compiled.

BN Chakravarty

Preface to Volume 1

Since ART became popular in the treatment of infertility, volumes of literature are accumulating in various fields of reproductive medicine.

Many unexplored areas of human reproduction are being explored adding new information to our existing knowledge of this newly developing science. A few of these areas have been included in volume 1 of *Clinics in Reproductive Medicine and Assisted Reproductive Technology*. The areas covered in this volume are: Male infertility, low ovarian reserve, primary amenorrhoea and sexual ambiguity.

Male infertility is a current subject of interest which is responsible for 40–45% cases of failure of normal human reproduction. The precise background of etiological factors and the exact treatment in many areas of male infertility are still very vague. Attempt has been made to clarify some of these grey areas through clinical approach backed up by basic science and wherever appropriate at molecular level. The different aspects of male infertility covering etiology, investigation and management including ICSI have been dealt with in eight different subchapters. In this endeavour, I have been immensely supported by Dr Ratna Chattopadhyay, Chief Embryologist, IRM, who had been the backbone in writing two chapters in male infertility. These chapters are 'Reactive Oxygen Species' and 'Role of Nutraceuticals in Male Infertility'. She was actively supported by Dr Sanghamitra Ghosh, our chief sonologist, who helped constantly in compiling these chapters. In addition, all the manuscripts in the first volume of the book have been meticulously scrutinised by two of my FNB students, Dr Radhika L Kandula and Dr Geetha Rani BS, and valuable additions and information have been added to most of the chapters published in this volume. Dr Rita Modi, another FNB student of mine, now in Mumbai, has also contributed some new information in some of the chapters of this book.

'Low ovarian reserve' is another difficult subject in infertility and an obstinate problem to treat. This subject has also been dealt with in three different chapters, viz. 'Genesis', 'Predictors' and 'Management' of low ovarian reserve. I express may sincere appreciation and heartfelt thanks to Dr SK Goswami, Chief Clinician, IVF Unit, who gave valuable suggestions and made careful scrutiny of the chapters on low ovarian reserve.

Before starting my career in IVF, I was deeply committed to two very challenging but fascinating topics in gynaecology closely related to human reproduction. The topics are primary amenorrhoea, sexual ambiguity and intersex disorders. I did these works in collaboration with one of the most renowned colleagues of mine, Late Prof Subhas Mukherjee, and some of our observations have been published in prestigious international journals like *Lancet, American Journal of Obstetrics and Gynecology*, etc. In our endeavour we received active support from our geneticist Dr NJ Gupta, Prof Lalji Singh and Dr Thangaraj from CCMB, Hyderabad. Some of our original works related to these topics have been included in these two chapters of the book.

Last but not the least I must acknowledge the sincere support I received from Prof Gita Ganguly Mukherjee, Prof HL Konar, Prof BB Hore, Prof Subir Kumar Dutta and Dr Biman Kumar Ghosh, Dr Anwesha Ghosh, Dr Saktirupa Chakrabarty and many others for their constant encouragement for compilation of this volume of the book. I also sincerely thank

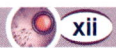

Mr Ashis Shit, Mr Arup Ranjan Sarkar and Ms Ria Chakraborty for their painstaking effort in repeated correction and typing of the manuscript.

I also express my deep sense of appreciation to my beloved wife Dr M Chakravarty, who helped me silently and provided courage to continue my professional and academic activities sparing me from the complexities of domestic duties.

The book is primarily written for the benefit of students undertaking training for fellowship and PhD degree in reproductive medicine in different universities and National Board. In addition, the book will also help young specialists who are aspiring to take up reproductive medicine as a superspecialty in their research and professional career. The chapters of the book have been outlined more on conventionally accepted facts than on controversy. Therefore, a list of too many references at the end of each chapter has been avoided. In a few chapters, in place of references a few relevant articles or the title of related textbooks have been cited for further review.

I shall feel very happy, if the contents of the book fulfill the purpose for which this has been written.

BN Chakravarty

The author appreciates the services and active support received from his following students during the course of the preparation of the manuscript of this volume.

Dr Ratna Chattopadhyay

Dr Sourendra Kanta Goswami

Dr Sanghamitra Ghosh

Dr Radhika L Kundula

Contents

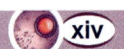

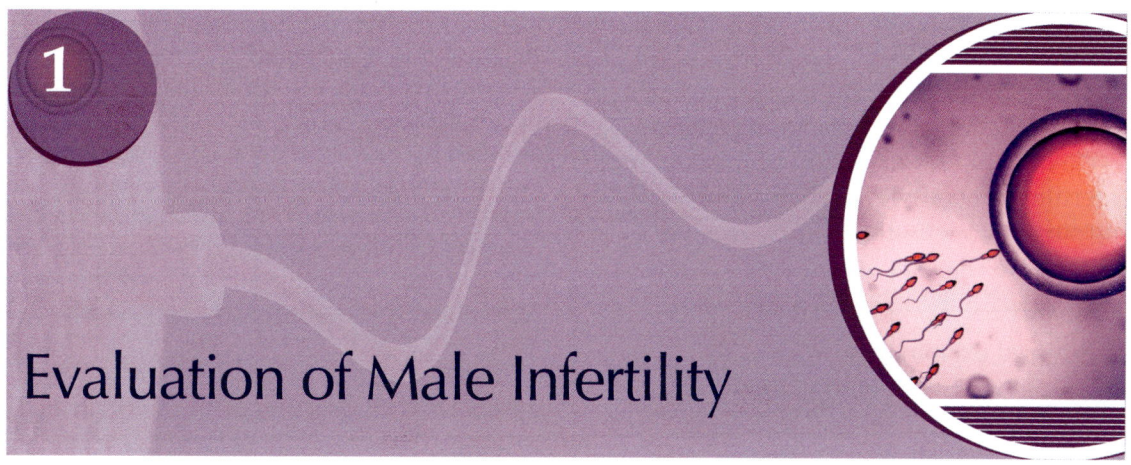

Evaluation of Male Infertility

INTRODUCTION

Infertility is a common yet complex problem affecting approximately 10–15% of couples attempting to conceive a baby. In more than one-third of couples having difficulty in getting pregnant, the problem is at least in part related to male reproductive issues which have certainly increased in recent years.

Infertility is defined as the inability to achieve conception despite one year of regular, unprotected intercourse.[1] For healthy young couples, the probability of achieving pregnancy within the first year of fertility-focused sexual activity is 84%.[2] Traditionally (and very wrongly), it is the woman who is always blamed when a couple cannot beget a child.

Incidence of infertility (even male infertility) is increasing globally. Increase is both apparent and real. Apparent—because in recent years, scope of investigation and treatment has increased. At the same time there are also reasons for real increase in the incidence of male infertility.

The common causes of such real increase are:
a. Advanced age of marriage of both partners
b. Changing lifestyle and dietary habits
c. Stress of modern society
d. Use of synthetic dyes in green vegetables
e. Consumption of poultry chickens—fattened with oestrogens
f. Use of pesticides

Reduced male fertility can be the result of congenital and acquired urogenital abnormalities, infections of the genital tract, increased scrotal temperature (varicocele), endocrine disturbances, genetic abnormalities and immunological factors.[3] No causal factor is found in 60–75% of cases (idiopathic male infertility).

With advancing age, there is telomeric deletion of chromosomes; this may reduce chromosomal integrity affecting spermatozoal viability. Telomeres are structures attached to terminal ends of each chromosome. Their function is to protect the chromosome in order to prevent loss of genetic material. Similarly, stress induced ACTH through its anti-gonadotropic effect may impair functional integrity of testes. Some of the pesticides like DDT have direct gametotoxic effect.

In addition to numerical and structural defects of spermatozoa, functional male partner defects like—erectile and ejaculatory dysfunctions have also increased tremendously in the recent years.

The current increase in demand for infertility services has been attributed to a greater awareness of diagnostic modalities and treatment options, increased acceptance of infertility, and a trend towards delayed marriage and childbirth leading to more fertility issues.[2]

It is hence essential that both women and men be assessed to pinpoint the treatable

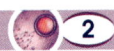

or untreatable causes of this heartbreaking health issue.

This chapter proposes to deal exclusively with evaluation of male factor infertility.

Currently, reported incidence of male infertility is about 40%, whereas incidence in our institute is around 48%.

Evaluation consists of

a. History
b. Physical examination
c. Special focused investigations

HISTORY

A detailed history either from the male partner or from his parents may directly or indirectly indicate some of the causes of his subfertility. A variety of information may be elicited only through history. The relevant points in several categories of information (past and present) are detailed below.

Information about childhood illness/abnormalities and treatment performed: History of trauma, torsion or undescended testes may have an impact on fertility. Surgery for undescended testes (orchidopexy) or injection of hCG before the age of 12 years may indicate and result in a satisfactory outcome.

Occasionally, a husband may present with past history of treated testicular cancer. Disease itself may affect semen quality and quantity. Treatment of testicular cancer both with radio- or chemotherapy has an adverse effect on testicular function. With some chemotherapeutic agents, damage is permanent; while with usage of a few drugs, the effects may be temporary—lasting for three to five years. Following this period, improvement may be expected.

Similarly, following surgical treatment especially after retroperitoneal lymph node dissection—which interrupts sympathetic chain innervation, there may be erectile or ejaculatory dysfunction often resulting in retrograde ejaculation.

As survival rate following therapy of testicular cancer has improved miraculously during last few years, preservation of fertility potential of affected men is currently being considered very seriously.

With this idea, attempts are being made for cryopreservation of testicular tissue, followed by *In vitro* growth (IVG) and *In vitro* maturation (IVM) or autografting the tissue into the testis when the disease is cured. Cryopreservation of gonadal tissue instead of spermatozoa is being considered because there is no spermatogenesis in prepubertal child.

There is also a future thought of cryo-preservation of testicular stem cells instead of testicular tissue. Alternatively, hormonal manipulation with GnRH-a or adjuvant therapy along with chemotherapy is also being considered for fertility preservation.

History of Current or Past Relevant Illness other than Carcinoma (Related to Spermatogenetic Defect)

A. Medical Illness

a. Mumps orchitis in childhood—this may cause destruction of seminiferous tubules—leading to azoospermia. The resulting condition is known as 'Sertoli cell–only syndrome'.
b. *Respiratory tract infection*: A few chronic respiratory diseases like bronchitis, bronchiectasis and sinusitis are often associated with:
    i. *Immotile cilia syndrome*: Generalised absence of cilia including complete asthenospermia. This is known as Kartagener's syndrome.
    ii. *Cystic fibrosis syndrome*: Associated with complete absence of vas deferens (CAVD), leading to obstructive azoospermia.
    iii. *Young's syndrome*: Another syndrome associated with azoospermia.

What is Young's syndrome?

In addition to respiratory problems, the syndrome may be associated with obstructive azoospermia due to blockage of epididymis with inspissated debris (genetic autosomal defect).

What is cystic fibrosis?

Cystic fibrosis may or may not be associated with chronic respiratory tract infection, but is almost always associated with absence of vas deferens. This also has a strong correlation with mutation of cystic fibrosis transmembrane receptor gene (CFTR).

Other medical illnesses with impact on semen profile

History of sexually transmitted diseases (STD)—a positive history with sperm abnormality suggests stricture of urethra, vas deferens or epididymis.

Similarly, history of genitourinary tuberculosis may also suggest obstruction of vas deferens and epididymis.

Acute viral fever may also cause temporary suppression of testicular function, but reversibility of spermatogenesis is expected within 3 months.

Other Relevant Points in History

B. Endocrine Dysfunction

a. *Diabetes*: Long-standing diabetes may cause erectile dysfunction due to diabetic neuropathy or vasculopathy. Diabetes may also be responsible for disturbance of emission or retrograde ejaculation (neurological dysfunction).

b. *Hypogonadotropic hypogonadism*: This is one of the important causes of delayed puberty and cryptorchidism. One important example is Kallmann's syndrome.

Kallmann's syndrome is a *variety of hypogonadotropic hypogonadism. This is an autosomal genetic defect—leading to defective embryogenesis of olfactory bulb and hypothalamus. The condition is also known as anosmia-azoospermia syndrome. Pregnancy is possible through testicular stimulation with exogenous gonadotropin.* Women may have similar problem resulting in anosmia and amenorrhoea (Kallmann's syndrome in women).

c. Another rare endocrine cause may be pituitary adenoma with clinical features of visual defects, disturbance in libido, hyperprolactinaemia and galactorrhoea. This is also correctable with or without surgical excision of adenoma. Congenital adrenal hyperplasia though rare, may also be responsible for delayed puberty and impaired fertility.

C. Environmental Toxin

a. *Pesticides*: Professionals having contact with nematocides, lead, ethylene dibromide, carbaril, etc. may suffer from effects of spermatogenetic damage.

b. *Similarly*, individuals involved in professions like agriculture, welding, factory workers working with ceramics may be victims of similar consequences of seminal defect.

Factory workers may have an additional risk of exposure of the scrotal area to hyperthermia. Hyperthermia has an adverse effect on spermatogenesis.

D. Lifestyle Factors

a. Modern lifestyle, including professional stress, results in excess adrenocorticotropic hormone release which has an adverse impact on gonadotropic hormone.

b. In addition, tight undergarments, sauna baths and long distance cycling may also cause spermatozoal abnormalities by creating scrotal hyperthermia and trauma.

E. Addiction and Male Infertility

a. Heavy smoking causes oxidative DNA damage of spermatozoa. This may result in sperm abnormalities, birth defects and increased cancer risk in the offspring.

b. Similar effects have also been observed following intake of marijuana, opiates and cocaine.

c. However, moderate alcoholism has no effect.

d. It has been observed that spermatogenesis is impaired following consumption of coffee in excess (caffeine—more than 2 cups coffee per day) than tea intake.

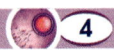

F. Impact of Steroids

a. Anabolic steroids used by body builders have direct gonadotropic toxic effects. These drugs have negative impact on hypothalamic-pituitary-gonadal axis.

b. Use of testosterone supplementation for hypogonadotropic conditions may further suppress gonadotropic action on gonadal spermatogenesis. Previous concept of rebound action of gonadotropin following cessation of testosterone therapy has not been authentically substantiated.

G. Chemotherapeutic Regimens

a. Almost all chemotherapeutic agents are gonadotoxic. Some are more detrimental than others.

b. Recovery is better with doxorubicin, methotrexate, oestrogens and androgens.

c. Chance of recovery is poor after bleomycin, etoposide, cisplatin, chlorambucil, pro-carbazine, vincristine.

d. Therefore, before using chemotherapeutic agents in general, cryopreservation of testicular tissue or spermatogonial stem cells should be seriously considered in young individuals—desiring preservation of fertility potential.

H. Other Commonly Used Drugs

a. Antihypertensive drugs

i. In general, all drugs have adverse effect on erection; worst are non-selective β-blockers, e.g. propanolol.

ii. Calcium channel blockers interfere with capacitation and acrosome reaction.

iii. α-blockers cause prostatic smooth muscle relaxation; may thereby cause retrograde ejaculation in approximately 10% of patients.

iv. However, no adverse effects has been observed with the use of ACE (angio-tensin-converting enzyme) inhibitors (like enalapril and lisinopril).

b. Antipsychotic and antidepressant drugs

i. In general, all drugs can inhibit erectile function. These drugs act through central dopamine pathways—suppress HPO axis—thereby suppress libido.

ii. Selective serotonin reuptake inhibitors—like fluoxetine (prozac), paroxetine (praxil) and sertranile (zoloft). These drugs may impair libido, delay ejaculation or may lead to anejaculation.

iii. Lastly, all these drugs may cause hyperprolactinaemia, impair sexual function and also the semen quality.

c. Antibiotics

i. High dose of nitrofurantoin may affect sperm maturation.

ii. Prolonged use of erythromycin and teracycline may impair sperm motility.

iii. Gentamicin and neomycin may also inhibit spermatogenesis.

d. A few commonly used drugs may also have adverse effects

i. Cimetidine—inhibits pulsatile release of LH.

ii. Colchicine—the drug used for gout impairs sperm-ovum binding during fertilisation.

iii. Sulfasalazine—also decreases sperm density, motility and morphology.

iv. Statins are the commonly used cholesterol lowering agents. But cholesterol is an essential component for spermatogenesis.

PHYSICAL EXAMINATION

Andrological examination is indicated, if semen analysis shows abnormalities specially in azoospermic individuals. Because semen analysis still forms the basis of important decisions concerning appropriate work up and management, local examination is always indicated in azoospermic individuals (undescended testes), history of failure to deposit semen in vagina (hypospadias) or clinical appearance suggestive of hypogonadotropism.

Inspection: Features of hypogonadism or Klienfelter syndrome can be easily recognised when clinical features are remarkably diagnostic.

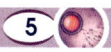

These include absence of beard, moustache and occasionally presence of gynaecomastia. Klinefelter's syndrome individuals are usually tall and sometimes well-built.

Local examination: This includes examination of penis, scrotum and testes.

   i. Examination of penis: Curvature of the penis, position of external urethral meatus to rule out hypospadias

  ii. Examination of scrotal sac and testes: Examination should be performed in erect position.

iii. Palpation of testes:

Length	: Should be more than 4 cm
Volume	: More than 20 ml (with such volume, 85% testes have normal spermatogenesis)
Vas deferens and varicocele	: Vas deferens should be palpated and varicocele is to be excluded; vas deferens may be congenitally absent in 1 to 1.5% of infertile men.

What is the significance of varicocele?

The subject of varicocele has generated controversy amongst the andrological community since the Edinburgh urologist Tulloch (1952)[4] first reported the beneficial effects of treatment apparently. Prevalence rate of about 5 out of 25 have been reported in surveys of apparently healthy men.[5] In contrast, amongst men attending the infertility clinics, varicocele affects about 11% of men with normal semen parameters and about 25% with abnormal semen.[6] It is hence difficult to establish the effect of varicocele on spermatogenesis and more importantly whether or not its treatment improves fertility. There is some evidences in favour of treatment[7, 8] especially in grades II and III varicocele and a few suggesting that it is of no benefit.[9, 10]

  iv. Rectal examination: This is not usually performed as a routine. In suspected obstructive azoospermia or in asthenospermia of infective origin, rectal examination may be indicated to exclude enlarged prostate or midline prostate cyst. If suspected, a transrectal ultrasound scan is advised.

Investigations

Routine investigations include semen analysis and when indicated—hormonal determinations. Other investigations are indicated according to the individual situation (Table 1.1).

Table 1.1: Investigation based on history

Relevant history	Provisional diagnosis	Investigation suggested
Cancer—radiation, chemotherapy	After some varieties of chemotherapy—irreversible damage may occur. In others—semen profile may be normal	Semen analysis (azoospermia) Normal investigations and sperm function test
Surgery for cancer	Injury to sympathetic chain— Loss of erection Loss of ejaculation Retrograde ejaculation	Semen analysis (azoospermia)— Postcoital urine (for evidence of sperm)
History of surgery for inguinal hernia (pre-pubertal)	Undescended testis	Semen analysis of FSH, LH
Surgery for neck gland biopsy	Obstructive azoospermia—may be tubercular	Blood for Hb%, TC, DC and ESR; chest X-ray Semen plasma—PCR Mantoux test—controversial

(Contd...)

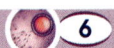 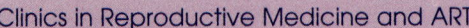
Table 1.1: Investigation based on history *(Contd...)*

Relevant history	*Provisional diagnosis*	*Investigation suggested*
Laparotomy in childhood for abdominal lump, intestinal obstruction, etc.	Tubercular	Relevant investigation including PCR of seminal plasma
Medical illness specially mumps or other viral infection	Mumps orchitis	Azoospermia (Sertoli-cell–only syndrome)
H/o diabetes—personal in the patient or in patient's family	Long-standing diabetes, leading to neuropathy or vasculopathy—sexual dysfunction	Blood sugar, semen analysis, post-coital urine
H/o STD	Obstructive azoospermia	Semen analysis of FSH, LH
Absence of smell sensation (anosmia)	Kallmann's syndrome	Serum FSH, LH semen analysis
Headache Visual disturbance Obesity Loss of libido	Hyperprolactinaemia Intracranial SOL Adenoma Craniopharyngioma	Semen analysis Serum TSH, PRL Skull X-ray CT scan of brain
Gross obesity Mental retardation	Prader-Willi syndrome	Semen analysis
H/o recurrent upper respiratory tract infection	Young's syndrome Prune-belly syndrome (rare)	Semen analysis, obstructive azoospermia Congenital absence of vas deferens (genetic evaluation)
H/o intake of drugs: Antihyperprolactinaemic Antipsychotic Anticholesterol, etc.	Seminopathy, diminished libido	Semen analysis
Erectile dysfunction	*May be functional or organic: Differentiation*: Presence of morning stiffness—functional No morning stiffness—organic	Diabetic neuropathy or vasculopathy
Ejaculatory dysfunction	*May be functional or organic: Differentiation*: Nocturnal emission (+ve)—functional Nocturnal emission (–ve)—organic	Diabetic neuropathy or vasculopathy; USG scan (rectal probe) for cyst in the region of prostatic utricle
Loss of libido, erectile or ejaculatory dysfunction	–	Serum prolactin, TSH, testosterone, PP blood sugar, and if PRL is elevated—CT scan of brain

Semen Analysis

The first test in the evaluation of the infertile male is the semen analysis. This test is inexpensive, easy to perform and gives valuable information.

A perfectly normal semen analysis report generally precludes a significant male factor component in etiology of infertility.

In azoospermia (non-obstructive type), when semen analysis shows normal ejaculate volume and azoospermia after repeated analysis, recommended method is semen centrifugation at 600 g for 10 min and thorough microscopic examination of the pellet (× 600). The upper fluid is then re-centrifuged (800 g) for an additional 10 min

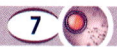

and examined. All samples can be stained and reexamined under the microscope.[11] This is suggested for confirmation of diagnosis of azoospermia.

Endocrine Assay: Role of Assay of Serum FSH and LH in Azoospermic Men

Generally, the levels of follicle-stimulating hormone (FSH) are mainly correlated with the number of spermatogonia. When these cells are absent or markedly diminished, FSH values are usually elevated. When the number of spermatogonia is normal, but there is complete spermatocyte or spermatid blockage, FSH values are within normal range. However, on an individual patient basis, FSH levels do not provide an accurate prediction of the status of spermatogenesis.[12–14] Preliminary data indicates a stronger correlation between low inhibin-B level and spermatogenic damage.[15] Estimation of LH, serum testosterone are indicated when hypogonadotropism is suspected. In sexual dysfunction, estimation of prolactin and postprandial blood sugar may help to ascertain the cause.

Testicular Biopsy

Currently, testicular biopsy is not usually performed for investigation of azoospermic men. A diagnostic testicular biopsy may be indicated in azoospermic men without causative factors (normal FSH and normal testicular volume) to differentiate between obstructive and non-obstructive azoospermia (NOA).

Testicular biopsy can also be performed as part of a therapeutic process in patients with clinical evidence of NOA who decide to undergo intracytoplasmic sperm injection (ICSI). Spermatogenesis may be focal. In these cases, one or more seminiferous tubules are involved in spermatogenesis while others are not.[16, 17] About 50–60% of men with NOA have some seminiferous tubules with spermatozoa that can be used for ICSI. The procedure of sperm retrieval has been recently modified with the use of microscopic TESE.

However, we do not recommend testicular biopsy as the first method of investigation. When ICSI has been decided, and testicular volume appears to be smaller than normal, fine needle aspiration cytology (FNAC) would be better alternative than testicular biopsy. The objective is to avoid trauma to the already compromised testicular function.

Relevant investigations are decided based on the findings of history and physical examination.

Investigations based on Findings of Physical Examination

Some of the examples are given below:

General

i. Tall, absent beard and moustache—may have gynaecomastia—these features are present typically in individuals with Klinefelter's syndrome. Karyotype (47XXY) confirms a diagnosis.

ii. Palpable neck gland or glands in other area of body—investigation for tuberculosis should be suggested.

Local

i. Empty scrotal sac (unilateral or bilateral)—indicates undescended testis. USG scan of inguinal region or lower abdomen should be advised.

ii. Presence of varicocele should be examined in standing position and should be confirmed by ultrasound.

iii. Any urethral discharge with or without history of recurrent urinary tract infection—prostatic smear should be suggested for bacteriological examination.

iv. Size and consistency of testes (to be discussed in detail in subsequent part of this chapter)

v. On rectal examination—if prostate is enlarged or a cyst is palpated, confirmation should be done by USG scan preferably by transrectal sonography.

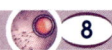

Management Outline of Azoospermic Husband

Summary of the current approach of management of azoospermic husband

Testicular sperm extraction (TESE) and ICSI were introduced in 1993 for treatment of obstructive azoospermia.[18–20] It was soon discovered that this technique could also be used for azoospermic men who appeared to have disturbed spermatogenesis.[21] If spermatozoa are detected in the testicular biopsy, ICSI with either cryopreserved or fresh spermatozoa can be proposed to the couple.

A karyotype (if not performed previously) and Yq deletions screening are indicated to analyse any therapeutic consequence for the newborn child. If genetic anomalies are detected, the couple has to be properly informed and counseled.

In case of azoospermia or ejaculatory failure not responding to vibro- or electro-ejaculation, spermatozoa can be harvested surgically for ICSI. The surgical technique depends on the cause of the azoospermia:

- In NOA, TESE is needed to retrieve spermatozoa.
- In obstructive azoospermia (OA), micro-surgical or percutaneous epididymal sperm aspiration (MESA/PESA) can be applied. If no spermatozoa are found in the epididymal fluid, TESE is recommended.
- In an ejaculation unresponsive to vibration or electroejaculation, TESE or seminal tract washout can be applied.

In NOA, the only good predictor of successful retrieval is testicular histology.[22] No clear relation was found with FSH, inhibin-B or testicular volume. In case of AZFa and AZFb microdeletions no spermatozoa can be retrieved.[23, 24] TESE is the technique of choice and shows excellent repeatability:[25] TESE results in retrievals in 50–60% of cases.[26, 27] Microsurgical TESE may increase retrieval rates[26–29] with lower complications than that with classical TESE:[30] Fluid from large caliber tubules is aspirated with the aid of the operating microscope. Positive retrievals are reported even in conditions such as Sertoli-cell–only syndrome.[26]

In OA (obstructive azoospermia), surgical retrieval can be combined with reconstruction of the seminal tract. TESE is usually successful and allows retrieval of a large number of spermatozoa suitable for cryopreservation. However, when epididymal tubules are enlarged, MESA enables both quantitatively and qualitatively better recovery of motile spermatozoa, with excellent chances for successful cryopreservation.

The results of ICSI are worse when using sperm retrieved in men with non-obstructive azoospermia as compared to obstructive azoospermia:[31–33] Birth rates of 19% in NOA versus 28% in OA[34] with significantly lower fertilisation and implantation rates[35] and higher miscarriage rates (11.5% vs 2.5%).[36] In OA, no significant difference in ICSI results was found between testicular or epididymal sperm.[37] Also no significant differences in ICSI results between the use of fresh and frozen-thawed sperm have been reported.[34, 37–41]

But all patients cannot afford ART (ICSI). Moreover, even for ART, specific clinical situation in which individual treatment protocol is indicated are detailed below. Therefore, specific individualised treatment can be planned depending on:

a. FSH level and testes size

b. Fructose in seminal plasma.

Management based on FSH Level and Testes Size

a. Testes size small or nearly normal; FSH is elevated

Azoospermia is usually non-obstructive; may be due to genetic, immunologic or some other causes. TESA/PESA/ICSI may not be possible. So counseling is very important. Adoption or artificial insemination with donor semen (AID) may be suggested. In rare cases sperm (immature) may be found in one of the four quadrants of testicular biopsy with which ICSI may be attempted.

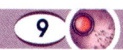

b. *Testes size small or nearly normal, but FSH level is low (hypogonadotropic hypogonadism)*

Gonadotropin replacement may be possible, but is expensive and often ineffective. Alternatively trial PESA with multiple biopsy followed by recovery of immature to mature sperm is sometimes possible. If sperms are available, ICSI may be performed. Alternative treatment is AID.

c. *Testes size normal and FSH level is also normal*

In these cases epididymis may or may not be distended which may be clinically palpable. If found distended, PESA/ICSI is possible. In expert hands VEA (vasoepididymal anastomosis) may be possible. On the other hand, if epididymis is not distended, PESA/TESE-ICSI is a treatment of choice. If the expensive treatment is not affordable, alternative choice is AID.

The entire management is diagrammatically represented in Fig. 1.1.

Management based on Fructose in Seminal Plasma

The biochemical evaluation of seminal plasma may reveal presence or absence of fructose. When present, the possible diagnosis is primary testicular failure. However, obstruction at the level of rete testis and epididymis cannot be excluded because fructose originates in seminal vesicles.

On the other hand, in azoospermic semen sample, if fructose is absent, the obstruction may be at the level of seminal vesicle (absence) vas deferens or ejaculatory duct.

It is important to note that in obstructive azoospermia, obstruction is usually found at four regions of seminal pathway: (i) Rete testis (ii) epididymis (iii) vas deferens, and (iv) ejaculatory duct. Rarely absent seminal vesicles may also be the cause of obstructive azoospermia.

Also it should be noted that absent fructose in azoospermic sample is almost always an evidence of obstructive azoospermia (seminal vesicle, vas deferens, ejaculatory duct), whereas presence of fructose in azoospermic subject may be related to 50% obstructive (rete testis and epididymis) and 50% non-obstructive causes (primary testicular failure, hypogonadotropic hypogonadism).

Approach to diagnosis and management is as follows

a. Fructose negative: The vas is to be examined. When vas is not palpable, the situation indicates congenital absence of vas deferens (may be associated with cystic fibrosis). The treatment options are: (i) PESA/ICSI after genetic counseling, (ii) donor insemination and (iii) adoption.

On the other hand, when vas is palpable with azoospermic sample, suspicion arises about ejaculatory duct obstruction. In these cases transrectal ultrasound scan is indicated. This may reveal a dilated or non-dilated seminal vesicle. Dilated seminal vesicles indicate a cyst in the region of prostatic utricle (müllerian remnant). Treatment consists of ultrasound guided transurethral removal of the cyst and dilation of ejaculatory duct. Alternative treatment is ICSI.

On the other hand, if seminal vesicle is not dilated, it indicates absence of seminal vesicle. The treatment is PESA/ICSI.

b. Fructose positive: As has already been mentioned this situation is encountered in

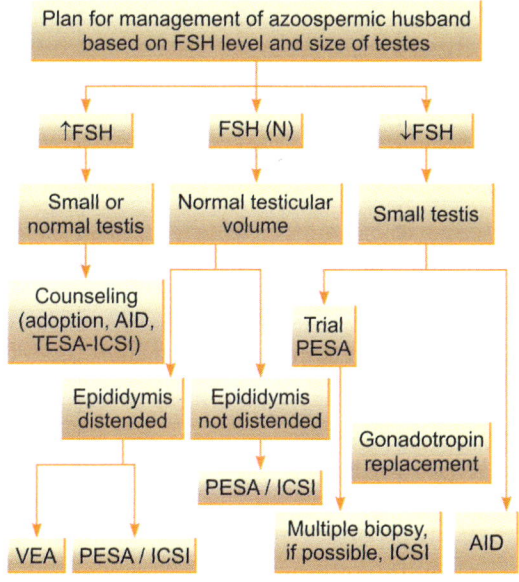

Fig. 1.1: Management based on FSH level and size of testes

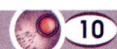

men with 50% obstructive and 50% non-obstructive azoospermia. The management depends on the size of testes and level of FSH:

  i. Testes small—FSH low or high—may be due to primary testicular failure or hypogonadotropic hypogonadism. TESE/ICSI may be possible with multiple biopsy of the testes. Alternatively donor insemination or adoption may be advised.

  ii. FSH normal—testes normal—in this situation (i) epididymis may be distended and (ii) may not be distended or size of epididymis may remain doubtful.

When distended, the treatment is PESA and ICSI. If epididymis is not distended, the treatment is TESE/ICSI. When in doubt, a scrotal exploration is done followed by epididymal aspiration. If sperm is found, ICSI is planned. If sperm is not found, TESE followed by ICSI is a treatment of choice. In expert hands when epididymis is distended, vaso-epididymal anastomosis (VEA) or vasovasal anastomosis (VVA) may offer good results.

Causes of azoospermia in relation to presence and absence of fructose are summarised as follows:

Fructose absent	Fructose present
Congenital absence of seminal vesicle or vas deferens	Obstruction in rete testis, epididymis
Ejaculatory duct obstruction	Primary testicular failure Hypogonadotropic hypogonadism

If these treatments are not affordable, the alternative management is insemination with donor semen sample.

Surgical Management

The scope of surgical treatment in male infertility is limited to a few conditions. They are:

  i. Varicocelectomy
  ii. VEA (vasoepididymal anastomosis)
  iii. VVA (vasovasal anastomosis)
  iv. Resection of müllerian cyst (in prostatic urethra)
  v. Transurethral resection.

Surgical treatment of male infertility has been further described in detail in a separate chapter.

In **male infertility,** some of the conditions described above and in addition a few to be described below are mostly due to chromosomal and genetic anomalies.

The subsequent part of this chapter has been reproduced in a separate chapter of this book (Sperm Abnormalities, Chapter 5). The information provided herein have been repeated only to maintain the sequence of information which is similar in both the chapters.

Chromosomal and genetic anomalies associated with male infertility

A thorough knowledge of genetic abnormalities in infertility is essential to every consultant dealing with male infertility in order to offer an appropriate advice and counseling to the couples seeking fertility treatment. With the advances in management options like IVF, ICSI and TESE, men with very low sperm count can be given a reasonable chance of paternity. However, this also increases the possibility of passing genetic abnormalities on to the next generation because the sperm of infertile men shows an increase in aneuploidy, other genetic abnormalities and DNA damage. Although there are prospects for screening of sperm,[42] current routine clinical practice is based on the screening of peripheral blood samples.

Chromosomal Abnormalities

They can be numerical or structural. Overall incidence is 5.8%;[43] of these, sex chromosomal anomalies account for 4.2% and autosomal anomalies exist in 1.5% individuals.

Apart from this, majority (30–40%) of idiopathic male infertility may have genetic anomalies.

Types of anomalies:

The types can be broadly classified into two groups:
  a. Chromosomal—which may be of two subtypes:
      i. Numerical
      ii. Structural

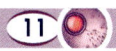

b. Genetic—which may affect:
  i. Pretesticular
  ii. Testicular
  iii. Posttesticular areas

Chromosomal: Numerical Anomalies

In male infertility, three types of anomalies have been observed.

a. 47XXY—Klinefelter's syndrome. This is the most frequent sex chromosomal abnormality and has been observed in about 14% of azoospermic men. They are usually tall with small soft testes devoid of germ cells, obesity and sometimes gynaecomastia.

  A special variety of Klinefelter's syndrome (mosaic variety, XXY/XY) patients have an increased chance of producing 47XXY spermatozoa. When IVF/ICSI is performed, pre-implantation diagnosis should be used, or if not available amniocentesis and karyotype analysis is to be performed. Embryos with known Klinefelter's karyotype should not be probably transferred.

b. 47XYY—this is rarely observed. They have increased height and low IQ. Usually these individuals are antisocial and they have impaired spermatogenesis.

c. 45X/46XY mosaic—these individuals are examples of mixed gonadal dysgenesis. Their phenotype may be male or female with ambiguous genitalia. They may have intra-abdominal testis and they almost always run a risk of gonadal malignancy, hence the gonads are to be removed. They also have defective sperm function and sperm production.

Chromosomal: Structural Anomalies (Deletions, Inversions or Translocations)

Reciprocal balanced translocations occur in 1 in 500 individuals. A person with a balanced translocation has a complete set of genetic information and is normal. However, when he or she has children, the child receives unbalanced genetic information, getting either too much or too little genetic material. A parental balanced translocation involving chromosome 21 is one of the causes of Down's syndrome. When IVF/ICSI is performed for men with translocations, pre-implantation genetic diagnosis should be used or, if not available, amniocentesis and karyotype analysis is to be performed. Embryos with known unbalanced translocation should not be probably transferred.

The commonest structural anomaly in azoospermic subject is found as micro-deletions of Y chromosome which is detectable through PCR.

The common regions affected in Y chromosome are—SRY and DAZ regions. Other areas of the Y chromosome which are affected in azoosperima are—AZF-A, AZF-B and AZF-C.

One more chromosomal structural anomaly which has been found associated with azoospermia is 46XX male. These individuals are phenotypically male and in 90% external genitalia is masculine. In about 10% individuals the external genitalia is ambiguous.

The molecular cause of this specific abnormality (46XX male) is translocation of SRY segment on one arm of X chromosome at the time of fertilisation.

Genetic Defect

The types of genetic defects detected in various types of male infertility are—deletions, mutation or polymorphic expansion.

Different areas are affected which may lead to spermatogenetic or seminal pathway abnormalities which are:

• Pretesticular abnormalities
• Testicular abnormalities
• Posttesticular abnormalities

Pretesticular defect

The affected genes lead to dysfunction of hypothalamic-pituitary-testicular axis. The commonest X-linked disorder in infertility practice is Kallmann's syndrome. The predominant form is an X-linked recessive disorder caused by a mutation in the KAL1 gene on Xp22.3.[44] Rarer forms of this syndrome include an autosomal dominant form.[45]

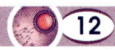
Patients with Kallmann's syndrome have hypogonadotropic hypogonadism and may have other clinical features, including anosmia, facial asymmetry, cleft palate, colour blindness, deafness, maldescended testes and renal abnormalities. It is important to note that some men with Kallmann's syndrome have an isolated gonadotropin deficiency without any other phenotypic abnormalities and may present *de novo* with infertility. It is often possible to stimulate spermatogenesis with replacement therapy.[46]

Posttesticular defect

The commonest example is mutation or deletion in cystic fibrosis gene or cystic fibrosis transmembrane receptor (CFTR) gene. The clinical consequence is hypoplastic, non-functional or absence of vas deferens and seminal vesicles. These individuals may have respiratory problem.

Another similar, but less commonly detected in clinical practice is Young's syndrome. This is also an example of posttesticular genetic defect. They also have respiratory tract anomaly with chronic sinusitis and bronchiectasis, spina bifida, ejaculatory failure due to epidydimal obstruction and defective spermatogenesis.

Combined testicular and posttesticular defects

One of the rarest varieties is prune-belly syndrome. They have bilateral cryptorchidism with bladder exostrophy (epispadias). They rarely survive through the neonatal life and hence not seen in the reproductive years.

Another rare variety of genetic testicular dysfunction is muscular dystrophy. This disease may cause seminiferous tubule destruction leading to azoospermia. This condition may also lead to impaired sperm motility resulting in situation like Kartagener's syndrome. They may also suffer from sinusitis, bronchiectasis and deafness. In these cases ICSI may be tried.

Genetic systemic disorders

Indirectly some genetic disorders may interfere with testicular and hypothalamic pituitary functions. The diseases concerned are thalassaemia and sickle cell anaemia.

These diseases by themselves do not cause infertility. Treatment with iron and multiple blood transfusions causes increased total body iron which is deposited in testes and pituitary. This causes haemochromatosis which may result in dysfunction of these organs leading to male infertility.

Based on these investigations the aetiology of common sperm abnormalities has been illustrated in the following Flowcharts 1.1 and 1.2.

Flowchart 1.1

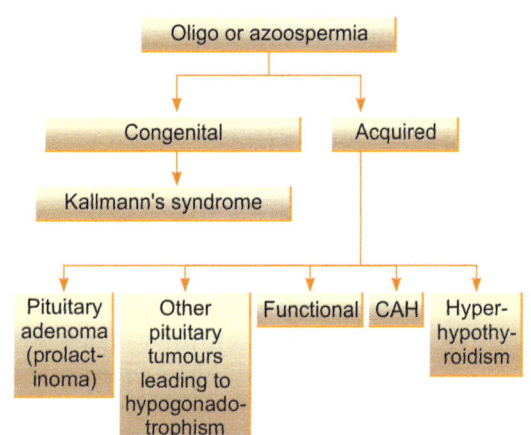

Flowchart 1.2

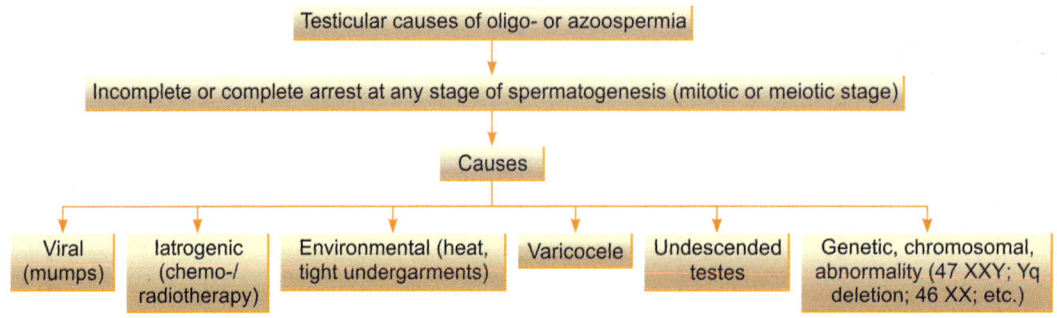

The classification has been designed with regard to pretesticular, posttesticular and testicular etiologies. The common sperm abnormalities discussed in the flowchart are:

a. Oligospermia and azoospermia
b. Isolated asthenospermia including (globozoospermia)
c. OTA syndrome.

In addition to the numerous functional and structural defects of spermatozoa, discussed above, there may be other embryologic or biochemical defects which will be further discussed in detail in subsequent chapters.

Medical management and management by ART in male infertility have been discussed in separate chapters.

Summary

During last 15–20 years incidence of male infertility has increased significantly. The increase in incidence is both real and apparent. The real increase may be due to advanced age of marriage, changing lifestyle and dietary habits, stress of modern society, use of synthetic dye in green vegetables, consumption of poultry chicken, use of pesticides, etc. The cause of apparent increase may be attributed to awareness of wider availability of facilities of diagnostic modalities and advanced treatment options.

The evaluation consists of history, physical examination and focused investigations.

History of medical illness, surgical intervention on genitourinary tract, urinary tract infection, recurrent respiratory tract infection (suggestive of CAVD or Young's syndrome), history of anosmia (Kallmann's syndrome), history of endocrine disorders (diabetes) may suggest a clue for diagnosis of specific cause of infertility in the male partner. While eliciting history, impact of environmental toxins like pesticides or professional stress, tight undergarments which may have their individual effect on spermatogenesis should be clearly noted.

Amongst drugs, not only chemotherapeutic agents, but many antihypertensives, antipsychotic drugs, a few antibiotics, steroids and statins may have antispermatogenic or gametotoxic effect.

Physical examination is indicated when semen analysis reveals abnormalities—specially azoospermia or when general appearance indicates features of hypogonadism. Presence/absence, size/consistency/volume of testes, presence/absence of varicocele (examine in erect position of the patient), position of urethral opening (to exclude hypospadias) are the areas to be carefully examined during physical examination.

Semen analysis is the first and foremost investigation in the evaluation parameters of male infertility workup. Relevant hormone analysis like FSH, LH, prolactin, TSH and imaging including CT scan of brain and chromosomal analysis depend on subjective symptom and objective signs elicited from individual patient.

Management protocol of azoospermic husband consists of PESA/TESE and ICSI both for obstructive and non-obstructive azoospermia. But all patients cannot accept this treatment. Therefore, the management for them may still be individualised depending on FSH level, testes size and fructose level in seminal plasma. Depending on clinical findings of testicular size and serum level of FSH the place of individual treatment including surgical correction by vasoepididymal anastomosis, if possible, may be planned.

In majority of idiopathic male infertility, either chromosomal or genetic factor may be involved. Chromosomal defect may be either numerical or structural. Example of numerical defect is Klinefelter's syndrome (47XXY) and that of structural defect is q deletion in Y chromosome (found in azoospermic individuals). Similarly, genetic defect may be pretesticular, testicular and posttesticular. Examples are—Kallmann's syndrome (pre-testicular, Xp 22.3), testicular (prune-belly syndrome) and posttesticular (deletion of cystic fibrosis transreceptor gene, CFTR) leading to azoospermia due to congenital absence of vas deferens.

REFERENCES

1. Frey KA. Male reproductive health and infertility. *Prim Care Clin Office Pract*. 2010; 37: 643–652.
2. Esteves SC, Miyaoka R, Agarwal A. An update on the clinical assessment of the infertile male. *Clinics*. 2011; 66: 691–700.

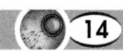
3. World Health Organisation. WHO Manual for the Standardised Investigation and Diagnosis of the Infertile Couple. Cambridge: Cambridge University Press, 2000.

4. Tulloch WS (1952). A consideration of sterility factors in the light of subsequent pregnancies: subfertility in the male. *Trans. Edinb. Obstet. Soc.* 52: 29–34.

5. Hargreave TB (1994). Varicocele. In Hargreave TB (ed.), Male Infertility. Springer-Verlag, London, 249–267.

6. World Health Organisation (1992a). The influence of varicocele on parameters of fertility in a large group of men presenting to infertility clinics. *Fertil. Steril*, 57, 1289–1293.

7. Laven JS, Haans LC, Mali WP et al (1992). Effects of varicocele treatment in adolescents: A randomized study. *Fertil. Steril.* 58, 756–762.

8. Madgar I, Weissenberg R, Lunenfeld B, et al (1995). Controlled trial of high spermatic vein ligation for varicocele in infertile men. *Fertil. Steril.*, 63, 120–124.

9. Baker HW, Burger HG, de Kretser, DM et al. Testicular vein ligation and fertility in men with varicoceles. *Br. Med. J.*, 291, 1678–1680.

10. Nieschlag E, Hertle L, Fischedick, A and Behre HM (1995). Treatment of varicocele: Counselling as effective as occlusion of the vena spermatica. *Hum. Reprod.*, 10, 347–353.

11. World Health Organisation. WHO Manual for the Examination of Human semen and sperm-cervical mucus interaction 4th edition, Cambridge: Cambridge University Press, 1999.

12. Hauser R, Temple-Simth PD, Southwick GJ, de Kretser DM. Fertility in cases of hypergonadotrophic azoospermia. *Fert Steril* 1995; 63(3): 631–36.

13. Martin-du Pan RC, Bischof P. Increased follicle-stimulating hormone in infertile men. Is increased plasma FSH always due to damaged germinal epithelium? *Hum Reprod.* 1995; 10(8): 1940–45.

14. De Kretser DM, Burger HG, Hudson B. The relationship between germinal cells and serum FSH in males with infertility. *J Clin Endocrinol Metab.* 1974; 38(5): 787–93.

15. Pierik FH, Vreeburg JT, Stijnen T, De Jong FH, Weber RF. Serum inhibin B as a marker of spermatogenesis. *J Clin Endocrinol Metab.* 1988; 83(9): 3110–3114.

16. Turek PJ, Kim M, Gilbaugh JH, Lipshultz LI. The clinical characteristics of 82 patients with Sertoli-cell–only testis histology. *Fertil Steril.* 1995; 64(6): 1197–1200.

17. Silber SJ, Nagy Z, Devroy P, Tournaye H, Van Steirteghem AC. Distribution of spermatogenesis in the testicles of azoospermic men: The presence or absence of spermatids in the testis of men with germinal failure. *Hum Reprod.* 1997; 12 (11); 2422–2428. *Erratum in Hum Reprod.* 1998; 13(3): 780.

18. Schoysman R, Vanderzwalmen P, Nijs M, Segal L, Segal-Bertin G, Geerts L, van Roosendaal E, Schoysman D. Pregnancy after fertilisation with human testicular spermatozoa. *Lancet* 1993; 342(8881): 1237.

19. Devroey P, Liu J, Nagy Z, Tournaye H, Silber SJ, Van Steirteghem AC. Normal fertilisation of human oocytes after testicular sperm extraction and intracytoplasmic sperm injection. *Fertil Steril.* 1994; 62(2): 639–641.

20. Silber SJ, Van Steirteghem AC, Liu J, Nagy Z, Tournaye H, Devroey P. High fertilisation and pregnancy rate after intracytoplasmic sperm injection with spermatozoa obtained from testicle biopsy. *Hum Reprod.* 1995; 10(1): 148–152.

21. Devroey P, Nagy P, Tournaye H, Liu J, Silber S, Van Steirteghem A. Outcome of intracytoplasmic sperm injection with testicular spermatozoa in obstructive and non-obstructive azoospermia. *Hum Reprod.* 1996; 11(5): 1015–1018.

22. Zheng J, Huang X, Li C. Predictive factors for successful sperm recovery in azoospermia patients. *Zhonghua Wai Ke Za Zhi.* 2000; 38 (5): 366–368.

23. Foresta C., Ferlin A, Rossi A, Salata E, Tessari A. [Alteration of spermatogenesis and Y chromosome microdeletions. Analysis of the DAZ gene family.] *Minerva Endocrinol.* 2002; 27(3): 193–207.

24. Hopps CV, Mielnik A, Goldstein M, Palermo GD, Rosenwaks Z, Schlegel PN. Detection of sperm in men with Y chromosome microdeletions of the AZF-a, AZF-b, and AZF-c regions. *Hum Reprod* 2003; 18(8): 1660–1665.

25. Amer M, Haggar SE, Moustafa T, Abd El-Naser, Zohdy W. Testicular sperm extraction: Impact to testicular histology on outcome, number of biopsies to be performed and optional time for repetition. *Hum Reprod.* 1999; 14 (12): 3030–3034.

26. Colpi GM, Piediferro G, Nerva F, Giacchetta D, Colpi EM, Piatti E. Sperm retrieval for intra-cytoplasmic sperm injection in non-obstructive azoospermia. *Minerva Urol Nefrol.* 2005; 57 (2): 99–107.

27. Vernaeve V, Verheyen G, Goossens A, Van Steirteghem A, Devroey P, Tournaye H. How

successful is repeat testicular sperm extraction in patients with azoospermia? *Hum Reprod* 2006; 21(6): 1551–1554.

28. Schlegel PN. Testicular sperm extraction: Microdissection improves sperm yield with minimal tissue excision. *Hum Reprod.* 1999; 14(1): 131–135.

29. Okada H, Dobashi M, Yamazaki T, Hara I, Fujisawa M, Arakawa S, Kamidono S. Conventional versus microdissection testicular sperm extraction for non-obstructive azoospermia. *J Urol* 2002; 168(3): 1063–1067.

30. Dardashti K, Williams RH, Goldstein M. Microsurgical testis biopsy: A novel technique for retrieval of testicular tissue. *J Urol.* 2000; 163 (4): 1206–1207.

31. Monzo A, Kondylis F, Lynch D, Mayer J, Jones E, Nehchiri F, Morshedi M, Schuffner, Muasher S, Gibbons W, Oehninger S. Outcome of intracytoplasmic sperm injection in azoospermic patients: Stressing the liaison between the urologist and reproductive medicine specialist. *Urology* 2001; 58(1): 69–75.

32. Vernaeve V, Tournaye H, Osmanagaoglu K, Verheyen G, Van Steirteghem A, Devroey P. Intracytoplasmic sperm injection with testicular spermatozoa is less successful in men with non-obstructive azoospermia than in men with obstructive azoospermia. *Fertil Steril* 2003; 79(3): 529–533.

33. Silber S, Munné S. Chromosomal abnormalities in embryos derived from testicular sperm extraction (tese) in men with non-obstructive azoospermia. Proceedings EAA International Symposium "Genetics of Male Infertility: From Research to Clinic", 2003, October 2–4, Florence, Italy.

34. Schwarzer J, Friedler K, Hertwig I, Krusmann G, Wurfel W, Schleyer M, Muhlen B, Pickl U, Lochner Ernst D. Sperm retrieval procedures and intracytoplasmatic spermatozoa injection with epididymal and testicular sperms. *Urol Int.* 2003; 70(2): 119–123.

35. Ghanem M, Bakr NI, Elgayaar MA, El Mongy S, Fathy H, Ibrahim AH. Comparison of the outcome of intracytoplasmic sperm injection in obstructive and non-obstructive azoospermia in the first cycle: A report of case series and meta-analysis. *Int J Androl.* 2005; 28(1): 16–21.

36. Borges E Jr, Rossi-Ferragut LM, Pasqualotto FF, dos Santos DR, Rocha CC, Iaconelli A Jr. Testicular sperm results in elevated miscarriage rates compared to epididymal sperm in azoospermic

patients. *Sao Paulo Med J.* 2002; 120(4): 122–126.

37. Gil Salom M. [Spermatic recovery techniques for intracytoplasmic spermatozoid injection (ICSI) in male infertility]. *Arch Esp Urol.* 2004; 57(9): 1035–1046.

38. Ben-Yosef D, Yogev L, Hauser R, Yavetz H, Azem F, Yovel I, Lessing JB, Amit A. Testicular sperm retrieval and cryopreservation prior to initiating ovarian stimulation as the first line approach in patients with non-obstructive azoospermia. *Hum Reprod.* 1999; 14(7): 1794–1801.

39. Gil-Salom M, Romero J, Rubio C, Ruiz A, Remohi J, Pellicer A. Intracytoplasmic sperm injection with cryopreserved testicular spermatozoa. *Mol Cell Endocrinol.* 2000; 169(1–2): 15–19.

40. Sousa M, Cremades N, Silva J, Oliveira C, Ferraz L, Teixeira da Silva J, Viana P, Barros A. Predictive value of testicular histology in secretory azoospermic subgroups and clinical outcomes after microinjection of fresh and frozen-thawed sperm and spermatids. *Hum Reprod.* 2002; 17(7): 1800–1810.

41. Hauser R, Yogev L, Amit A, Yavetz H, Botchan A, Azem F, Lessing JB, Ben-Yosef D. Severe hypospermatogenesis in case of nonobstructive azoospermia: Should we use fresh or frozen testicular spermatozoa? *J Androl.* 2005; 26(6): 772–778.

42. Griffin DK, Finch KA. The genetic and cytogenetic basis of male infertility. *Human Fertil.* 2005; 8(1): 19–26.

43. Johnson MD. Genetic risks of intracytoplasmic sperm injection in the treatment of male infertility: Recommendations for genetic counseling and screening. *Fertil Steril.* 1998; 70(3): 397–411.

44. Franco B, Guioli S, Pragliola A, Incerti B, Bardoni B, Tonlorenzi R, Carrozzo R, Maestrini E, Pieretti M, Taillon-Miller P et al. A gene deleted in Kallmann's syndrome shares homology with neural cell adhesion and axonal path-finding molecules. *Nature.* 1991; 353(6344): 529–536.

45. Santen RJ, Paulsen CA. Hypogonadotropic eunuchoidism. I. Clinical study of the mode of inheritance. *J Clin Endocrinol Metab.* 1973; 36(1): 47–54.

46. Miyagawa Y, Tsujimura A, Matsumiya K, Takao T, Tohda A, Koga M, Takeyama M, Fujioka H, Takada S, Koide T, Okuyama A. Outcome of gonadotropin therapy for male hypogonadotropic hypogonadism at university affiliated male infertility centres: A 30-year retrospective study. *J Urol.* 2005; 173(6): 2072–2075.

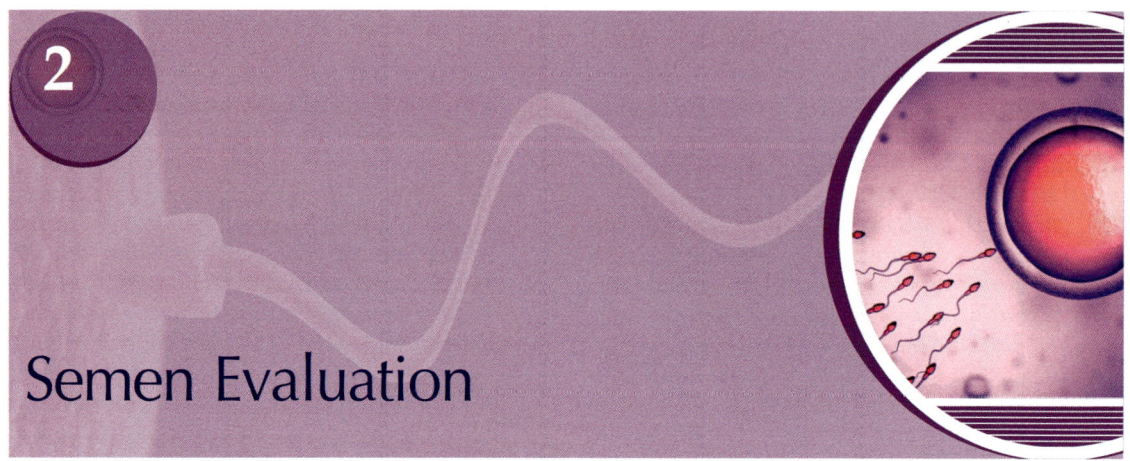

Semen Evaluation

Significant Historical Landmarks

In 1677

The scientific approach to semen analysis was started with van Leeuwenhoek's letter to the 'Royal Society of London', describing the discovery of spermatozoa by 'Johan Ham'.

In 1866

Sims performed postcoital examination on endocervical fluid and observed the importance of the presence of sperm in endocervical fluid for conception to occur.

In 1940

Weisman stated 'semen analysis was not completed until and unless its volume, sperm concentration, motility and morphology were determined'. Minimal requirement for semen analysis and semen parameter standards were published in 1951 by American Fertility Society.

INTRODUCTION

A standard infertility workup includes medical and sexual history followed by physical examinations of both partners. Subsequent evaluation should be conducted in a systematic, and cost-effective manner so as to identify all relevant factors with initial emphasis on the least invasive methods for detection of the most common cause of infertility. One such least invasive, rapid and most important step is semen analysis. It is said to be the 'Gateway' test for male infertility. If the analysis is performed skillfully and the results interpreted intelligently, it will provide a wide range of informations reflecting the spermatogenetic and endocrinologic functions of the testes with functional state of secondary sex glands.

Therefore, semen analysis reflects not only the activity of testes, but also provides information about many functions of endocrine organs and accessory sex glands, each requiring different technologies and skills.[1] Apart from mature and immature spermatozoa originating in the testes, semen contains fluids with composite biochemical elements contributed by different accessory sex organs. The important constituents are:

a. Small amount of mucoid secretion of bulbourethral (Cowper's) glands which normally lubricate the urethra and neutralise any residual acidic urine.

successful is repeat testicular sperm extraction in patients with azoospermia? *Hum Reprod* 2006; 21(6): 1551–1554.

28. Schlegel PN. Testicular sperm extraction: Microdissection improves sperm yield with minimal tissue excision. *Hum Reprod.* 1999; 14(1): 131–135.

29. Okada H, Dobashi M, Yamazaki T, Hara I, Fujisawa M, Arakawa S, Kamidono S. Conventional versus microdissection testicular sperm extraction for non-obstructive azoospermia. *J Urol* 2002; 168(3): 1063–1067.

30. Dardashti K, Williams RH, Goldstein M. Microsurgical testis biopsy: A novel technique for retrieval of testicular tissue. *J Urol.* 2000; 163 (4): 1206–1207.

31. Monzo A, Kondylis F, Lynch D, Mayer J, Jones E, Nehchiri F, Morshedi M, Schuffner, Muasher S, Gibbons W, Oehninger S. Outcome of intracytoplasmic sperm injection in azoospermic patients: Stressing the liaison between the urologist and reproductive medicine specialist. *Urology* 2001; 58(1): 69–75.

32. Vernaeve V, Tournaye H, Osmanagaoglu K, Verheyen G, Van Steirteghem A, Devroey P. Intracytoplasmic sperm injection with testicular spermatozoa is less successful in men with non-obstructive azoospermia than in men with obstructive azoospermia. *Fertil Steril* 2003; 79(3): 529–533.

33. Silber S, Munné S. Chromosomal abnormalities in embryos derived from testicular sperm extraction (tese) in men with non-obstructive azoospermia. Proceedings EAA International Symposium "Genetics of Male Infertility: From Research to Clinic", 2003, October 2–4, Florence, Italy.

34. Schwarzer J, Friedler K, Hertwig I, Krusmann G, Wurfel W, Schleyer M, Muhlen B, Pickl U, Lochner Ernst D. Sperm retrieval procedures and intracytoplasmatic spermatozoa injection with epididymal and testicular sperms. *Urol Int.* 2003; 70(2): 119–123.

35. Ghanem M, Bakr NI, Elgayaar MA, El Mongy S, Fathy H, Ibrahim AH. Comparison of the outcome of intracytoplasmic sperm injection in obstructive and non-obstructive azoospermia in the first cycle: A report of case series and meta-analysis. *Int J Androl.* 2005; 28(1): 16–21.

36. Borges E Jr, Rossi-Ferragut LM, Pasqualotto FF, dos Santos DR, Rocha CC, Iaconelli A Jr. Testicular sperm results in elevated miscarriage rates compared to epididymal sperm in azoospermic patients. *Sao Paulo Med J.* 2002; 120(4): 122–126.

37. Gil Salom M. [Spermatic recovery techniques for intracytoplasmic spermatozoid injection (ICSI) in male infertility]. *Arch Esp Urol.* 2004; 57(9): 1035–1046.

38. Ben-Yosef D, Yogev L, Hauser R, Yavetz H, Azem F, Yovel I, Lessing JB, Amit A. Testicular sperm retrieval and cryopreservation prior to initiating ovarian stimulation as the first line approach in patients with non-obstructive azoospermia. *Hum Reprod.* 1999; 14(7): 1794–1801.

39. Gil-Salom M, Romero J, Rubio C, Ruiz A, Remohi J, Pellicer A. Intracytoplasmic sperm injection with cryopreserved testicular spermatozoa. *Mol Cell Endocrinol.* 2000; 169(1–2): 15–19.

40. Sousa M, Cremades N, Silva J, Oliveira C, Ferraz L, Teixeira da Silva J, Viana P, Barros A. Predictive value of testicular histology in secretory azoospermic subgroups and clinical outcomes after microinjection of fresh and frozen-thawed sperm and spermatids. *Hum Reprod.* 2002; 17(7): 1800–1810.

41. Hauser R, Yogev L, Amit A, Yavetz H, Botchan A, Azem F, Lessing JB, Ben-Yosef D. Severe hypospermatogenesis in case of nonobstructive azoospermia: Should we use fresh or frozen testicular spermatozoa? *J Androl.* 2005; 26(6): 772–778.

42. Griffin DK, Finch KA. The genetic and cytogenetic basis of male infertility. *Human Fertil.* 2005; 8(1): 19–26.

43. Johnson MD. Genetic risks of intracytoplasmic sperm injection in the treatment of male infertility: Recommendations for genetic counseling and screening. *Fertil Steril.* 1998; 70(3): 397–411.

44. Franco B, Guioli S, Pragliola A, Incerti B, Bardoni B, Tonlorenzi R, Carrozzo R, Maestrini E, Pieretti M, Taillon-Miller P et al. A gene deleted in Kallmann's syndrome shares homology with neural cell adhesion and axonal path-finding molecules. *Nature.* 1991; 353(6344): 529–536.

45. Santen RJ, Paulsen CA. Hypogonadotropic eunuchoidism. I. Clinical study of the mode of inheritance. *J Clin Endocrinol Metab.* 1973; 36(1): 47–54.

46. Miyagawa Y, Tsujimura A, Matsumiya K, Takao T, Tohda A, Koga M, Takeyama M, Fujioka H, Takada S, Koide T, Okuyama A. Outcome of gonadotropin therapy for male hypogonadotropic hypogonadism at university affiliated male infertility centres: A 30-year retrospective study. *J Urol.* 2005; 173(6): 2072–2075.

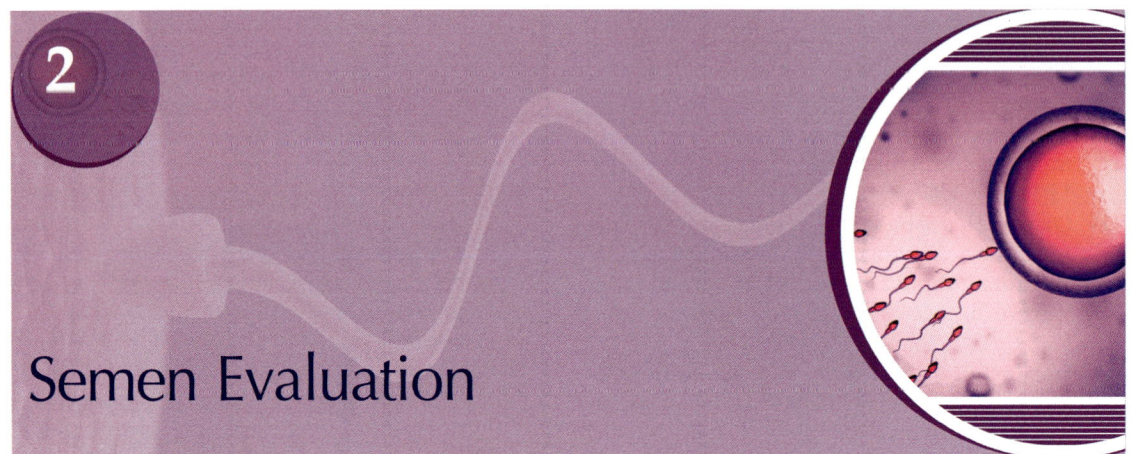

Semen Evaluation

INTRODUCTION

A standard infertility workup includes medical and sexual history followed by physical examinations of both partners. Subsequent evaluation should be conducted in a systematic, and cost-effective manner so as to identify all relevant factors with initial emphasis on the least invasive methods for detection of the most common cause of infertility. One such least invasive, rapid and most important step is semen analysis. It is said to be the 'Gateway' test for male infertility. If the analysis is performed skillfully and the results interpreted intelligently, it will provide a wide range of informations reflecting the spermatogenetic and endocrinologic functions of the testes with functional state of secondary sex glands.

Therefore, semen analysis reflects not only the activity of testes, but also provides information about many functions of endocrine organs and accessory sex glands, each requiring different technologies and skills.[1] Apart from mature and immature spermatozoa originating in the testes, semen contains fluids with composite biochemical elements contributed by different accessory sex organs. The important constituents are:

a. Small amount of mucoid secretion of bulbourethral (Cowper's) glands which normally lubricate the urethra and neutralise any residual acidic urine.

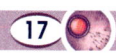

b. Some amount of acidic secretions from prostate which contains zinc, citric acid, acid phosphatase and prostate specific antigen (PSA).

c. Secretions from cauda epididymis and vas deferens which contains spermatozoa.

d. The major portion of seminal fluid originates in seminal vesicles. This is an alkaline secretion and contains fructose, prostaglandins and seminogelin proteins.

Semen analysis is generally performed in two types of settings:

i. In clinical pathology laboratories where most of the initial screening is performed

ii. In andrology and fertility clinics for more intensive analysis in infertility treatment settings

An incorrect report on semen analysis may result in unnecessary expensive and invasive treatment or inappropriate focus in investigating the wrong partner.[2]

Routine semen evaluation should include:

a. Background data during collection of sample

b. Physical characteristics

c. Microscopic analysis

d. Biochemical profile. Additional procedures like sperm function tests, evaluation of ROS, cytogenetic and immunologic defects have been discussed in some other chapters of this book.

BACKGROUND DATA FOR COLLECTION

Interpretation of semen analysis cannot be perfect until certain background data are known.

a. Abstinence: At least 2–5 days abstinence is essential for proper evaluation. Prolonged abstinence may result in accumulation of more number of morphologically abnormal spermatozoa,[3] whereas shorter duration of abstinence may be responsible for quantitatively less volume of semen and reduced number of spermatozoa per ejaculate.

b. Method of sample collection: How, when and where semen was collected matters a lot

for correct interpretation and final outcome. Ideally semen should be collected in a well-equipped room ensuring complete privacy, adjacent to the laboratory where semen analysis, semen preparation and sperm function tests are performed. A relationship can be built with the patients by this method. Information, such as exact time of collection, whether the first part was missed or not, injury during collection is easy to obtain and his queries can be answered accordingly.

The commonest and most acceptable method of collection is by masturbation. This method permits complete collection of specimen in a suitable wide-mouthed container and avoids contamination. Withdrawal method is not very reliable, since first part of the sample which contains the most vigorously motile spermatozoa may be lost during withdrawal and there may be contamination of the specimen with vaginal secretion. Laboratory collection is ideal since the semen is available for immediate evaluation. However, it may be less embarrassing to produce semen at patient's own home. Domiciliary collection is acceptable provided the sample can be delivered to the laboratory within 45 minutes or collected in a sterile container containing sperm wash media (or some other less expensive nutrient medium). In the second instance, the interval between collection and delivery of the sample may be extended to 2 to 3 hours. Semen should be collected in media in case of liquefaction problem and antisperm antibody. Advice should be given while collecting by masturbation, that the glans penis should be washed properly with normal water (preferably saline) and not with soap or antiseptic.

The history should be elicited about medical illness while the sample was collected for evaluation. Material of the container in which semen should preferably be collected is polypropylene and not a glass jar or polystyrene container. Because with the latter container there is increased risk of viscosity or viral infection.

Sildenafil derivatives may be prescribed in persons having difficulty in producing semen.

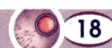

Vibrator can be used in case of failed collection during ART procedure.

PHYSICAL EVALUATION

The characteristics to be noted are:

A. **Temporary coagulation:** This occurs immediately after ejaculation. This is a normal feature. Coagulation is due to protein kinase secreted by seminal vesicles seminogelin protein.[4, 5] Absence of coagulation suggests absence of seminal vesicles and vas deferens. Absence of coagulation is usually associated with absence of fructose in seminal plasma.

B. **Liquefaction:** Following coagulation, there is liquefaction. Normal liquefaction time is 20 to 30 minutes. Period longer than 30 minutes is considered abnormal. Liquefaction is caused by proteolytic enzyme fibrinolysin, fibrinogenase and aminopeptidase secreted by prostate. Normal liquefaction is an indication of normal prostatic function. Delayed liquefaction or non-liquefaction is a sign of abnormal prostrate function usually due to prostatitis. Non-liquefaction may be a cause of primary infertility as majority of sperm is not released from the coagulum.

C. **Viscosity:** Following liquefaction, semen achieves a viscous state. Increased viscosity may be the result of abnormal prostatic function or due to infection in the genital tract—prostate or seminal vesicle. Increased viscosity has adverse impact on available sperm concentration and motility. This is an indication of 'postcoital' test in infertility workup.

A viscous sample is homogenous, whereas a non-liquefied sample is heterogenous.

D. **Volume:** Most of the seminal plasma is from seminal vesicles. Low volume of seminal plasma leads to impairment of fertilising capacity because of low vesicle function and biochemical interaction of sperm cells, whereas high volume of seminal plasma results in dilution of sperm cells; consequently the fertilising potential of a sperm cell is reduced.

Normal volume of ejaculate after 2 to 5 days of sexual abstinence is 1.5 to 5 ml.

Depending upon the volume, a person may be:

a. *Aspermic*—no semen at all even after orgasm, common in retrograde ejaculation.

b. *Hypospermic*—when the volume of the ejaculate < 1.5 ml:

   i. Loss during collection, or androgen deficiency

   ii. Partial retrograde ejaculation due to obstruction by infection or mucus plug

   iii. Congenital absence of vas deferens or seminal vesicles (fructose may be absent)

   iv. Too short abstinence period.

c. *Hyperspermic*—when the volume of the ejaculate > 5 ml:

   i. Prolonged period of abstinence

   ii. Accessory sex glands over secretion.

E. **pH:** Normal pH is between 7.2 and 7.8. pH is elevated (more than 8.0) in acute infections like prostatitis, vesiculitis or bilateral epididymitis. pH is low (below 7.2) in obstruction of ejaculatory duct; and may be less than 6.6 in chronic infection of these organs. Because the seminal plasma contains only prostatic fluid secretion which is acidic, low pH with azoospermia indicates bilateral congenital absence of vas deferens.

F. **Colour:** Normal colour of semen is opaque or grayish.

Yellowish semen indicates prolonged abstinence, presence of lots of pus cells or pyospermia and jaundice.

Reddish or brownish colour indicates fresh or old blood. Injury during collection or any pathology in male reproductive path should be eliminated.

Watery semen—due to less cellular elements as in azoospermia.

A few medicines like pyridium or methylene blue cause colouration of semen.

MICROSCOPIC EXAMINATION OF SEMEN

Sperm count: This typically refers to the sperm density reported as millions of sperm per ml of semen. The other parameter reported under the same category is total sperm count. This term indicates the total number of sperm within the whole ejaculate. This is obtained by multiplying the sperm concentration by the seminal volume. There are a number of methods to determine sperm concentration. The majority utilises counting chambers in which the sperms are counted within a grid. *A sample should be considered as azoospermic, if after 15 min centrifugation at 3,000 RPM, the pellet reveals no spermatozoa.*

Because sperm production is not tightly regulated for blood cells or hormone production, concentration is not a measure with much clinical relevance. The total sperm output is a more important parameter, and it depends on testicular size, a variable that is almost never known to the laboratory and often not known even to the treating physician.[6] Unfortunately, the WHO and many authors perpetuate the use of concentration as a key parameter and till someone thinks about it seriously, the procedure of current reporting will continue. Sperm count alone is not an accurate indicator of male fertilisation potential. Only in azoospermic husband it is an absolute factor. Because so long a single sperm is present in ejaculate the possibility of fertilisation, however, remote almost always exist. *Nowadays different disposable counting chambers are available, but the most sensitive one is Makler's chamber.*

Motility: Motility refers to percentage of sperm demonstrating any movement, whereas forward progression is a qualitative assessment of the speed with which the sperm moves in forward direction. For assessment of movement, two scoring systems are used. In one, the rating has been graded as 0, indicating no motility; 1, indicating sluggish or non-progressive movement; 2, referring to sperm moving with slow forward progression; 3, indicating movement in a reasonably straight line in moderate speed and 4, indicating sperm movement with high speed in a straight line.[7]

An alternative system also classifies sperm movement in 4 categories:

Category A—indicates rapid progressive motility

Category B—represents sluggish or slowly progressive motility

Category C—motility that is not progressive

Category D—indicates lack of motility.[8]

Progressive motility is the percentage of number of motile sperms moving in a linear forward progression. 75% progressive motility is associated with higher fertilisation rate. Time and temperature have detrimental effect on sperm motility. Therefore, motility should be assessed within one hour of ejaculation and at standard room temperature (28–30°C).

Abnormal sperms never show good motility except headless or pin head sperms. Again sperms having abnormal DNA may look or behave like normal sperms, but show zero fertilisation potential. Therefore, it appears that all fertile sperms are naturally motile, but all motile sperms are not potentially fertile.

Occasionally, clumps of agglutinated sperm appear under the microscope with no forward movement. They signify antisperm antibodies.

Under wet mount microscopy, round cells without tails are commonly identified. These are termed as round cells. Both immature germ cells such as spermatocytes, and white blood cells may have the same appearance (Fig. 2.1).

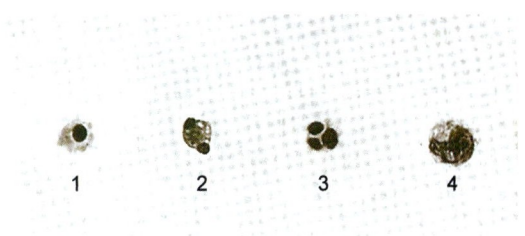

Fig. 2.1: Comparison of leukocytes and sperm precursors: (1) Spermatocyte; (2) spermatid; (3) polymorphonuclear leukocyte (PMN)—note nuclear bridges; (4) monocyte–note large U-shaped nucleus, foamy cytoplasm

Because non-motile sperm may be alive, the term "necrospermia' should not be used unless sperm viability assay has demonstrated as all sperms are non-viable. A high percentage of viable non-motile sperm suggests the presence of an ultrastructural abnormality such as primary ciliary dyskinesia. Electron microscope may help to confirm the diagnosis. *A person is considered to be asthenozoospermic, if his ejaculate displays < 32% of sperms moving in linear forward progression within 60 min of ejaculation.*

Morphology: Sperm morphology is one of the most predictive measures of assessment of fertility potential and therapeutic outcome.[9–14] Unfortunately, this is probably the most confusing component of semen analysis and extremely difficult part to interpret.[6, 15–17]

Over the last 50 years, 5 morphological classification systems have been used in clinical practice. The commonly quoted classification systems are: (a) Macleod,[16] (b) WHO manual— 2nd edition,[30] (c) WHO manual—3rd edition,[31] (d) ASCP,[18] 'strict' described by Menkveld[19, 20] and Krüger[14, 21] and (e) promoted by WHO manual—4th edition.

The latest WHO manual 2010, even described a further lower cut-off level of normal morphology as 4%. These controversies are probably due to disagreement amongst different observers about shape and size of different segments of spermatozoa, namely head, acrosome, cytoplasmic vacuoles, mid-piece and tail (Fig. 2.2).

Therefore, there are multiple morphology scoring systems currently in use with no consensus among laboratories. The reported lower limits of normal are 60%, 30%, 14% and 4%.

Recent studies recommend that the lower reference limit for 'strict' normal should be only 3%.[22] About the same time the Krüger's group published a lower reference value of 5%.[23] It is difficult to accept that in a normal fertile man, normal shape of spermatozoa decreases from 14 to 3% in a span of 10 years.[24] Comparison of methodology of classification between WHO 3rd and 4th edition/'strict' are detailed in Table 2.1.

Table 2.1: Comparison of methodology of classification between WHO 3rd and 4th edition/'strict' are detailed

	WHO 3rd edition	*Strict / WHO 4th edition*
Head Small	Large	*Borderline abnormal:* Slight deviation from oval
	Tapering Amorphous	*Abnormal:* Acrosome < 40% or > 70% of
	Double Pyriform Pin Round Vacuolated	head area round head small head tapered head double head large head diadem defect (vacuoles)
Mid-piece	Abnormal size Thickened Bent tail Missing tail CD present	*Borderline abnormal:* Slightly thick *Abnormal:* Abnormal length very thick bent tail missing tail CD present
Tail	Multiple tails Short tail Broken tail Hairpin Coiled tail Irregular width Terminal droplet	*Abnormal:* All tail defects

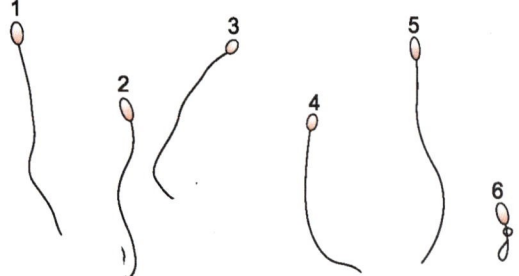

Fig. 2.2: Examples of normal and abnormal sperms: (1) Normal sperm; (2) normal sperm; (3) borderline abnormal head (normal for WHO 3rd, abnormal for WHO 4th); (4) abnormal head (small, small acrosome, irregular), normal mid-peice and tail; (5) abnormal mid-piece (thick), normal head and tail; (6) abnormal tail (coiled), normal head and mid-piece

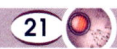

Therefore, interpretation of the morphology score in the semen analysis report requires that the physician is familiar with the individual laboratory specification systems.

The lower normal values have been utilised in 'strict' morphology criteria studied in patients undergoing IVF. What has become clear is that pregnancies are possible even when morphology scores are low, and therefore, morphology score should not be used in isolation and is only significant when used with other parameters.

BIOCHEMICAL ANALYSIS

Prostrate, seminal vesicle and epididymis produce chemical components specific to each accessory sex glands.

Zinc and acid phosphatase are products of prostrate , their level is decreased in chronic prostratitis.

Fructose is produced by seminal vesicle, absence of fructose indicates congenital absence of seminal vesicle/vas deferens or obstruction in ejaculatory duct. α-glucosidase is secreted by epididymis and is reduced in chronic epididymitis.

COMPUTER-ASSISTED SEMEN ANALYSIS

This is an effort to improve upon manual semen analysis. Computer-assisted semen analysis (CASA) is an automated semen analyser. Majority of the systems utilise videoclipped multiple frames which are then analysed to determine specific semen parameters. CASA systems are often used to measure hyperactivation which is a state obtained by sperm after capacitation.

Advantages claimed in CASA systems include the ability to obtain precise quantitative data as well as the potential for standardisation of semen analysis procedure. However, these advantages have been overshadowed by disadvantage like lack of standardisation and more importantly significant expenses of acquiring the equipment.[25] However, CASA still remains as a valuable research tool, but has not proved more useful in the clinical area than the manual semen analysis.[26-29]

FUNCTIONAL SEMEN ANALYSIS

Commonly performed sperm function tests are:
1. Hypo-osmotic swelling test (HOST)
2. Supravitality staining test
   - Clinical acrosin assay
   - Comet/tunel assay.

For details *see chapter on Sperm Function Defects*.

Normal Semen Parameters

While there is no universally accepted reference range for semen analysis, the WHO reference values have been utilised universally. The following table illustrates the reference range of normal semen parameters as published by WHO (2010).

Lower reference limits (5th centiles and their 95% confidence intervals) for semen characteristics are given in Table 2.2.

It is also important to keep in mind that the *semen parameters to be adequate for pregnancies by ART including IUI, should not be confused with those necessarily adequate for normal pregnancy rates by intercourse*. As sperm density is decreased, pregnancy rates by intercourse have also been

Table 2.2: Lower reference limits for semen characteristics

Parameter	Lower reference limit
Semen volume (ml)	1.5 (1.4–1.7)
Sperm concentration (10^6 per ml)	15 (12–16)
Total motility (PR + NP, %)	40 (38–42)
Progressive motility (PR, %)	32 (31–34)
Vitality (live spermatozoa, %)	58 (55–63)
Sperm morphology (normal forms, %)	4 (3.0–4.0)
Other consensus threshold values	
pH	≥7.2
Peroxidase-positive leukocytes (10^6 per ml)	< 1.0
MAR test (motile spermatozoa with bound particles, %)	< 50
Immunobead test (motile spermatozoa with bound beads, %)	< 50
Seminal zinc (μmol/ejaculate)	≥ 2.4
Seminal fructose (μmol/ejaculate)	≥ 13
Seminal neutral glucosidase (mU/ejaculate)	≥ 20

found to decrease. In addition both sperm motility and morphology have been reported to be as important, if not more important than sperm density. To obtain these information, it is significant to realise that, in general, a minimum of two semen analyses should be obtained from all patients who are considered to be subfertile men following semen evaluation.

Apart from number, motility and morphology of spermatozoa, detection of leukocyte is currently considered as a significant part of semen analysis. Sometimes it is difficult to identify and distinguish between leukocytes and germinal epithelial cells (also called round cells). Germinal epithelial cells are also found in fertile men instead of women and they must be identified separately from leukocytes. *Leukocytes are detected by peroxidase test which requires special solution for identification of leukocytes. Presence of $> 1 \times 10^6$ leukocytes/ml in the ejaculated semen suggests leukocytospermia.* In addition, monoclonal antibody test provides another detection method for identification of lymphocyte and monocyte in addition to granulocytes. But this is more laborious and sophisticated test.

Most basic way to detect WBC in semen sample is to examine under bright field light microscope with Papanicolaou or Leishman's staining. However, good quality staining and extensive experience is essential to differentiate between different subgroups of leukocytes and between leukocytes and immature germ cells.

Leukocytes may generate reactive oxygen species (ROS) in the semen sample. ROS may damage sperm nuclear DNA and also ROS may cause lipid peroxidation of sperm membrane which eventually leads to: (a) Reduced sperm motility (b) absence of acrosome reaction and (c) interference with sperm-zona binding and fertilisation. Hence, ROS leads to reduced motility and sperm dysfunction.

The impact of ROS on sperm function has been dealt with in detail in separate chapter (ROS in Male Infertility).

Summary

Apart from history and physical examination, semen evaluation is the first essential step not only for the evaluation of the male infertility but also for entire infertility workup. For all practical reasons, if semen parameters are normal and if no positive indication is elicited from the history, physical examination of the male is absolutely not essential. Semen evaluation, nowadays, is performed in two types of settings; one is general clinical pathological laboratory for overall broad assessment and the other one is specialised andrology and fertility clinics where more intensive analysis is performed.

Collection by masturbation in the laboratory is the best recommended method for proper semen analysis. Domiciliary collection is accepted provided the sample can be delivered within 1–2 hours. Sample should be collected in a polypropylene and not in a polystyrene container.

The important physical characteristics to be evaluated are volume, viscosity and liquefaction time. Average volume is between 1.5 ml and 5 ml, and liquefaction time should not exceed 20 to 30 minutes. Increased viscosity is an evidence of infection of accessory sex organs—prostate and seminal vesicle.

Microscopic examination includes count, motility and morphology of spermatozoa. Presence of leukocytes and immature germ cells are also noted. The minimum 'norms' of semen parameters are differently reported by different authors and even by WHO. A few years ago, the acceptable minimum 'norms' were total count as 20 million/ml, motility 30%—0 hour and morphology 14% and should be of normal shape. However, recent WHO report has reduced the lower 'cut-off' value of normal level to a very low limit—of which most striking reduction has been in the morphology ('strict' morphology) level to 4%. These figures have raised wide range of controversies.

Though biochemical analysis has no direct effect on sperm function, it helps to ascertain the health of secondary sex glands which has indirect effect on sperm parameters and function. Moreover, inclusion of functional semen analysis in abnormal situation may further localise the potential etiology.

REFERENCES

1. Kinzer DR, Rothmann SA. The Andrology Trainer, 2nd edn. Cleveland, OH: Fertility Solutions Inc., 2003.

2. McLachlan RI, Baker HW, Clarke GN, et al. Semen analysis: Its place in modern reproductive medical practice. *Pathology*. 2003; 35: 25–33.

3. Levitas E, unenfeld E, Weiss N, et al. Relationship between the duration of sexual abstinence and semen quality: Analysis of 9,489 semen samples. *Fert Steril*. 2005; 83: 1680–6.

4. Robert M, Gagnon C. Purification and characterisation of the active precursor of a human sperm motility inhibitor secreted by the seminal visicles: identity with semenogelin. *Biol Reprod*. 1996; 55: 813–21.

5. Robeert M, Gagnon C. Semenogelin I: A *coagulum* forming, multifunctional seminal vesicle protein. *CMLS Cell Mol Life Sci*. 1999; 55: 944–60.

6. Eliasson R. Basic semen analysis. In: Current Topics in Andrology. Perth: Ladybrook Publishing. 2003.

7. Davis RO, Gravance CG, Overstreet JW. A standardised test for visual analysis of humansperm morphology. *Fertil Steril*. 1995; 63: 1058–63.

8. Boyers SP, Davis RO, Katz DF. Automated semen analysis. *Curr Prob Obset Gynecol Fertil*. 1989; 12: 165–200.

9. Guzick DS, Overstreet J, Factor-Litvak P, et al. Sperm morphology, motility, and concentration in fertile and infertile men. *N Engl J Med*. 2001; 345: 1388–93.

10. MacLeod J, Gold RZ. The male factor in fertility and infertility. IV Sperm morphology in fertile and infertile marriage. *Fertil Steril*. 1951; 2: 394–414.

11. Mortimer 4 D, Menkveld R. Sperm morphology assessment: Historical perspectives and current opinions. *J Androl*. 2001; 22: 192–205.

12. MacLeod J. A possible factor in the etiology of human male infertility: Preliminary report. *Fertil Steril*. 1962; 13: 29–33.

13. MacLeod J. Human seminal cytology as a sensitive indicator of the germinal epithelium. *Int J Fertil*. 1964; 9: 281–95.

14. Kruger TF, Acosta AA, Simmons KF, et al. Predictive value of abnormal sperm morphology in *in vitro* fertilisation. *Fertil Steril*. 1988; 49: 112–17.

15. Nazerali H, Thapa S, Hays M, et al. Vasectomy effectiveness in Nepal: A retrospective study. *Contraception*. 2003; 67: 397–401.

16. Kaye MC, Schroeder-Jenkins M, Rothmann SA. Impairment of sperm dmotility by water-soluble lubricants as assessed by computer-assisted sperm analysis. *J Androl*. 1991; 12: 52.

17. MacLeod J. The semen examination. *Clin Obstet Gyn*. 1965; 8: 115–27.

18. Adelman MM, Cahil EM, eds. Atlas of sperm Morphology. Chicago, IL: ASCP Press, 1989.

19. Toft G, Rignell-Hydbom A, Tyrkiel E, Shvets M, Giwercman A. Quality control workshops in standardisation of sperm concentration and motility assessment in multicentre studies. *Int J Androl*. 2005; 15: 667–71.

20. Department of Health, and Human Services, Healthcare functioning administration. Clinical laboratory improvement amendments of 1988, Final Rule (42 CFR 493) Federal Register 1992 (Friday, Feb 28); 57: 7002–86.

21. College of American Pathologyists. Semen Analysis Survey SEM-B. Northfield, IL, 1999.

22. Menkveld R, Wong WY, Lombard Cj, et al. Semen parameters, including WHO and strict criteria morphology, in a fertile and subfertile population: An effort towards standardisation of *in vivo* thresholds. *Hum Reprod*. 2001; 16: 1165–71.

23. Gunalp S, Onculoglu C, Gurgan T, Kriger TF Lombard CJ. A study of semen parameters with emphasis on sperm morphology in a fertile population: An attempt to develop clinical thresholds. *Hum Reprod*. 2001; 16: 110–14.

24. Kruger TF, Franken DR. Atlas of Human Sperm Morphology Evaluation. London: Taylor and Francis, 2004.

25. Agarwal A, Sharma RK. Automation is the key to standardise semen analysis using the automated SQA-V sperm quality analyser. *Fertil Stertil*. 2007; 87: 156–62.

26. Medical Electronic Systems, Inc. Spermalite[TA] SQA –V User Guide. Version 245, 2005.

27. Akashi T, Mizuno I, Okumura A, d Fuse H. Usefulness of sperm quality analyser-V (SQA-V) for the assessment of sperm quality in infertile men. *Arch Androl*. 2005; 51: 437–42.

28. Rpyster MO, Lobdell DT, Mendola O, et al. Evaluation of a container for collection and shipment of semen with potential uses in population-based, clinical, and occupational settings. *J Androl.* 2000; 21: 478–84.

29. Martinez C, Mar C, Azcarate M, et al. Sperm motility index: A quick screening parameter from sperm quality analyser-IIB to rule out oligo- and asthenozoospermia in male fertility study. *Hum Reprod.* 2000; 15: 1727–33.

30. World Health Organisation. Laboratory Manual for the examination of Human Semen and Sperm—Cervical Mucus Interactions, 2nd edn. Cambridge: Cambridge University Press: 1987.

31. World Health Organisation. WHO Laboratory Manual for the Examination of Human Semen and Sperm—Cervical Mucus Interactions, 3rd edn. Cambridge: Cambridge University Press, UK, 1992.

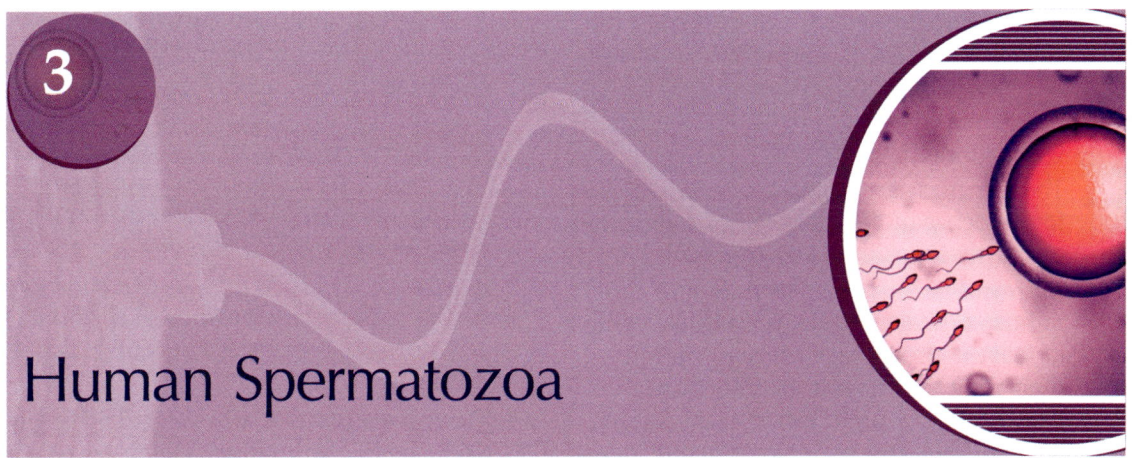

Human Spermatozoa

INTRODUCTION

The term spermatozoon is derived from the ancient Greek word "sperma" (meaning seed) and "zoon" (meaning living being) and more commonly known as a sperm cell. It is haploid cell and is the male gamete involved in reproduction.

There are three types of cells in our body, e.g. somatic cells, stem cells and germ cells.

Spermatogonia are the immature germ cells. They divide several times during the process of sperm development. The entire process of sperm formation and maturation takes about 9–10 weeks. The separate divisions that take place and what happens in each are described in detail in the later part of this chapter. Brief description of these events are as follows:

- **First division:** The first division is done by mitosis, and ensures a constant supply of *spermatocytes*, each with the diploid number of chromosomes.

- **Second division:** Spermatocytes then undergo a series of two cell divisions during meiosis to become *secondary spermatocytes*.

- **Third division:** Secondary Spermatocytes finally become *spermatids*. Spermatids which are haploid cells, differentiate morphologically into sperm by nuclear condensation, ejection of the cytoplasm and formation of the *acrosome* and *flagellum.* The

sperm is the main reproductive cell in males.

A uniflagellar sperm cell that is motile is referred to as a spermatozoon, whereas a non-motile sperm cell is referred to as a spermatium.

In humans, sperm cells consist of a flat, disc-shaped head 5 µm by 3 µm and a tail 50 µm long. The tail flagellates which propel the sperm cell (at about 1–3 mm/minute in humans) by whipping in an elliptical cone.

The spermatozoon is characterised by a minimum of cytoplasm and the most densely packed DNA.

Compared to mitotic chromosomes in somatic cells, sperm DNA is at least sixfold more highly condensed.

Human spermatozoa have some unique characteristics which are summarised below:

Unique characteristics of human spermatozoa:

a. Sperm cell is one of the smallest cells in the body; length of the sperm head being 4–5 µm and has a long tail.

b. These cells (adult sperm cells) do not grow or divide.

c. The sperm cells are the most polarised cells; head in front and flagellum at the rear part of the body.

d. They fulfil their function outside the body, in different individuals, e.g. in female genital tract.

e. Unlike somatic cells, the sperm head has a large nucleus, but lacks large cytoplasm.

f. Nucleus constitutes 65% of spermatozoal head and is composed of DNA conjugated with protein.

g. The sperm cells are unique among mammals for presence of plenty of abnormal forms of spermatozoa in the ejaculate.

Mammalian sperm DNA is the most tightly compacted eukaryotic DNA, being at least sixfold more highly condensed than the DNA in mitotic chromosomes. To achieve this high degree of packaging, sperm DNA interacts with protamines to form linear, side-by-side arrays of chromatin. This differs markedly from the builder DNA packaging of somatic cell nuclei and mitotic chromosomes, in which the DNA is coiled around histone octamers to form nucleosomes. The overall organisation of mammalian sperm DNA, however, resembles that of somatic cells in that both the linear arrays of sperm chromatin and the 30 nm solenoid filaments of somatic cell chromatin are organised into loop domains attached at their bases to a nuclear matrix. In addition to the sperm nuclear matrix, sperm nuclei contain a unique structure termed the sperm nuclear annulus to which the entire complement of DNA appears to be anchored.

The centromeres are located centrally and telomeres peripherally. Folding of chromosome p and q arms are flexible (Fig. 3.1). This specific chromosomal arrangement may be responsible for increased frequency of abnormal sperm shape and increased frequency of aneuploidy.

h. It has been observed that sex chromosome and G-group (chromosomes 21 and 22) are more susceptible to non-disjunction during spermatogenesis.

i. Morphologically abnormal sperms (large head, round head, etc.) have either numerical or structural abnormalities of chromosomes.

Anatomical segments of adult spermatozoa (Fig. 3.2): A mature human sperm cell has got the following parts—head, neck, middle piece and tail.

Head (Fig. 3.3): It is oval in shape consisting of large nucleus and a dome-shaped acrosome present on the nucleus.

The sperm head is oval-shaped and smooth on the surface. Length of the sperm head is 3–5 μm and the width is 2–3 μm. The coverings of the sperm head from outside are: (i) Plasma membrane; (ii) outer and inner acrosomal layers of membrane; (iii) acrosomal sac containing enzymes; (iv) nuclear cap and (v) nucleus.

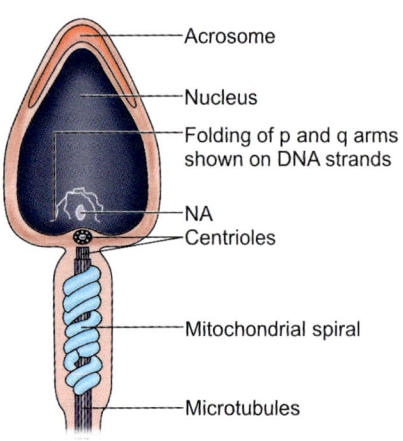

Fig. 3.1: Human spermatozoa

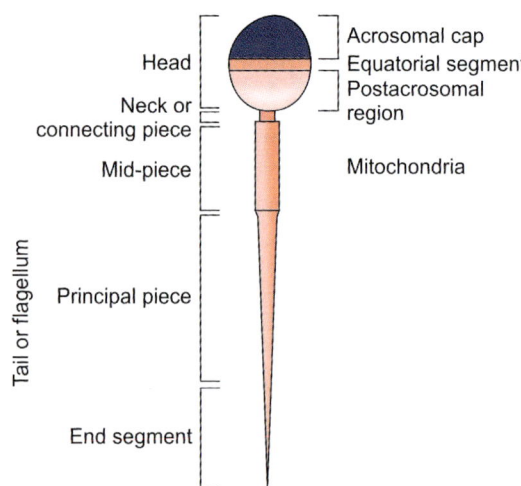

Fig. 3.2: Schematic diagram of different segments of spermatozoa

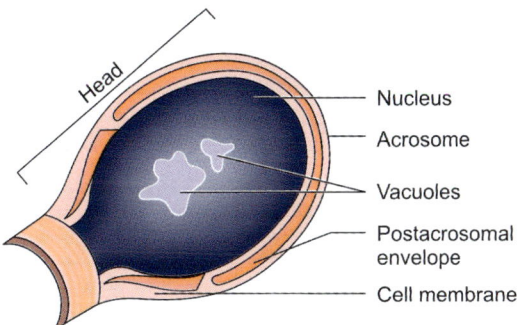

Fig. 3.3: Morphological anatomy of sperm head

Acrosome

This is found at the anterior tip of the sperm (derived from Greek term *"akron"* meaning extremity and *"soma"* meaning body). The acrosome forms a cap-like structure called the head cap. This occupies the space between anterior half of the nucleus and the plasma membrane of the sperm tip. In its origin (during spermatogenesis), the acrosome is formed from the Golgi complex.

The acrosome itself is bounded by a unit membrane. It consists of a number of hydrolytic enzymes such as acid phosphatase, hyaluronidase and others. These enzymes help in tissue lysis (dissolving) and this facilitates the penetration of the sperm into the egg membrane. The enzymes are proteolytic and help in dissolving the egg membrane.

Sperm Nucleus

The nucleus occupies most of the available space of the sperm head. It is the shape of the nucleus that ultimately decides the shape of the sperm head. Structurally, it is enveloped by a nuclear membrane. Sometimes, however, the posterior part of nuclear membrane (towards the body of the sperm) is somewhat depressed to accommodate the proximal centriole. The nucleus consists of DNA as well as basic proteins. There is no nucleolus or any fluid contents.

Function: Nucleus contains genetic information and half number of chromosomes. The acrosome releases an enzyme hyaluronidase which destroys the hyaluronic acid of the ovum and enters into the ovum.

Connecting piece or neck: It contains centrioles which are proximal centriole and distal centriole (Fig. 3.4).

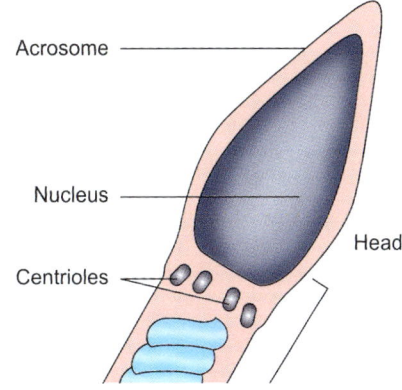

Fig. 3.4: Centriole in the connecting piece (neck)

Function: Distal centriole gives rise to axial filament of the sperm which runs up to the end of the tail. Centrioles help the zygotic division by forming the first mitotic spindle. The posterior or the distal centriole is responsible for the formation of the microtubules of the sperm tail.

Tail: It consists of three parts:
a. Mid-piece
b. Principal piece
c. End piece.

a. Mid-piece (Figs 3.5 and 3.6): It is a tubular structure in which mitochondria are spirally arranged. It has a pair of longitudinal fibres called β-fibres surrounded by a ring of nine pairs of longitudinal fibres called α-fibres. In human sperms, the α-fibres of axial filament are accompanied on the outside by 9, much thicker fibres called γ-fibres or coarse fibres. The α-, β-, and γ-fibres are the sites of various enzymes.

α-fibres have ATPase enzyme, while β-fibres have acetylcholine and succinic dehydrogenase. These fibres are anchored to the distal centrioles. The fibres are surrounded by the mitochondria. Very often the mitochondria are fused together and form a spiral sheet that surrounds the axonemal fibres. Around the periphery of mid-piece of the sperm is found a thin sheet of cytoplasm mainly

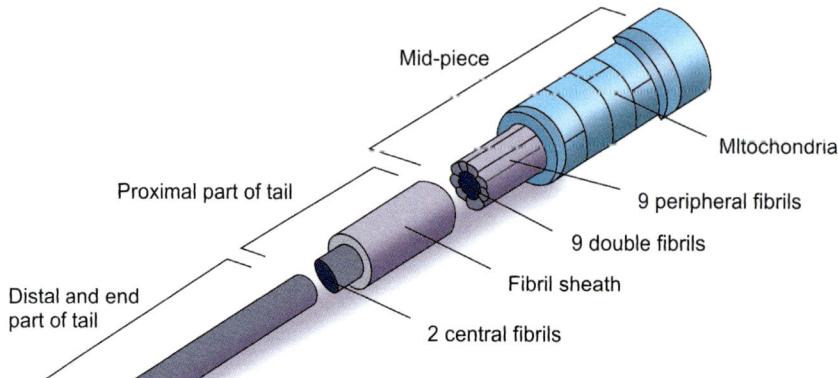

Fig. 3.5: Morphological anatomy of mid-piece

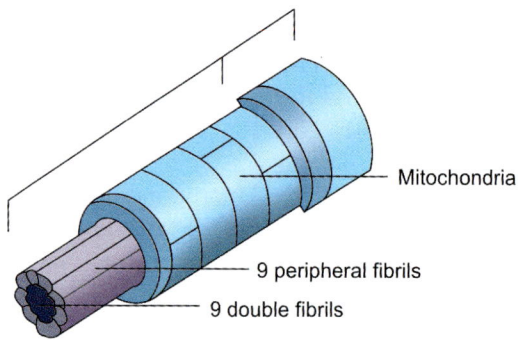

Fig. 3.6: Principal piece and end piece

composed of microtubules. This layer is called manchettee.

Function: Middle piece is called powerhouse of sperm because it gives energy to the sperm to traverse through the female genital tract.

b. Principal piece: It constitutes most of the length of tail consists of the central core made up of axial filaments with a (9 + 2) arrangement (2 central, 9 peripheral).

Surrounding this core is a fibrous tail sheath which often appears as semicircular ribs oriented at right angles to the long axis of the filament. Sometimes they appear as helical coils. In human beings, two of the γ-fibres are fused with the surrounding ribs to form anterior and posterior columns extending throughout the length of the principal piece.

This arrangement divides the principal piece into two functional compartments—one having three γ-fibres and the other containing four.

This symmetry is thought to help in a more powerful stroke of the tail in one direction. This is called the powerstroke. The end piece is a small tapering portion of the tail containing only the axial filament covered with cytoplasm and plasma membrane.

There is no stored food in the sperm. It also does not have cytoplasmic organelles such as ribosomes and endoplasmic reticulum.

Function: Tail helps the sperm to swim in the female genital tract. It is the main part of sperm that helps in movement through the female genital tract.

c. End piece: The principal piece terminates in the end piece, it is very narrow due to absence of outer fibre and sheaths and gradual disappearance of microtubules.

Plasma membrane occurring in the mid-piece is to be ruptured before ICSI for the release of cytosolic factor.

The morphological characteristics of these segments and their physiological functions are described below:

Molecular Functions of Different Segments of Spermatozoa

a. Functions of the head: The plasma membrane which constitutes the outer coat of the head consists of a very unstable fatty acid which is known as polyunsaturated fatty acid (PUFA). PUFA has both helpful and unwanted functions in reproduction. The helpful function consists of facilitating fusion and disintegration of plasma and acrosin membranes leading to exocytosis of the enzyme acrosin. This happens when the sperm head comes in contact with zona pellucida at the time of fertilisation. This procedure is known as 'acrosome reaction' and zona penetration which allows the sperm head to enter into the perivitelline space.

The undesirable reaction is due to excessive fluidity of plasma membrane due to presence of PUFA (unstable fatty acid) which may be responsible for premature disintegration and exocytosis of acrosome. This may happen when many leukocytes are present in seminal plasma, or due to presence of plenty of immature sperm cells, varicocele and excessive centrifugation.

Under normal conditions, the sperm head after zona penetration comes in contact with oocyte oolemma (outer coating of oocyte cytoplasm). This is known as cytoplasmic syngamy. Two important molecular events occur after cytoplasmic syngamy—(a) calcium oscillation and (b) cortical reaction. This happens due to oocyte activation through sperm head contact with oolemma.

Calcium oscillation: Calcium oscillation occurs due to calcium influx from cytoplasmic organelles (rich in calcium stores). The primary effect of calcium oscillation within oocyte cytoplasm is removal of inhibitory factor for completion of meiosis II which gets initiated with meiosis I (during intrauterine life). In other words, calcium oscillation induces MPF (maturation promoting factor) within oocyte cytoplasm which is necessary for release of

second polar body (completion of meiosis II). Following meiosis II, the oocyte nucleus is converted into a spindle (containing half of the maternal genetic material) and forms the female pronucleus. Before the female pronucleus is formed, calcium oscillation also helps in formation of male pronucleus. This is an interesting step. The male pronucleus is formed primarily by removal of nuclear cap of the sperm head, replacement of the special type of sperm head protein—protamine by histone migrating from the oocyte nucleus. This is followed by assembly of a new nuclear envelop—formation of male pronucleus. Pronuclear chromatin condenses to form nucleolar precursor body (NPB). These are also known as nucleoli. Arrangement and synchrony of male pronuclear nucleoli with regard to nucleoli of the female pronucleus are significant markers of good or bad pronuclei. (normal or abnormal fertilisation) (Fig. 3.7).

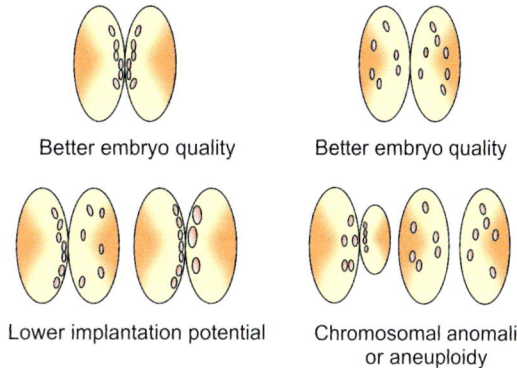

Better embryo quality   Better embryo quality

Lower implantation potential   Chromosomal anomalies or aneuploidy

Fig. 3.7: Morphological assessment of fertilisation through nuclear arrangement in pronuclei

b. Function of centriole in sperm neck: This helps in apposition of two pronuclei (male and female) by forming microtubules. These microtubules bring two pronuclei (male and female) in close proximity to complete the last stage of fertilisation, namely 'nuclear syngamy'.

When pronuclear differentiation and apposition have been completed, the respective pronuclear envelop degenerates—leading to exchange of paternal and maternal genetic material—the process is known as nuclear syngamy. Thereafter the first embryonic cell division begins by 'mitotic division'—leading to the formation of a zygote. This is the beginning of a new individual.

Examples of Sperm Abnormalities

a. Head—defects in shape and size—like large, small, tapering, pyriform, amorphous and vacuolated (more than 20% of head surface is occupied by vacuoles). There may be also double head or combination defect.

b. Neck and mid-piece abnormalities—this consists of absence, non-inserted, fractured, bent and thin mid-piece.

c. Tail abnormalities—tail abnormalities include short, multiple, hairpin, broken, coiled and tail with terminal droplets.

d. Cytoplasmic droplets in the head—cytoplasmic content of the sperm head is much less than the nuclear DNA content. Cytoplasmic area greater than 1/3rd of the area of normal sperm head is considered abnormal (Fig. 3.8).

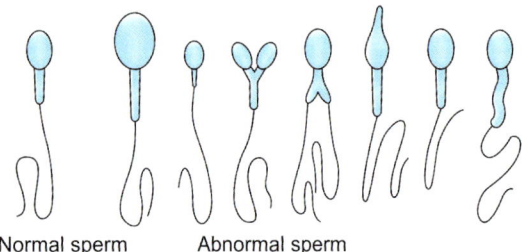

Normal sperm   Abnormal sperm

Fig. 3.8: Normal and abnormal sperms

e. Function of mid-piece, principal piece and end piece—the specific functions have been elaborated in the previous section of the chapter.

Spermatogenesis (Embryologic Development of Spermatozoa)

This can be discussed under two broad headings:

a. Molecular consideration
b. Anatomic consideration

Molecular Consideration

The origin of adult spermatozoa from spermatogonial germ cell passes through three molecular phases:

i. Proliferation and differentiation of diploid spermatogonial germ cell

ii. Phase of meiosis where chromosome pairing and genetic recombination occurs.

iii. Phase of spermiogenesis—this phase consists of a series of changes involving development of nuclear DNA, acrosomal cap, tail and ultimately resulting in development of an adult spermatozoa.

These events collectively, continue for a period of 74 days. Within this long period there may be numerous opportunities for introduction of damage to the genome of male gamete. *This knowledge provides the practical information that while performing ICSI with spermatid or secondary spermatocyte, there may be a risk of injecting a damaged spermatocyte.* This may lead to failure of fertilisation or development of an abnormal embryo.

Proliferation and differentiation of diploid spermatogonial cell

In the testis, the spermatogonial stem cells proliferate and differentiate producing three types of spermotogonia: (i) Population identical to spermatogonial stem cell (resting cell) and these do not differentiate towards adult spermatogonial cell; (ii) population trying to differentiate towards adult sperma-togonial cell—they are the precursors of future adult spermatozoa; and (iii) cells that are likely to undergo apoptosis.

During this phase, the spermotagonial cells are diploid, i.e. they contain two chromosomes each, and 2 chromatids (DNA strands) in each chromosome.

Phase of meiosis

During this phase, the diploid proliferating and differentiating stem cells are converted to haploid gamete. This is a critical and unique event of genetic recombination. Primary spermatocyte (spermatogonial stem cells) with DNA content equivalent to 2 chromatids in two chromosomes replicate into 4 distinct chromatids (DNA strands) initiating meiosis. (Fig. 3.9).

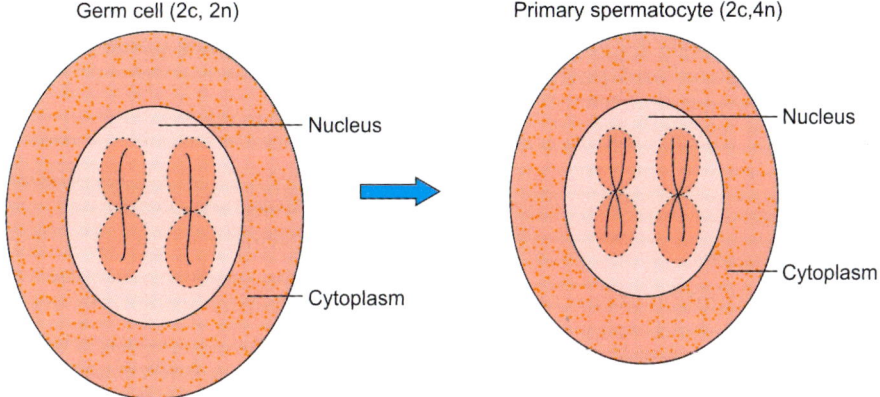

Fig. 3.9: First meiotic division

Chromosome segregation and crossing over of genes amongst DNA strands occurs during this phase. Crossing over is critical in gametogenesis —may lead to genetic defect and structural anomaly of sperm. Because during this phase of crossing over, there may be loss or defect in the genetic material.

After chromosomal pairing and crossing over the first meiotic division is completed, i.e. two secondary spermatocytes are formed. There is one chromosome and two chromatids (DNA strands) in each secondary spermatocyte. Therefore, the DNA content in each secondary spermatocyte is still diploid.

The second meiotic division (Fig. 3.10) starts where there is separation of two DNA strands in each chromosome—resulting in formation of four spermatids, each spermtaocyte having a haploid number of chromosome and a haploid DNA.

The diagrammatic representation of the entire process of spermatogenesis at molecular level is shown in Fig. 3.11.

Possible problems arising during the phase of meiosis

For comprehensive meiotic division to occur, meiotic cell contains many novel proteins and enzymes. These are essential for chromosome and DNA alignment, DNA breakage, recombination and DNA repair. Occasionally

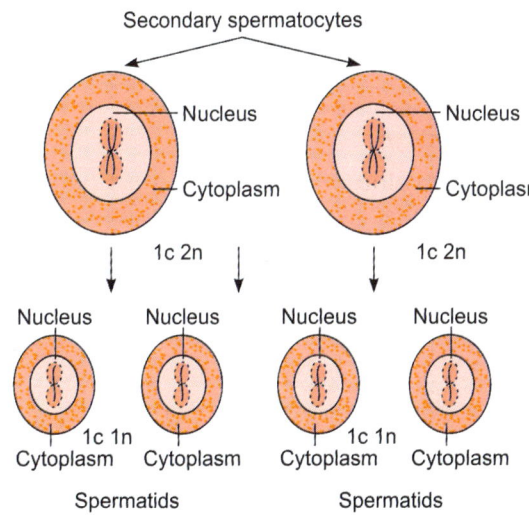

Fig. 3.10: Second meiotic division

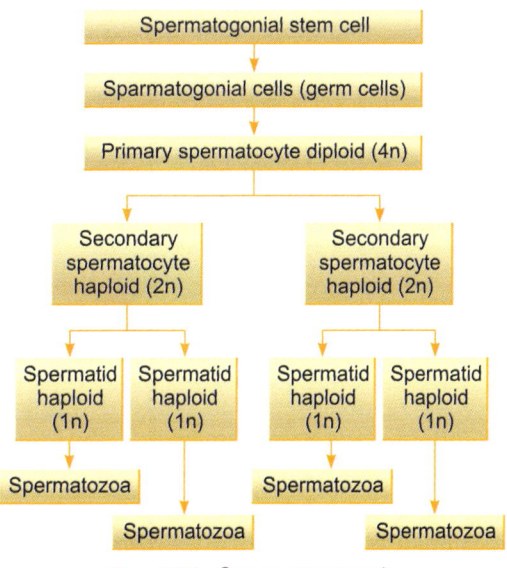

Fig. 3.11: Spermatogenesis

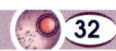

DNA repair mechanism in the phase of meiosis may be defective—there may be anomalies in chromosomal segregation and pairing and crossing over of genetic material. These defects may lead to germ cell differentiation arrest at the spermotocyte level either primary or secondary.

Phase of Spermiogenesis

During this phase, maturation of spermatozoa starts. From the stage of secondary spermatocyte a round-shaped spermatid forms followed by elongated spermatid and finally an adult spermatozoon develops.

During these transitional phases the specific changes which occur consist of: (a) Elongation of nucleus, (b) appearance of acrosomal sac containing proteolytic enzymes, (c) formation of neck and differentiation of the terminal part into three distinct segments like mid-piece, principal piece and end piece. These changes occur during six different stages; the stages have been designated as SA-1 and 2, SB-1 and 2 and SC-1 and 2.

Specific and remarkable changes during spermiogenesis

i. Head nuclear protein consisting of histone is replaced by protamin—producing a tightly compacted nucleus. Protamine is a stronger DNA compared to histone. Unlike all other somatic cells of the body where histone is the DNA in the nucleus, spermatozoon is the only cell which contains protamin to offer compactness of the sperm head nuclear DNA.

ii. Chromatin condensation during spermiogenesis results in DNA occupying nearly 70% of the total volume of sperm nucleus (somatic cell—only 5%).

iii. The adverse effect of displacement of histone and replacement by protamine may result in haploid genome damage (after secondary spermatocyte, the sperm cell genome becomes haploid).

iv. Repair capabilities during spermiogenesis phase is limited (unlike those during meiosis phase).

v. In addition to nuclear DNA structuring—axoneme, outer dense fibre and protein (dyenin) in mid-piece, principal piece and end piece develop.

vi. Mitochondria develops on the sheath of mid-piece as germ cell differentiation by spermiogenesis continues.

As a consequence of massive changes during spermiogenesis there may be tremendous load on 'haploid' spermatozoa, leading to germ cell arrest or blockage—thereby causing infertility in many individuals.

Defects in synthesis of mid-piece and tail mitochondria may result in structurally abnormal spermatozoa with poor motility. Also mutation in protein essential for compaction of sperm nuclear DNA may result in spermatozoa with abnormal head.

Minor genetic defects may not alter spermatozoa morphology, but may lead to production of genetically defective spermatid. This will be a great concern for spermatid injection which is sometimes performed in the procedure of ICSI (ROSNI-round spermatid nuclear injection).

Difference of Initiation of Meiosis in the Male and Female Gametes

In female, meiosis starts at 12 weeks of intra-uterine life, but remains arrested at meiosis I. This is completed at puberty with onset of LH surge. In male, spermatogonial cells (the stem cells) remain at rest till puberty—meiosis and spermiogenesis start after puberty.

Spermatogenesis—Anatomical Consideration

Sperms develop and mature within seminiferous tubules. Seminiferous tubules consist of basement membrane and lumen.

Basement Membrane

Basement membrane consists of two types of cells

Germ cells and Sertoli cells. Sertoli cells are triangular shaped cells with their apex projecting towards the lumen. The base of these triangular cells are situated peripherally. Apex of the Sertoli cells are interconnected by tight junction. This tightly interconnected apical junction forms 'blood-testes barrier'. Blood-testes barrier when intact does not allow seminal antigens to pass into the systemic circulation (reticuloendothelial system) to produce self-antibodies.

Germ cells lie in between the Sertoli cells—they are precursors of adult spermatozoa.

Lumen

Interconnected Sertoli cells divide the lumen of seminiferous tubules into two compartments: (a) Basal compartment and (b) Adluminal compartment.

Significance of Two Compartments

a. **Basal compartment:** In this compartment, maturation of early stages of spermatozoa occurs. This compartment is in direct contact with interstitial cells containing Leydig cell, blood vessels and lymphatics, and therefore, is directly exposed to immune phenomenon. But the tight interconnection of the apices of Sertoli cells which form the blood-testes barrier, prevents antigens crossing this barrier and prevents antibody formation. But when this blood-testes barrier is damaged as in infection, trauma, excessive exposure to heat and following vasectomy, antigens may cross-over allowing antibodies to develop in reticulo-endothelial system of the body. These antibodies then reenter the seminiferous tubules and damage the developing spermatozoa.

Basement membrane contains myofibrils which are under control of oxytocin. They help in forward sperm propulsion.

b. **Adluminal compartment:** Within the adluminal compartment, late stages of spermatozoal maturation continues. This is a sealed compartment, and therefore, not exposed to external or environmental trauma.

Final Maturation and Acquisition of Motility of Spermatozoa

This occurs through exposure of spermatozoa to many biochemical components while the sperm travels through the seminal pathway. The principal sites where the sperm acquires significant motility are—rete testes, epididymis, seminal vesicles and prostate. The important biochemical constituents which provide additional sources of sperm vitality, motility and integrity are carnitine, acid glycerophosphate from epididymis, fructose and coagulase from seminal vesicle, liquefying enzymes and acid phosphatase from prostate.

Endocrine Control of Spermatogenesis

Just like ovulatory control, spermatogenesis has also an endocrine control with feedback mechanism between hypothalamic pituitary control from one side and testicular control from the other side. FSH is secreted from the pituitary which stimulates Sertoli cell within the seminiferous tubules and Sertoli cells in turn produce two factors: (a) Inhibin which regulates the production of FSH from pituitary and (b) androgen binding globulin (ABG).

ABG transports testosterone produced by Leydig cells which exist outside the seminiferous tubules into the lumen of the seminiferous tubules allowing maturation of germ cells. LH also produced by pituitary stimulates Leydig cells to produce testosterone. Testosterone on one side helps maturation of germ cells and on the other hand regulates production of pituitary LH through negative feedback mechanism.

In addition to endocrine control there are other paracrine procedures which help in spermatogenesis. These paracrine factors consist of IGF-1, cytokines, proteins and enzymes (Fig. 3.12).

Summary

Spermatozoa is the male gamete which performs the function of reproduction.

There are a few unique characteristics of human spermatozoa; the important ones are: Adult sperm cells do not grow or divide; unlike other somatic cells sperm head has a large nucleus and lacks large cytoplasm and the sperm cells are unique for the presence of plenty of abnormal forms in the ejaculate. This

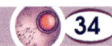

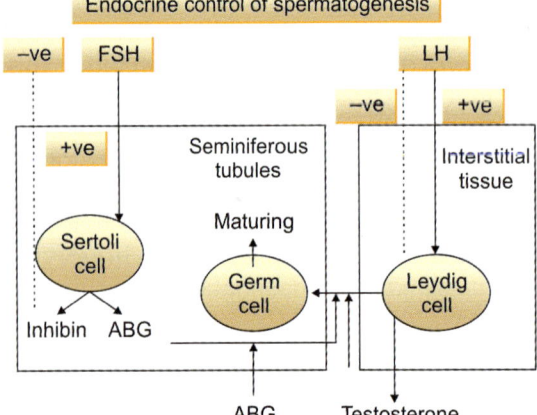

Fig. 3.12: Growth factor, cytokine, proteins, enzymes are the additional factors

is because of frequency of aneuploidy due to specific chromosomal arrangements in the nucleus.

There are four anatomical segments of adult spermatozoa, each with specific physiological function. The segments and their functions are: Head—involved in the main biological function of fertilisation; centriole—in the neck helping in the process of pronuclear apposition; while the mid-piece and tail maintain sperm vitality, metabolism, respiration and locomotion.

Spermatozoal developments occur within the testes from immature germ cells which are known as spermatogonial cells. There are three types of cells in our body, viz. somatic cells, stem cells and germ cells. All cells are diploid except adult spermatozoa which is haploid. The entire process of adult sperm (haploid) formation from immature sperm (diploid) takes about 9 to 10 weeks and passes through several phases of divisions. Broadly changes occur through three phases: (a) Proliferation and differentiation of diploid spermatogonial germ cells, (b) phase of meiosis—chromosomal pairing and genetic recombination, (c) phase of spermiogenesis—series of changes occur—involving development of nuclear DNA, acrosomal cap, etc. ultimately developing into a haploid adult spermatozoon. This long period of spermatogenesis provides enormous opportunities for morphological

and genetic abnormalities to occur in adult spermatozoa. This is one of the reasons for presence of large number of abnormal spermatozoa in the ejaculate.

Anatomically, germ cells exist in the basal compartment of seminiferous tubules. Seminiferous tubule is divided into two compartments—basal and adluminal, by tight apical junction of Sertoli cells. Germ cells lie in between Sertoli cells.

The primary development up to secondary spermatocyte occurs within basal compartment, whereas the final maturation occurs within the adluminal compartment. The biochemical environment for final maturation and acquisition of motility is provided by different molecular constituents available in the seminal pathway—epididymis, vas deferens, seminal vesicles, prostate, bulbourethral glands, etc.

Like endocrine control of ovulation, spermatogeneisis also has a similar mechanism of endocrine feedback regulation. The principal participants are: FSH, LH from pituitary and feedback control is provided through testosterone from Leydig cells and inhibin and androgen binding globulin (ABG) from Sertoli cells.

FURTHER READING

1. Bench GS, Friz AM, Corzett MH, et al. DNA and total protamine masses in individiual sperm from fertile mammalian subjecs. *Cytometry.* 1996; 23: 263–71.

2. C. Van Duijin Jnr. The structure of human spermatozoa F.R.M.S., Journal of the Royal Microscopcial Society Vol. 72, Issue 4, Pages 189–198, Du 1952.

3. Fuentes—Mascorro G. Serrano H, Rosado A. Sperm Chromatin. Arch Androl 45; 215–25, 2000.

4. Gatewood JM, Cook GR, Balhorn R, et al. Sequence specific packaging of DNA in human sperm chromatin. *Science.* 1987; 236:962–4.

5. Hormonal control of spermatogenesis R I McLachlan, NG. Wreford, D.M. Robbertson, DM De Kretser, Trends in Endocrinology and Metabolism, Vol 6, Issue 3,95–101, April 1995.

6. Irina A Zalenskaya, E. Morton Brabdury, Andrei O, Zalensky. Chromatin Structure of Telomere: Domain in Human Sperm. Biochemical and Biophysical Research Communications Vol 279, Issue 1; 213–218, 9 Dec 2000.

7. Johnson GD, Lalancette G, Linnemann AK, et al. The sperm nucleus: chromatin, RNA, and the nuclear matrix. Reproduction; 141: 21–36, 2011.

8. Oliva R, Castillo J. Proteomics and the genetics of sperm chromatin condensation. *Asian J Androl.* 2011; 13: 24–30.

9. Robert I, McLachlan, the endocrine control of spermatogenesis, Best practice and Research Clinical Endocrinology and Metabolism, Vol. 14, Issue 3, 345–362, Sept 2000,.

10. Sakkas D, Mariethoz E, Manicardi G, et al. Origin of DNA damage in ejaculated human spermatozoa. *Rev Reprod.* 1999; 4: 31–7.

11. Shettles, L.B. Nuclear structure of human spermatozoa, Nature. 186, 648 (1960).

12. Smith, DJ (2009). "Human sperm accumulation near surfaces: A simulation study". *Journal of Fluid Mechanics* 621: 295. doi:10.1017/S00 22112008004953. Retrieved 20 May 2012.

13. Solov'eva L, Svetlova M, Bodinski D, et al. Nature of telomere dimmers and chromosome looping in human spermatozoa. *Chromosome Res* 2004; 12: 817–23.

14. Spermatogenesis de Kretsner DM, Loveland KL, Meinhardt A, Simorangkir D and Wreford N, HUM Reprod 13 (Suppl 1): 1–8, 1998.

15. Sumio Ishijima, Shigeru Oshio, Hideo Mohri. *"Flagellar movement of human spermatozoa"*, *Gamete research*, Vol. 13, no. 3, pp. 185–197, 1986.

16. Ward WS, Coffey DS. "DNA packaging and organization in mammalian spermatozoa: comparison with somatic cells". *Biol. Reprod.* 44 (4): 569–74, 1991.

17. Ward WS, Coffey DS. DNA packaging and organisation in mammalian spermatozoa: Comparison with somatic cells. Biol Reprod 1991; 44: 569–74.

18. Ward WS, Zalensky AO. The unique complex organisation of the transcriptionally silent sperm chromatin. *Crit Rev Eukaryot Gene Expr* 1996; 6: 139–47.

19. Ward WS. Deoxyribonucleic acid loop-domain tertiary structure in mammalian spermatozoa. *Biol Reprod.* 1993; 48: 1193–201.

20. Zalensky AO, Allen MJ, Kobayashi A, et al. Well-defined genome architecture in the human sperm nucleus. *Chromosoma* 1995; 103: 577–90.

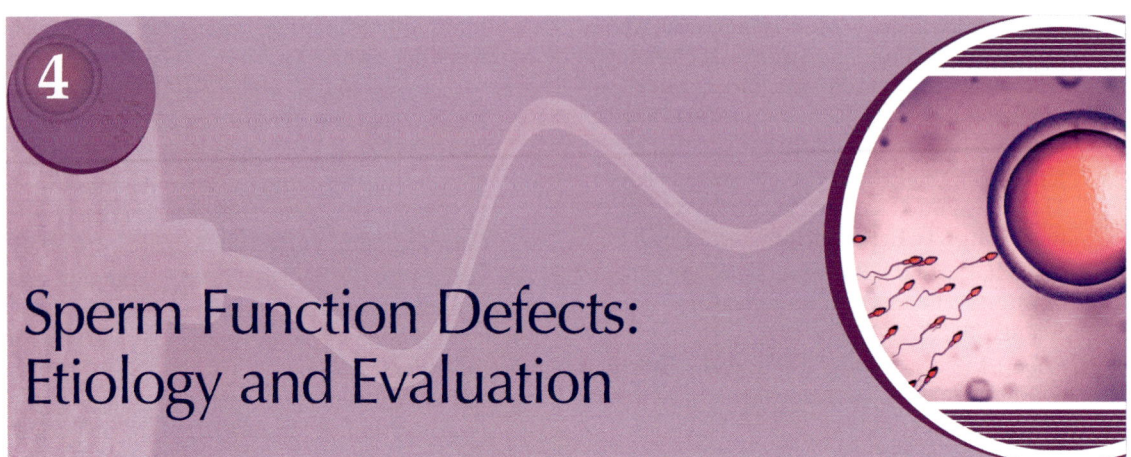

Sperm Function Defects: Etiology and Evaluation

INTRODUCTION

Infertility has been a major medical and social problem since the dawn of human evolution. Despite the enormous progress in research and reasoning, most of the blame for infertility until recently, was placed on the female. Only during the last 15–20 years, advances in understanding of gonadal/sperm function and dysfunction led to a dramatic increase in our knowledge of male infertility. Defective sperm function is the most prevalent cause of male infertility and a difficult condition to treat.[1]

Many environmental, physiological and genetic factors have been implicated as etiological factors for poor sperm function and infertility. Although techniques like intracytoplasmic sperm injection (ICSI) offer considerable promise to such male factor patients, the indiscriminate use of such assisted fertility treatments, especially when the etiology of sperm dysfunction is poorly understood is not warranted. Thus it is very important to identify the factors/conditions which affect normal sperm function.

The ultimate goal of a spermatozoon is the successful fertilisation of ovum resulting in normal conception. In order to achieve this, the spermatozoa after spermiation must mature within the male genital tract, travel through the female reproductive system, undergo capacitation and acrosome reaction,

bind to and penetrate the zona pellucida of the ova as well as the oolemma, and finally DNA of sperm head nucleus should fuse with the spindle (precursor of the female pronucleus) to form a zygote. Normal spermatozoa should properly undergo or go through all of these steps in order to fertilise the ova. However, many men who demonstrate normal parameters on standard semen analysis remain infertile.[2] This suggests that the routine semen analysis (assessment of seminal volume, spermatozoal motility, density, viability and morphology) does not necessarily provide complete diagnostic information.[3]

With the technological advancements in assisted reproductive treatment, it is now feasible to cause fertilisation and pregnancy by injection of a single spermatozoon into the oocyte via the ICSI method. The ultimate goal in this respect is the selection of a spermatozoon that has genetic and cellular attributes comparable to those sperms that interact with the zona pellucida under physiological or conventional IVF fertilisation conditions.

In functional defects, available medical treatments are not very effective. Semen samples containing plenty of functionally abnormal sperms are also not suitable for ICSI. They often lead to fertilisation failure. Donor insemination may not be acceptable by many couples. Moreover, in recent years the number of voluntary donors is also declining because of the new law in 'Human Rights' stating that maintenance of anonymity of sperm donor is not mandatory. Children born through sperm donation, after the age of 18, shall have the right to know the name of his/her genetic father. Obviously this has inflicted an adverse influence on sperm donation.

With these background facts, this chapter emphasises on:

a. Normal function at molecular level of different anatomical segments of spermatozoa

b. Common functional abnormalities; their assessment

c. Additional tests for functional abnormalities

d. Immunological defects; their impact on functional integrity

e. Impact of infection

f. Future thoughts—stem cell culture for production of germ cells which may help men with uncorrectable sperm abnormalities in their own spermatozoa to achieve a pregnancy.

ANATOMICAL SEGMENTS OF SPERMATOZOA AND THEIR FUNCTIONS

Anatomically human spermatozoon consists of four segments (Fig. 4.1). Each segment contains specific biochemical components for performing physiological functions either in the sperm itself or in the host system. The different spermatozoal segments, their biochemical components and the related physiological functions are detailed below:

Head: This is the most important segment of spermatozoa. Head performs the major biological function of fertilisation in the host (female partner). For successful fertilisation of oocyte, sperm head contains a set of vital components which are essential to complete the different molecular events of fertilisation. The related components and their functions are:

a. *Outermost covering of the sperm head known as 'plasma membrane'*: Macromolecular

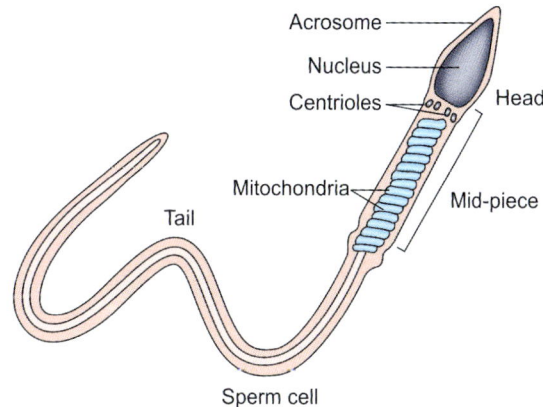

Fig. 4.1: Sperm cell

substances on the surface of the membrane undergo specific changes. This is known as capacitation. Capacitation occurs when sperm comes in contact with periovulatory fluid in the uterine cavity. 'Capacitation' is a process of hyperactivation which is essential for spermatozoa before the next step of fertilisation, i.e. acrosome reaction and zona penetration.

b. *Acrosomal sac with outer and inner layer membranes:* When the sperm head comes in contact with zona pellucida, the plasma membrane fuses with outer acrosome membrane and then disintegrates. This leads to release of acrosin from acrosomal sac which allows sperm head to penetrate zona pellucida and enter into ooplasm. The process is known as "acrosome reaction". Without capacitation, acrosome reaction does not occur.

c. After penetrating zona pellucida, the sperm head comes in contact with oocyte cytoplasmic membrane—oolemma. While in contact with oolemma, the "activated" sperm head generates 'Ca-wave' in ooplasm. 'Ca-wave' or 'Ca-oscillation' is essential for series of molecular events to occur for successful fertilisation. This event is known as 'cytoplasmic syngamy'

d. Sperm head enters into oocyte cytoplasm known as "ooplasm". While inside "ooplasm" and "Ca-oscillation" in the

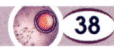

ooplasm already generated, further molecular events of fertilisation continue to follow. Briefly these events are:

i. 'Extrusion of second polar body from oocyte nucleus—leaving behind the mitotic spindle in oocyte cytoplasm—precursor of female pronucleus.

ii. Disintegration of sperm nuclear membrane; change of sperm nuclear DNA from protamine to histone; formation of pronuclear membrane—precursor of male pronucleus.

iii. Formation of microtubules from sperm neck 'Centriole'.

iv. Apposition of two pronuclear membranes—formation of pro-nuclear bodies (PNB); dissolution of pronuclear membrane—exchange of genetic material between male and female pronuclei.

v. The process is known as "nuclear syngamy"—formation of new individual zygote—by mitotic division.

Mid-segment: Consists of mitochondrial sheath which is involved in spermatozoal metabolism and respiration. Mitochondrial sheath contains many trace elements, viz. selenium, zinc, magnesium, etc.

Tail: Tail contains a specific protein known as 'dyenin' which confers propellary force for spermatozoa.

For further details—see Chapter 3 on "Human Spermatozoa"

Assessment of Functional Abnormalities of Spermatozoa

Three types of functional abnormalities are currently being assessed. These tests are performed when normal semen analysis reveals decreased or abnormal motility, abnormal morphology or repeated fertilisation failure in IVF or ICSI. Specific functional tests performed are: (a) Tests for viability are performed when there is poor progressive motility or higher percentage of immotile sperms, (b) test for acrosomal integrity and (c) tests for nuclear DNA fragmentation.

a. Test for absence of motility in viable or nonviable sperms: A sperm may be living, but immotile and also a sperm may be dead and immotile. These two conditions can be differentiated by hypo-osmotic swelling test[4] (HOST) (Fig. 4.2). In this test, the sperms are placed in hypo-osmotic solution mixed with media (modified HOS test) and incubated in CO_2 incubator for half an hour. After incubation, if more than 58% (WHO Lab Manual, 2010) of sperms exhibit 'swelling' and 'coiling' of the mid-piece or tail (Fig. 4.3), then it can be assumed that the sperms are living but immotile. On the other hand, if less than 58% of the sperms exhibit these changes, then the conclusion is that most of the sperms are dead and immotile. Such a sample cannot be used for IVF or ICSI.

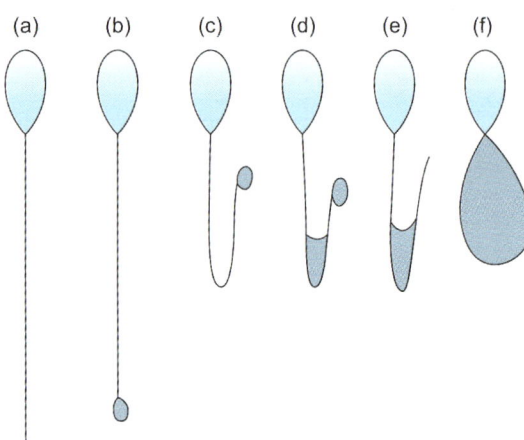

(a)   (b)   (c)   (d)   (e)   (f)

Fig. 4.2: Hypo-osmotic swelling test (HOST)

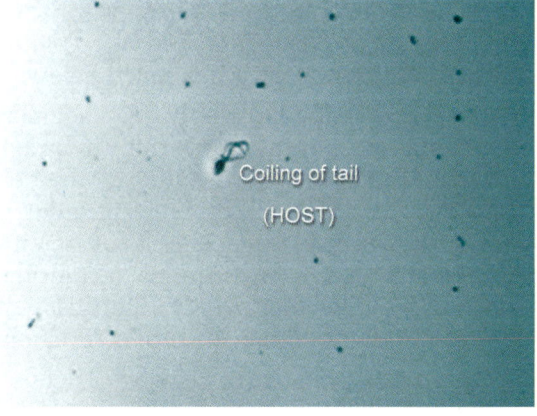

Coiling of tail (HOST)

Fig. 4.3: HOST as seen under microscope

b. Test for acrosomal integrity: It is well-known that acrosome reaction (AR) or exocytosis of acrosin from acrosomal sac should occur when the sperm head is in contact with zona pellucida (Fig. 4.4a). But, if acrosomal leakage has occurred before the sperm head reaches the zona then there will be fertilisation failure. This abnormality can be assessed either by biochemical test or by polscopic evaluation.

Biochemical tests for acrosome content can be performed by: (a) Triple stain technique, (b) monoclonal antibodies to acrosomal contents, (c) pisum sativam agglutinin and fluorescent stain technique, (d) radioimmunoassay and (e) clinical acrosin assay.

These tests involve treating the spermatozoa with some chemicals. Therefore, any sperm from the sample tested biochemically for acrosin, reacted or non-reacted, cannot be used for ICSI.

But polscopic evaluation aids in identifying acrosome reacted sperms that can also be used for ICSI. The acrosome reacted sperm appears with a birefringent[5] head (Fig. 4.4b). Obviously the sperm with birefringent head can be directly used for ICSI. The following photographs illustrate acrosome reacted and acrosome non-reacted sperms.

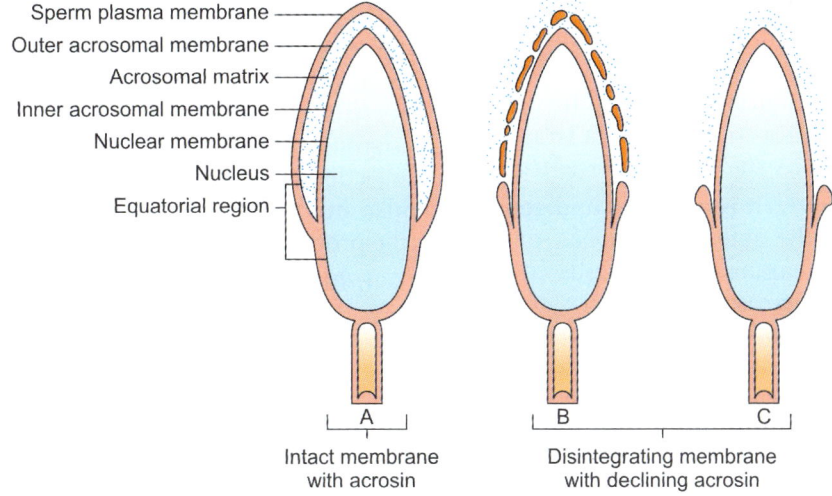

Sperm plasma membrane
Outer acrosomal membrane
Acrosomal matrix
Inner acrosomal membrane
Nuclear membrane
Nucleus
Equatorial region

A — Intact membrane with acrosin

B C — Disintegrating membrane with declining acrosin

Fig. 4.4a: AR under electron microscope

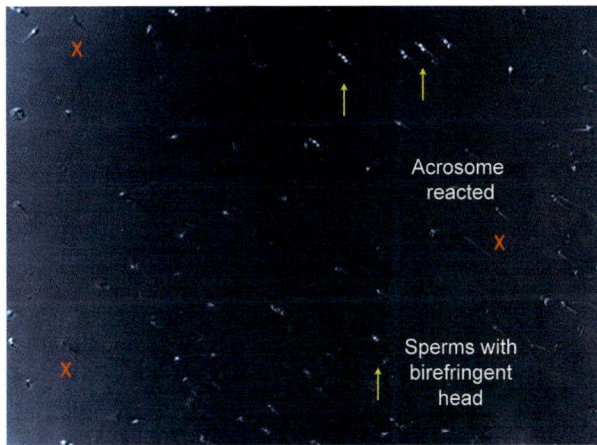

Acrosome reacted

Sperms with birefringent head

Fig. 4.4b: AR under Polscope

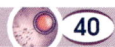
c. Tests for nuclear DNA fragmentation: The commonly used methods to estimate sperm DNA damage are:

1. TUNEL assay
2. COMET assay
3. HALO sperm test

TUNEL (Terminal deoxynucleotidyl transferase dUTP nick end labeling) assay:[6–9] It is a method of detecting DNA fragmentation resulting from apoptosis signaling cascades by labeling the terminal end of nucleic acids. The assay relies on the presence of nicks in the DNA which can be identified by an enzyme, terminal deoxynucleotide transferase (TdT). The process itself is lengthy and the reagents used in this method may cause apoptosis.

Results of TUNEL is analysed by FACS flow cytometry:

Sperm with normal DNA have only background fluorescence while those with fragmented DNA *fluorescence brightly.*

COMET assay:[8, 9] It is a simple and sensitive technique for the detection of DNA damage. It involves encapsulation of cells in a low melting point agarose suspension, lysis of the cells in neutral or alkaline (pH > 13) conditions and electrophoresis of the suspended lysed cells. Normal sperm cells look round whereas sperm with damaged DNA look like a *comet* under fluorescence microscope (Fig. 4.5a).

HALO sperm test: It is a simple method to evaluate sperm DNA health by commercially available 'HALO sperm test kit'.

Sperm nuclei containing elevated DNA fragmentation generate small or no halos of DNA dispersion. Whereas sperm with no or low level of DNA fragmentation release DNA loops in an area surrounding the sperm head, forming large halos (Fig. 4.5b).

DFI (DNA fragmentation index): DFI[9] indicates the cut-off value of extent of nuclear fragmentation—beyond which, pregnancy even by ICSI is not possible. The cut-off value has been estimated as 19%. If the level exceeds 20%, the semen sample is unsuitable for fertilisation.

Special methods of sperm selection for ICSI: Two special methods are now sometimes used for selecting functionally efficient sperm for injection in ICSI procedure. These tests are performed specially when there are repeated fertilisation failures in ICSI. They help in identification of a fertilisable spermatozoon for injection in the ICSI procedure. The procedures also involve additional requirements during the procedure of sperm injection. They are:

i. **PICSI ("Physiologic" ICSI):** The test is performed in special types of petridish coated with hyaluronan[10]—in this type of petridish, there are some wells coated with hyaluronan (Fig. 4.6a). These special petridishes are available commercially. The most efficient sperm is attracted and attached to this hyaluronan-coated wells. These sperms are the most efficient sperms which are to be used for ICSI.

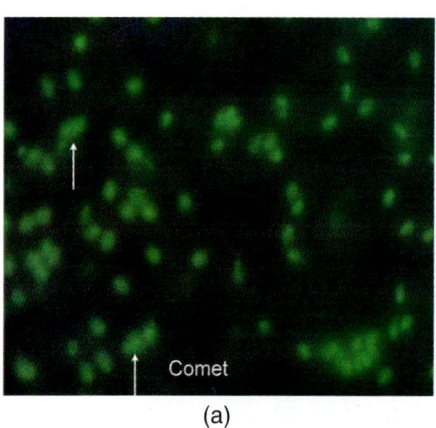

(a)

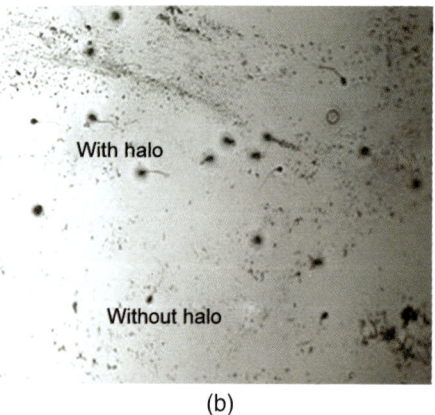

With halo

Without halo

(b)

Figs 4.5a and b: AR under electron microscope

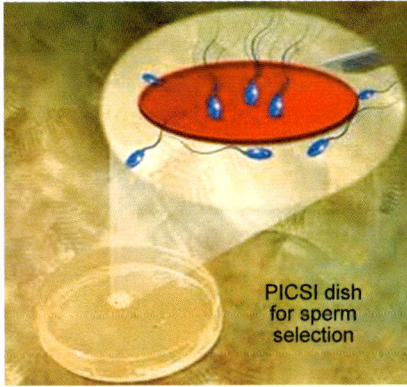

Fig. 4.6a: PICSI

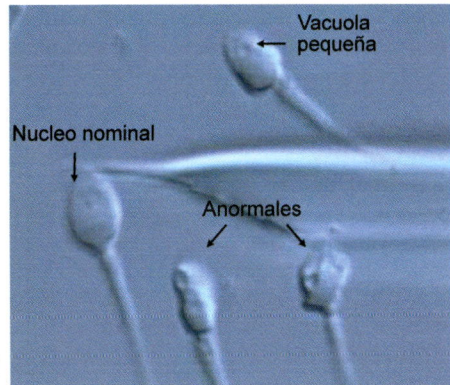

Fig. 4.6b

ii. IMSI (Intra cytoplasmic morphologically selected sperm injection):[11] In this procedure, a special attachment is fixed to the micromanipulator which allows a magnification × 8000. The details of sperm morphology (vacuoles, fragmentation, etc.) including biochemical anatomy are clearly visualised and the most efficient looking sperm can be selected for ICSI. Sperm nucleus having one big vacuole >0.84 μm or many small vacuoles should not be aspirated for ICSI to avoid failed or abnormal fertilisation (Fig. 4.6b).

ADDITIONAL SPERM FUNCTION TEST

Apart from the tests which have been described above, additional sperm function tests include: (i) strict morphology, (ii) computer-assisted semen analysis (CASA), (iii) cervical mucous-sperm interaction assay and (iv) sperm capacitation. Of these, strict sperm morphology is an important test which is also an integral sperm parameter, always assessed before IVF or ICSI.

Cervical Mucous-sperm Interaction Test

Cervical mucous-sperm interaction test is not performed as a routine in assisted reproduction. This is a screening test in the conventional infertility evaluation.

Other less commonly performed sperm function tests include sperm capacitation assay, Hemizona binding assay and sperm penetration assay. These tests are rarely performed nowadays.

Strict Morphology

The 'strict criteria'[12] with clinically significant threshold of 14% normal forms is an important predictor for IVF success. Fertilisation in IVF with these criteria is expected to be 94.3%. Fertilisation rate sharply declines when normal sperm morphology is less than 4%.

The criteria for defining normal morphology are (Fig. 4.7):
a. Smooth and oval head
b. No defects in mid-piece, neck and tail
c. No cytoplasmic droplets larger than half the size of sperm head
d. Acrosome should comprise 40–70% of the sperm head
e. Large vacuoles in sperm nucleus is associated with significantly lower pregnancy rate and higher early embryo death rate.[13]

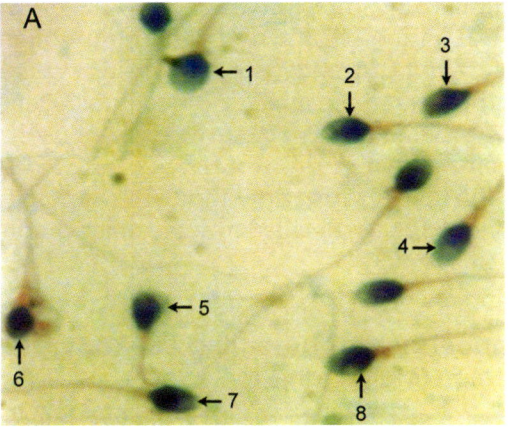

Fig. 4.7: Diff-Quik staining method

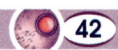

Sperm morphology is an indicator of germinal epithelial function. Presence of cytoplasmic droplets reflects a defect in epididymal maturation. Currently, computer-assisted semen analysis (CASA) is very promising to classify sperm morphology.

Computer-assisted Semen Analysis (CASA)[14]

The procedure provides sperm motility variables. In addition, it helps in assessment of amplitude of lateral head movement. Average velocity is positively correlated with fertilisation capacity of spermatozoa. It is a useful instrument for diagnosis of abnormalities of sperm function. Though a powerful instrument, it appears to be an expensive and complex research tool. The benefits achieved by the use of this instrument is not very cost-effective.

IMMUNOLOGICAL DEFECT

Antisperm antibodies can also impair the sperm function.[15] There are about 36 types of antigens in seminal plasma and on the surface of spermatozoa. But only 6 are sperm-specific; they can produce antibodies either in the host (autoimmunity) or in the female partner (isoimmunity).

Autoimmunity develops either as a result of trauma, infection, use of tight undergarments, varicocele or following vasectomy. Isoimmunity develops either in the cervical mucous or systemically in the wife's serum.

However, presence of antisperm antibodies circulating is not a sufficient proof of immunologic infertility. Sperm surface ASA (local antibody) may indicate immunologic infertility. Currently, sperm is being washed and prepared for all ART procedures. Hence the problem of sperm surface antibody has been eliminated.

Further information about immunologic defect has been detailed in some other chapter of this book.

IMPORTANCE OF INFECTION[16, 17]

Importance of Detecting Leukocytes in Semen (More than 6 to 7 in hpf)

They may generate reactive oxygen species (ROS). ROS may damage sperm nuclear DNA and may cause lipid peroxidation of sperm membrane which eventually leads to:

  i. Reduced sperm motility
 ii. Absence of acrosome reaction
iii. Interference with sperm zona binding and fertilisation failure.

ROS—what are they?

A variety of metabolic products derived from metabolism of molecular oxygen at different cellular levels including sperm cells. These metabolites damage the sperm cells thereby generating reactive oxygen species (ROS) (mechanism of generating ROS has already been described in some other chapter).

Clinical Consequences of Generation of ROS

ROS leads to production of either (a) morphologically abnormal spermatozoa or (b) morphologically normal, but functionally abnormal spermatozoa.

Protective Mechanism Against ROS

ROS generated in the seminal plasma are always being scavenged out thereby preventing excessive sperm damage. Not only leukocytes but also there are other agents or factors which are responsible for generating ROS in the seminal plasma. These are: (a) Cytoplasmic droplets, (b) abnormal spermatozoa and (c) excessive centrifugation. While ROS is being generated, the scavenging system in the seminal plasma is trying to wash it out, sparing the spermatozoa from damage. The scavenging system consists of: (a) Superoxide dismutase (SOD), (b) catalase, (c) glutathaione peroxidase (GPX), (d) vitamin A, Vitamin C, Vitamin E and (e) coenzyme Q10. When the balance between the two is more in favour of ROS generating system, it is known as 'oxidative stress'. 'Stress' damages functional potential of spermatozoa and in addition causes sperm head nuclear damage (Fig. 4.8).

FUTURE THOUGHTS

Creating sperm cells in the laboratory through stem cell culture: Over the past few years the number of sperm donors is declining.

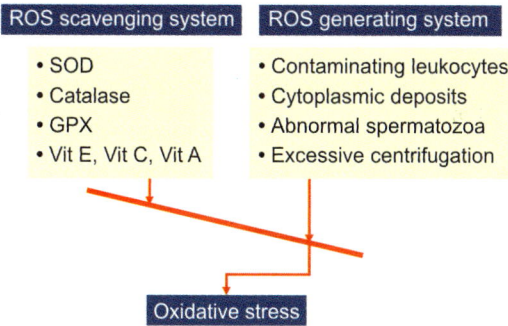

ROS scavenging system	ROS generating system
• SOD • Catalase • GPX • Vit E, Vit C, Vit A	• Contaminating leukocytes • Cytoplasmic deposits • Abnormal spermatozoa • Excessive centrifugation

Oxidative stress

Fig. 4.8: Balance between ROS generating system and scavenging system

Attempt has already been made, based on animal experiments, to produce human male and female germ cells and the following ideas have been proposed.

   a. From ES cells through embryoid bodies — Geijessen[18], et al. *Nature*, 427; 148–54 (2004).

   b. From spermatogonial stem cells (adult stem cells)—Hiroshi Kubuta.[19] *Proc National Acad of Science* (2001).

   c. From ovarian stem cells[20] (Adult stem cells)—Bokovsky, et al. *Rep Biol Endocrin* 2005.

Origin of Germ Cell from Embryonic Stem Cell

While culturing embryonic stem cell in the specialised culture, some cells were identified which had a 'genetic signature' of primordial germ cell (PGC). These are known as embryoid bodies. These cells were continuously grown in specialised culture and it is proposed that both egg cell and sperm cell can be generated from primordial germ cell looking embryoid bodies (Fig. 4.9).

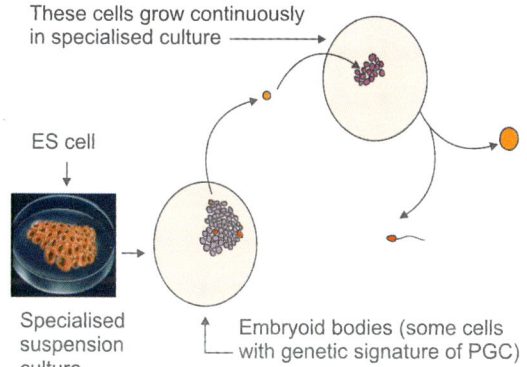

These cells grow continuously in specialised culture

ES cell

Specialised suspension culture

Embryoid bodies (some cells with genetic signature of PGC)

Fig. 4.9: Diagrammatic representation of production of germ cell through stem cell culture

Immediate Benefits Following Creation of Human Eggs and Sperms from Stem Cells

This avoids use of donor sperm or eggs in assisted reproduction. This also helps in preservation of fertility in men and women awaiting chemotherapy.

Instead of getting embryonic stem cell for creating human sperm and egg, it may also be possible to get the adult stem cell from ovarian tissue or testicular cortical tissue in order to create egg and sperm.

Freezing sperm stem cell or ovarian stem cell is better than freezing the spermatozoa or testicular and ovarian tissue. Because the stem cells are diploid they can withstand the freezing better than haploid spermatozoa.

Lastly, sperm stem cells may enhance survival of endangered species of animals or valuable livestock.

In conclusion, it may be said that spermiology is a rapidly developing science. Many areas of reproduction are likely to be explored with further understanding of molecular physiology and genetics of human spermatozoa.

REFERENCES

1. Hull M, Glazener C, Kelly N, Conway D, Foster P, Hunton R, Coulson C, Lambert P, Watt E, and Desai K: Population study of causes, treatment and outcome of infertility. *Br Med J* 291, 1693–7 (1985).

2. WHO laboratory manual for the examination of human semen and sperm-cervical mucus interaction. Cambridge Univ Press, Cambridge, 3rd Edition (1992).

3. Sigman M, Lipshultz L, Howards S. Evaluation of the subfertile male. In: *Infertility in the male*. Eds: Lipshultz LA, Howards SS: Chuchill Livingstone, NY (1991).

4. Susan Avery, Bolton Virginia N, Mason Bridgett A. An evaluation of the hypo-osmotic sperm swelling test as a predictor of fertilizing capacity *in vitro*. International Journal of Andrology; 1990: Volume 13, Issue 2; 93–99.

5. Ghosh S, et al. Selection of birefringent spermatozoa under Polscope: Effect on intracytoplasmic sperm injection outcome: 2012; Andrologia; 03/07/2012.

6. Gorczyca W, Gong J, Darzynkiewicz Z. Detection of DNA strand breaks in individual apoptotic

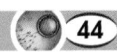
cells by the *in situ* terminal deoxynucleotidyl transferase and nick translation assays. *Cancer Res.* 1993a; 53: 945–951.

7. Gorczyca W, Traganos F, Jesionowska H, Darzynkiewicz Z. Presence of DNA strand breaks and increased sensitivity of DNA in situ to denaturation in abnormal human sperm cells: analogy to apoptosis of somatic cells. *Exp Cell Res.* 1993b; 207: 202–205.

8. Hughes CM, Lewis SE, McKelvey-Martin VJ, Thompson W. A comparison of baseline and induced DNA damage in human spermatozoa from fertile and infertile men using a modified comet assay. *Mol Hum Reprod.* 1996; 2 : 613–619.

9. Jose Luis Fernández, Lourdes Muriel, Maria Teresa Rivero, Vicente Goyanes, Rosana Vazquez, Juan G. Alvarez: The Sperm Chromatin Dispersion Test: A Simple Method for the Determination of Sperm DNA Fragmentation. Journal of Andrology; 2003:24; 1:59–66.

10. Lodovico Parmegiani, Graciela Estela Cognigni, Silvia Bernardi, Enzo Troilo, Walter Ciampaglia, Marco Filicori. "Physiologic ICSI": Hyaluronic acid (HA) favors selection of spermatozoa without DNA fragmentation and with normal nucleus, resulting in improvement of embryo quality: Fertility and Sterility; 2010: 93; 2, 598–604.

11. Martin Wilding, Gianfranco Coppola, Loredana di Matteo, Antonio Palagiano, Enrico Fusco, Brian Dale. Intracytoplasmic injection of morphologically selected spermatozoa (IMSI) improves outcome after assisted reproduction by deselecting physiologically poor quality spermatozoa; Journal of Assisted Reproduction and Genetics: 2011:28:3; 253–262.

12. Menkveld Roelof, Stander Frik SH, Theunis JVW Kotze, Kruger Thinus F, van Zyl Johannes A. The evaluation of morphological characteristics of human spermatozoa according to stricter criteria: Hum. Reprod: 1990: 5; 5, 586–592.

13. Arie Berkovitz, Fina Eltes, Adrian Ellenbogen, Sigal Peer, Dov Feldberg, Benjamin Bartoov. Does the presence of nuclear vacuoles in human sperm selected for ICSI affect pregnancy outcome? Human Reproduction: 2006: 21; 7; 1787–1790.

14. Vantman D, Koukoulis G, Dennison L, Zinaman M, Sherins RJ. Computer-assisted semen analysis: Evaluation of method and assessment of the influence of sperm concentration on linear velocity determination. Fertility and Sterility; 1988; 49; 3:510–515.

15. Claudia Bohring Walter Krause. Immune infertility: Towards a better understanding of sperm auto-immunity. The value of proteomic analysis. Human Reproduction; 2003:18; 5:915–924.

16. Ralf Henkel. ROS and semen quality. Studies on men's health and fertility; oxidative stress in applied basic research and clinical practice; 2012; 301–323.

17. Weidner W, Pilatz A, Diemer Th, Schuppe HC, Rusz A, Wagenlehner F. Male urogenital infections: Impact of infection and inflammation on ejaculate parameters. World Journal of Urology; 2013; 31; 4; 717–723.

18. Geijessen, et al. Nature 427; 148–54 (2004)

19. Hiroshi Kubota, Avarbock Mary R, Brinster Ralph L. Spermatogonial stem cells share some, but not all, phenotypic and functional characteristics with other stem cells. Proceedings of the National Academy of sciences of the United States of America. 2003; 100; 11: 6487–6492.

20. Bukovsky A, Svetlikova M, Caudle MR. Oogenesis in cultures derived from adult human ovaries. Reprod Biol Endocrinol, 2005; 3; 17.

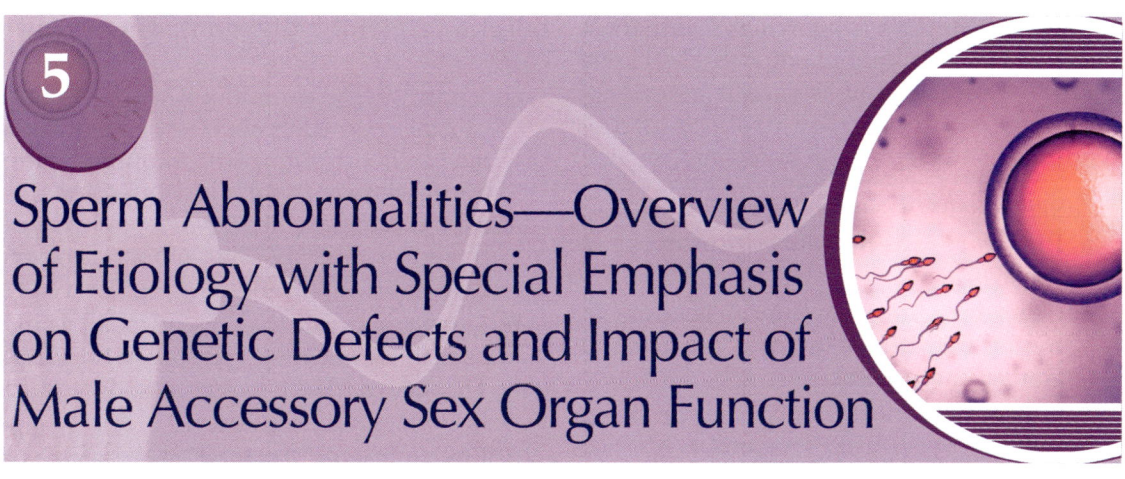

Sperm Abnormalities—Overview of Etiology with Special Emphasis on Genetic Defects and Impact of Male Accessory Sex Organ Function

INTRODUCTION

This chapter deals with etiological factors of sperm abnormalities with special emphasis on impact of genetic defects and influence of male accessory sex organ function. The details of seminal plasma defects, like pH, viscosity, liquefaction time, etc. have been detailed in other chapters of this book. However, a brief description of structural and biochemical abnormalities like plasma membrane defects or nuclear fragmentation leading to functional defect have also been included in this chapter.

Contents of this chapter are

a. Types of abnormalities commonly encountered
b. Etiological background of the defects either individually or collectively
c. Brief description of structural and bio-chemical abnormalities leading to sperm function defect
d. Genetic anomalies associated with sperm abnormalities
e. Impact of male accessory sex organs
f. Areas affected in obstructive azoospermia.

TYPES OF ABNORMALITIES COMMONLY DETECTED

i. Oligospermia or azoospermia
ii. Isolated asthenozoospermia
iii. Only teratozoospermia—is not common

iv. Oligoasthenospermia
v. Oligoasthenoteratozoospermia (OAT syndrome)
vi. Common sites of obstruction in obstructive azoospermia

Etiological Background of Oligo- or Azoospermia

Etiological factors can be broadly classified into: (a) Pretesticular, (b) Testicular and (c) Post-testicular causes.

Broad classification of etiological factors of oligo-or azoospermia (Flowchart 5.1)

Flowchart 5.1

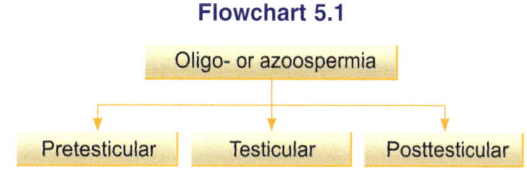

Pretesticular Causes

The commonest pretesticular cause of oligo-or azoospermia is endocrine dysfunction. Endocrine dysfunction may be of two types: (i) Congenital and (ii) Acquired.

Congenital endocrine defect leading to azoospermia is due to embryologically determined (genetic background) endocrine defect at the level of hypothalamus and pituitary. This leads to hypogonadotropic

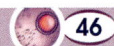

hypogonadism. This is known as Kallmann's syndrome. It affects about one in 8,000–10,000 males.[1, 2] The syndrome is usually associated with anosmia. Infertility problem of the syndrome is treatable with hormones.

Acquired endocrine defect may be due to

a. Pituitary adenoma; commonest is prolactinoma[3, 4]
b. Other rare pituitary tumour leading to hypogonadotropism may be due to craniopharyngioma
c. Functional (anorexia nervosa) or stress induced hyperprolactinaemia.

Other acquired endocrine defects consist of

a. Congenital adrenal hyperplasia (↑ACTH counteracts gonadotropin)
b. Hyper- or hypothyroidism may also lead to oligo- or asthenospermia by alteration of metabolism or direct action of TRH (thyroid-releasing hormone) at the level of hypothalamus or pituitary (for details *see* Chapter 14 on Primary Amenorrhoea).

The etiological factors described above under pretesticular causes are summarized in Flowchart 5.2.

Flowchart 5.2

```
              Oligo or azoospermia
                      │
          ┌───────────┴───────────┐
     Congenital                Acquired
          │
  Kallmann's syndrome
          │
  ┌──────┬───────┬──────────┬──────┬────────┐
Pituitary  Other  Functional  CAH  Hyper-
adenoma    pituitary               hypothy-
(prolact-  tumours                 roidism
inoma)     leading to
           hypogonado-
           trophism
```

Testicular Causes

Testicular causes of oligo- or azoospermia are commonly due to incomplete or complete arrest at any stage of spermatogenesis (during mitotic or meiotic division). The specific causes are:

i. **Viral:**[21–23] The commonest viral infection causing spermatozoal defect or destruction is childhood mumps or mumps during adolescence. Other viral infections or even mumps orchitis beyond adolescence have less, but positive impact on spermatogenic maturation.

ii. **Iatrogenic:** Chemotherapy and radiotherapy have the worst impact on spermatogenesis. The causes have been discussed in detail in some other chapters.

iii. **Environmental factors:**[8–10] Exposure of testicular area to high temperature as in factory workers, usage of tight undergarments, diet consisting of vegetables coloured with synthetic dye, poultry chicken.

iv. **Varicocele[5–7] Grade II or Grade III:** Due to rise in local temperature[8–10]

v. Undescended testes is a congenital defect which is responsible for azoospermia. If detected before puberty, treatment is possible either by surgery (Orchidopexy) or by hCG injection.[11–16]

vi. Genetic or chromosomal abnormalities like—47XXY; Yq deletion; 46XX male; etc.[17–20]

Genetic/chromosomal cause is the commonest testicular cause of oligo- or azoospermia. Flowchart 5.3 illustrates the summary of the testicular causes of oligo- or azoospermia.

Posttesticular Causes

These may be:

i. **Congenital:**[24–27] For example, absence of vas deferens commonly associated with, cystic fibrosis gene mutation.

ii. **Infective:** May be due to tubercular, gonococcal or *Chlamydia* infection

iii. **Retrograde ejaculation:** In this situation not only azoospermia but also absence of ejaculation is a subjective symptom. Occasionally there may be ejaculation— but small amount of ejaculate which comes out is from the bulbourethral or

Flowchart 5.3

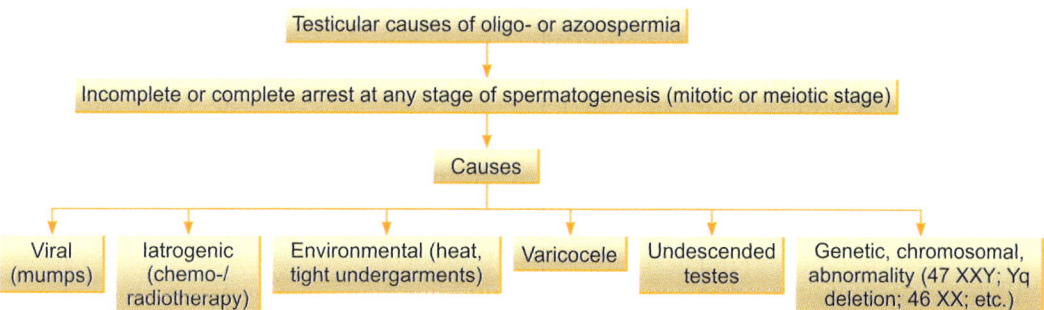

Cowper's glands. Major portion of the ejaculate goes back into the bladder. The easiest way to differentiate between 'functional' and 'organic' retrograde ejaculation may be through a leading question to the male partner—the occurrence of nocturnal emission. Absence of nocturnal emissions suggests an underlying organic defect. On the other hand, history of nocturnal emissions goes in favour of functional retrograde ejaculation.

The organic causes of retrograde ejaculation may be due to accidental postsurgical injury of sympathetic plexus—during bladder neck surgery or following preaortic and para-aortic lymphadenectomy. Alternatively, such defect may also occur in long-standing diabetic neuropathy or vasculopathy.

Flowchart 5.4 illustrates posttesticular etiologies of oligo- or azoospermia.

Etiology of Isolated Asthenospermia

The common causes are:

i. **Infective:**[28] More than 6–8 leukocytes/hpf indicate active infection in the seminal plasma. They may cause asthenospermia or oligoasthenospermia by generating reactive oxygen species (ROS) in the seminal plasma. The production of ROS depends on the presence of the scavenging antioxidants in the seminal plasma. The balance between pro-oxidants (leukocytes generating ROS) and antioxidants (superoxide dismutase, catalase and glutathionase) results in presence or absence of oxidative stress (OS). If on the positive side, the consequence is defective sperm function in morphologically normal looking spermatozoa. The details have been described in some other chapter of this book.

ii. **Antisperm antibodies:**[29, 30] The seminal plasma and spermatozoa contain various types of antigens, of which six are sperm specific. Spermatogonial antigens can produce antibodies which can react with their own antigens leading to 'autoimmunity'. On the other hand, these antigens, when the sperms are deposited in the female genital tract can provoke production of antibodies in the female partner. These are known as isoantibodies. Local isoantibodies present in the

Flowchart 5.4

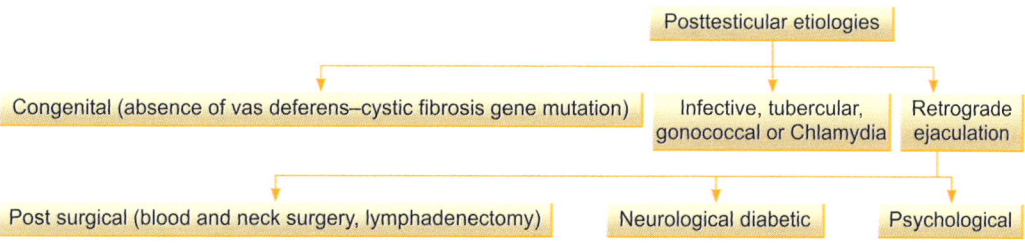

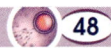

cervical mucous (IGG, IGA variety) can produce immunological infertility by interfering with sperm motility and transport. For autoimmunity to develop (self-antibodies) the blood-testes barrier has to be broken either by trauma, infection or production of high local temperature. This may be the reason for reduced motility of spermatozoa (for details see chapter on Functional Defect of Spermatozoa).

iii. **Anatomic segmental defect:** Three areas of the spermatozoa are primarily involved with sperm vitality (metabolism) and motility (propellary function). The areas concerned are—axoneme defect ("dyenin deficiency"sperm propellary defect), mitochondrial defect (metabolic dysfunction), centriolar dysfunction (problem during fertilisation—defect in nuclear syngamy).

iv. **Epididymal pathology:** Epididymis normally contains many biochemical constituents of which carnitine is important for preservation of sperm viability, motility and continuing maturation. Infection of epididymis impairs this physiological function and leads to asthenospermia.

v. **Genetic:** One of the commonest genetic causes of isolated asthenospermia is immotile cilia syndrome—Kartagener's syndrome. This is a generalized ciliary defect affecting all the ciliated epithelia of the body, namely the bronchus, sinus, fallopian tube, etc. When this affects spermatozoa, there will be 100% spermatozoal immotility.

vi. **Iatrogenic:** This is a rare apparent cause of asthenospermia. This may be due to improper handling of the semen sample and contaminating normal samples with infected samples.

The etiological factors described above are summarized in Flowchart 5.5.

OTA Syndrome

Oligoteratoasthenozoospermia (OTA) is an extreme degree of spermatozoal abnormality—involving count, motility and morphology. Apart from infection, the other etiology of OTA syndrome may be an accidental defect of the proceedings of the Spermatogenesis. The defect may occur at the level of meiotic or mitotic division in the stages of:

a. Spermatogonial type-B mitotic division
b. The stage of meiosis (crossing over of genes) or
c. In the stage of spermiogenesis.

In the OTA syndrome the sperm head may be acrosomeless—round-headed sperm or globozoospermia. These sperms are not very suitable for ICSI, though pregnancies have been reported following injection of globozoospermic sperm.

Structural or Biochemical Sperm Abnormalities

The abnormalities are summarized below (for details see Chapter on Functional Sperm Abnormalities).

Flowchart 5.5

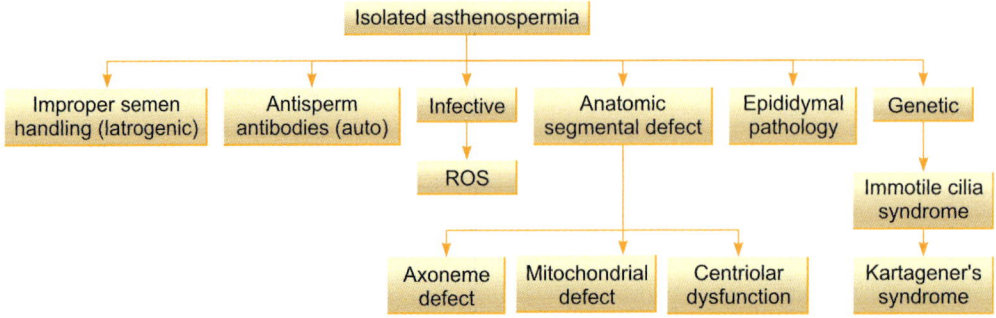

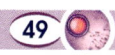

The commonest abnormality is plasma membrane defect. The consequences of these abnormalities lead to premature lipid peroxidation of the membranes resulting in exocytosis of acrosin before the sperm head reaches the zona pellucida. This leads to failure of fertilisation and nuclear chromatin decondensation.

The second common biochemical abnormality is nuclear chromatin aberrations. This occurs at the stage of spermiogenesis when the nuclear DNA material replacement occurs from histone to protamine. Protamin is more compact DNA than histone. As a result of imperfect replacement there may be DNA fragmentation of the sperm head nucleus leading to abnormal fertilisation.

As it has been described earlier, there is scanty cytoplasm and more DNA material in the sperm head nucleus. As a result of excessive ROS production, too many cytoplasmic vacuoles may be produced in the sperm head nucleus which may again be a cause of failure of fertilisation.

Lastly, biochemical abnormalities of the mid-piece, principal piece and end piece (tail of spermatozoa) lead to disturbance of function of mitochondria and the fibrous sheath of the mid-piece. Mitochondria of the mid-piece controls metabolic and respiratory functions of spermatozoa, whereas the axoneme of the end piece provides propellary sperm function. Therefore, abnormalities in these areas may be responsible for abnormal motility and vitality of the sper-matozoa.

CHROMOSOMAL AND GENETIC ANOMALIES ASSOCIATED WITH MALE INFERTILITY

Majority of idiopathic (30–40%) male infertility is associated with genetic anomalies of the spermatozoa. These defects cannot be detected by karyotyping only.

Overall chromosomal abnormality associated with male infertility is 5.8%; of which sex chromosome abnormality comprises 4.2% and autosomal anomaly is around 1.5%.

Types of Anomalies

Two types of anomalies are commonly found

a. Chromosomal—may be of two types:
   i. Numerical
   ii. Structural.
b. Genetic—affecting:
   i. Pretesticular
   ii. Testicular
   iii. Postesticular areas.

CHROMOSOMAL

Numerical anomalies: These anomalies may be of three types:

i. **47XXY:** Klinefelter's syndrome —14% of azoospermic men will have Klinefelter's syndrome. The clinical features are very obvious in majority. They are tall with small soft testes, may or may not have gynaecomastia and obesity. Invariably they have scanty or absent beard and moustaches.

ii. **47XYY:** The incidence of this variety of anomaly in general population is very rare. They are also tall and have low IQ (intelligence quotient). More often they are antisocial and will have impaired spermatogenesis.

iii. **45X/46XY:** This group of individuals have mixed gonadal dysgenesis, thereby meaning that they may have ambigious genitalia. Depending on the number of cell types (more 46XY cells or more 45XO cells) their phenotype is either male or female because individuals with absence of Y chromosome have a female phenotype. In individuals with male phenotype, the gonads (testes) may be located within the abdomen. Under such conditions there is a risk of malignancy and the gonads are to be removed. The gonads in the abdominal cavity either do not produce spermatozoa at all or spermatozoa, if produced, are invariably defective in function and morphology. Therefore, the ectopic gonads should always be removed.

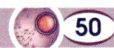
Structural anomalies: These anomalies affect genes on Y chromosome of an azoospermic male individual. The specific anomalies are:

i. Microdeletion of the gene on Y chromosome.[30] This is the commonest anomaly which can be detected only through PCR. The common genes which are affected are located at SRY and DAZ regions. Other genes may also be affected, they are—AZF-A, AZF-B and AZF-C.

ii. One rare variety of structural anomalies leading to azoospermia is 'translocation' of SRY segment from Y chromosome to one of the X chromosomes in 46XX individuals. Although the chromosomal pattern of these individuals is 46XX the phenotype is typically male. They are known as 46XX male just like 46XY female where the phenotypic pattern of the individual is typically female (testicular feminization).

The reason for male phenotype in 46XX azoospermic individual is because of existence of translocated SRY gene in one of the segments of X chromosome. External genitalia is masculine in 90%, whereas the genitalia may be ambigious in 10% of the individuals. The accidental translocation occurs at the time of fertilisation when SRY segment of the father's Y chromosome is accidentally translocated to nondysjuncted X chromosome of the developing zygote (Fig. 5.1).

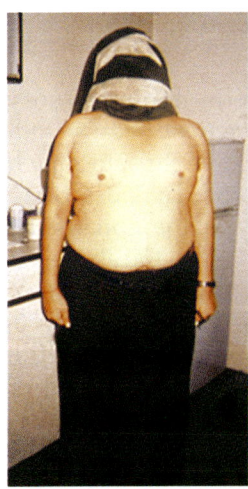

Fig. 5.1: 46XX male SRY gene in Xp 3.1

GENETIC

As stated, genetic anomalies may affect pretesticular, testicular and posttesticular areas. The types of defect commonly observed consist of deletion, mutation or polymorphic expansion of the genes. The specific defects in different areas are briefly discussed below:

Pretesticular Defect

Azoospermia due to pretesticular defect of genes mainly involves the function of hypothalamic pituitary ovarian (HPO) axis. The commonest clinical condition encountered with this type of defect is X-linked disorder—Kallmann's syndrome. Mutation involves Kal-1 gene. The incidence is one in 10,000 to 60,000 births.[31] This type of genetic defect leads to some types of embryologic disorder involving olfactory area and hypothalamus (*for details see other chapter*)

The physical stigma in Kallmann's syndrome consists of tall stature, delayed puberty, small testes, micro-penis, **anosmia** and sometimes cryptorchidism. Anosmia is a prominent symptom of Kallmann's syndrome which sometimes may have to be elicited through a leading question.

This condition (Kallmann's syndrome), however is amenable to treatment with testosterone and gonadotropin.

Posttesticular and Testicular Defects

The commonest defect observed in clinical practice is the defect or deletion in cystic fibrosis gene leading to hypoplastic, nonfunctional or absent vas deferens and seminal vesicles. These individuals may have respiratory problems as well. In this syndrome there is mutation in cystic fibrosis transmembrane receptor (CFTR) gene.[24–27]

There is another syndrome similar to the previous one which is known as Young's syndrome.[32] The clinical features are respiratory tract anomaly, chronic sinusitis with or without bronchiectasis and spina bifida. Spermatozoal anomalies in this syndrome consist of defective spermatogenesis in addition to ejaculatory failure due to epididymal obstruction.

A third and very rare type of defect leading to sperm abnormalities may be associated with 'prune-belly' syndrome.[33] This syndrome is associated with features of respiratory tract anomalies and more importantly another major congenital defect (exstrophy with epispadias) may coexist in this syndrome. Cryptorchidism is also commonly observed in these individuals. They usually do not survive up to the childbearing age.

Testicular affection leading to sperm abnormality may also be associated with some systemic genetic abnormalities. One of such abnormalities is muscular dystrophy. In this genetic disorder, there is extensive seminiferous tubular dysfunction and destruction. Consequently, there may be azoospermia or impaired sperm motility like Kartagener's syndrome.[34] Systemic manifestation of this disorder may also cause sinusitis, bronchiectasis and deafness. However, ICSI may be attempted.

Systemic genetic disorders may affect testicular and pituitary function in an indirect way. The specific disorders referred to are thalassaemia and sickle cell anaemia. These diseases by themselves do not cause infertility. Treatment with iron and multiple blood transfusions cause increased total body iron which is deposited in testes and pituitary leading to haematochromatosis. This situation may result in male infertility.

SEMINAL PATHWAY AND ACCESSORY SEX ORGAN—IMPACT OF BIOCHEMICAL COMPONENTS ON SPERM FUNCTION ABNORMALITIES

Seminal pathway begins in testes and ends at penile urethra. The components concerned with spermatogenesis and maintenance of sperm viability and fertilisability (Fig. 5.2) are:

a. Interstitial tissue
b. Leydig cell
c. Seminiferous tubules
d. Rete testis
e. Epididymis
f. Vas deferens
g. Ampulla of vas
h. Seminal vesicles
i. Ejaculatory duct
j. Prostate
k. Cowper's gland

A brief description of each segment with its biochemical component and sperm function is discussed below:

Interstitial tissue: This is located in the space in between adjacent seminiferous tubules. It contains blood and lymph vessels, fibroblastic supporting cells, macrophages,

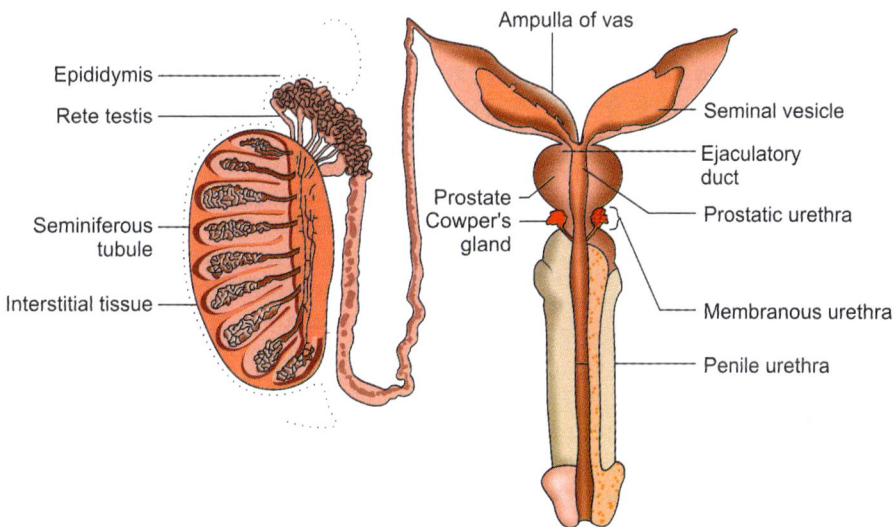

Fig. 5.2: Seminal pathway, accessory sex organs and areas affected in obstructive azoospermia

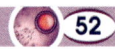

mast cells and Leydig cells. The interstitial tissue occupies 34% of testes volume.

Leydig cell: These cells are located outside the seminiferous tubules and within the interstitial tissues. They constitute 5 to 15% of total volume of testes. These cells are the sources of androgen production. The number of Leydig cells in a 20-year-old boy is around 700 million. With advancing age there is gradual apoptosis of the Leydig cell. At the age of 60, the number of Leydig cells is reduced to 300 million. Androgens produced by Leydig cell are carried inside the seminiferous tubule by androgen-binding globulin (ABG) produced by Sertoli cell inside the seminiferous tubule.

Seminiferous tubule: There are about 600 to 1200 seminiferous tubules within each testis. Estimated total length is about 250 meters. The lumen of each seminiferous tubule is lined by basement membrane and contains two types of cells—germ cells and Sertoli cells. The adjacent Sertoli cells by their tightly connected apical junction divide the lumen of seminiferous tubules into two compartments — basal towards the basement membrane and adluminal towards the lumen of the seminiferous tubule. In between the Sertoli cells the germ cells (primary spermatocytes) are located. The earlier phases of sperm maturation—from spermatogonial type B stem cells to primary spermatocytes occur within the basal compartment of seminiferous tubules. The subsequent maturation of the sperm cells—from primary to secondary spermatocyte to spermatid (round and elongated)—and finally to adult spermatozoa takes place in the adluminal compartment. Adluminal compartment is sealed off from basal compartment by tight interconnected apical junctions of Sertoli cell. This barrier (interconnected Sertoli cell junction) is known as 'blood-testes barrier'. The barrier prevents toxins or oxidative stress generated by infection within the interstitial tissue of the testes to enter into the adluminal compartment where final maturation of spermatozoa is occurring. But under abnormal conditions, like infection, trauma and excessive heat this blood-testes barrier is broken. The impact of infection or other noxious elements in the interstitial tissue may enter into adluminal compartment when this blood-testes barrier is damaged. Damage of blood-testes barrier may also allow sperm antigens to enter into general circulation and produce antibodies. The antibodies in turn may reenter the adluminal compartment and adversely affect the spermatozoal function and vitality.

Rete testis: Rete testis is the junctional area between the terminal end of seminiferous tubules and the head of the epididymis. The epithelium covering lumen of rete testis may have some secretory activities. Their exact function is not known. In obstructive azoospermia this area is sometimes affected.

Epididymis: It is functionally an important organ contributing ingradients for sperm maturity, motility and vitality. It extends from cranial to caudal pole of the testis. On one side, it is connected with efferent ducts (rete testis) and on the other side, it continues up to vas deferens. Epididymis consists of three segments—caput, corpus and cauda. The length is about 5 to 6 meters. The biochemical contributions are—synthesis and production of protein, carnitine, lipids, glycerylphosphorylcholine (GPC), carbohydrate, steroids, etc. Of these, carnitine and GPC are the most significant constituents which provide energy for sperm viability and motility. Carnitine is the marker of epididymal function.

Vas deferens: Vas begins from the cauda of epididymis encircles seminal vesicle and at its terminal part dilates in a glandular enlargement to form ampulla of the vas and finally fuses with terminal part of seminal vesicle to form the ejaculatory duct. The function of the vas is to supplement constituents for continuation of sperm maturation initiated at seminiferous tubules and epididymis. Vas also helps in sperm transport for emission.

Ejaculatory duct: It opens into the floor of prostatic urethra at the level of verumontanum (prostatic utricle—müllerian remnant). Ampulla of vas produces fructose. This helps in continuation of maturation of spermatozoa which started in epididymis.

Seminal vesicles: These are paired pyriform accessory sex glands. 70% of ejaculate originates in seminal vesicles. Fructose and prostaglandins are the main biochemical constituents. Vesiculase enzyme contributes to seminal plasma viscosity. Control of seminal vesicle function is maintained by a number of hormones namely testosterone, estrogen, prolactin and vasopressin. Semen immediately after ejaculation clots (become more viscid) due to vesiculase enzyme. Unless the coagulum is liquefied sperm transport through female genital tract does not occur leading to infertility. This may be cause of infertility. Prostatic enzyme—plasminogen activator causes lysis of seminal clot and allows the sperm transport.

Prostate: This is the largest accessory sex gland. 3–4 cm in length and 20 gm in weight. Two ejaculatory ducts pierce prostate obliquely and open into the prostatic urethra at the region of prostatic utricle. The prostate contributes many biochemical constituents which are vital for sperm vitality and obviously for fertilisability. The important micronutrient elements are zinc, magnesium and calcium. Plasminogen activator (PA— already referred) for causing seminal clot lysis is an important constituent for maintaining sperm motility. Prostaglandin is also an important constituent of prostatic fluid which prevents formation of antibodies in seminal plasma. Acid phosphatase and prostate specific antigen (PSA) are markers of prostatic function.

Cowper's glands: Cowper's glands are located one on each side; the openings are located between membranous and cavernous portions of the urethra. The secretion of these glands occurs during penile erection and possibly during ejaculation and helps in lubrication of glans penis. The function of the gland is under the control of testosterone.

AREAS AFFECTED IN OBSTRUCTIVE AZOOSPERMIA

Obstructive azoospermia occurs mostly due to infection and rarely due to agenesis or developmental defects. The following areas are commonly affected: (a) Rete testis, (b) epididymis, (c) vas deferens and (d) ejaculatory duct. The commonest developmental anomaly leading to obstructive azoospermia is müllerian cyst at the region of opening of ejaculatory duct at the floor of prostatic urethra (prostatic utricle).

Summary

Etiologies of common sperm abnormalities have been discussed.

The causes of azoo- or oligospermia have been broadly classified under three main headings—pretesticular, testicular and post-testicular. Endocrine disorder either congenital or acquired is the commonest pre-testicular background, of which Kallmann's syndrome has been frequently associated with pretesticular causes of azoospermia.

Amongst testicular causes, spermatogenetic arrest at any stage (meiotic or mitotic) has been found to be commonly associated with azoospermia.

In most posttesticular causes of azoospermia, genetic (cystic fibrosis gene mutation), infective (obstructive) or retrograde ejaculation are the common etiological factors.

The common cause of isolated astheno-zoospermia is leukocytospermia—resulting in oxidative stress. Other less common causes are antisperm antibodies and sperm anatomical segmental defects, affecting centriole in neck, mitochondrial sheath in the mid-piece and axoneme in the end piece.

OTA syndrome involves spermatozoal defect in count, motility and morphology. Defect may arise in any stage of spermatogenesis.

Structural or biochemical abnormalities include plasma membrane defect, nuclear chromatin aberration or disturbance in the function of mitochondria or axoneme leading to impairment of sperm metabolic, respiratory or propellary function.

Chromosomal anomalies may exist in two forms, namely numerical and structural. Klinefelter's syndrome and microdeletions are the examples of these two types of defect. Genetic defect is responsible for sperm abnormalities and may have their impact in

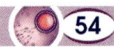
three areas, namely pretesticular, testicular and posttesticular areas.

Biochemical components of seminal pathway and accessory sex gland fluids have their individual and collaborative contribution for each embryologic step of spermatogenesis, maintenance of viability, motility and lastly for effective fertilisability. Abnormalities of this area lead to either numerical, structural or functional abnormality of spermatozoal morphology and function.

The areas affected in obstructive azoospermia are—rete testis, epididymis, vas deferens and ejaculatory duct.

REFERENCES

1. Dodé C, Hardelin JP. Kallmann syndrome. Eur J Hum Genet. 2009; 17: 139–46.

2. Fechner A, Fong S, McGovern P. A review of Kallmann syndrome: Genetics, pathophysiology, and clinical management. Obstet Gynecol Surv. 2008; 63(3): 189–94.

3. Buvat J. Hyperprolactinemia and sexual function in men: A short review. Int J Impot Res. 2003; 15 (5): 373–7.

4. Carter JN, Tyson JE, Tolis G, et al. Prolactin-screening tumors and hypogonadism in 22 men. N Engl J Med. 1978; 299(16): 847–52.

5. World Health Organization. The influence of varicocele on parameters of fertility in a large group of men presenting to infertility clinics. Fertil Steril. 1992; 57: 1289–93.

6. MacLeod J. Seminal cytology in the presence of varicocele. Fertil Steril. 1965; 16(6): 735–57.

7. Paduch DA, Niedzielski J. Semen analysis in young men with varicocele: preliminary study. J Urol. 1996; 156: 778–90.

8. Hjollund NH, Storgaard L, Ernst E, et al. The relation between daily activities and scrotal temperature. Reprod Toxicol. 2002; 16(3): 209–14.

9. Ivell R. Lifestyle impact and the biology of the human scrotum. Reprod Biol Endocrinol. 2007; 5: 15.

10. Dada R, Gupta NP, Kucheria K. Spermatogenic arrest in men with testicular hyperthermia. Teratog Carcinog Mutagen. 2003; S1: 235–43.

11. Trsinar B, Muravec UR. Fertility potential after unilateral and bilateral orchidopexy for cryptorchidism. World J Urol. 2009; 27 (4): 513–9.

12. Gracia J, Sánchez Zalabardo J, Sánchez García J, et al. Clinical, physical, sperm and hormonal data in 251 adults operated on for cryptorchidism in childhood. BJU Int. 2000; 85(9): 1100–3.

13. Lee PA, O'Leary LA, Songer NJ, et al. Paternity after unilateral cryptorchidism: a controlled study. Pediatrics. 1996; 98: 676–9.

14. Lee PA, O'Leary LA, Songer NJ, et al. Paternity after bilateral cryptorchidism. A controlled study. Arch Pediatr Adolesc Med. 1997; 151 (3): 260–3.

15. Canavese F, Mussa A, Manenti M, et al. Sperm count of young men surgically treated for cryptorchidism in the first and second year of life: fertility is better in children treated at a younger age. Eur J Pediatr Surg. 2009; 19(6): 388–91.

16. Wiser A, Raviv G, Weissenberg R, et al. Does age at orchidopexy impact on the results of testicular sperm extraction? Reprod Biomed Online. 2009; 19(6): 778–83.

17. Ferlin A, Raicu F, Gatta V, Zuccarello D, Palka G, Foresta C. Male infertility: Role of genetic background. Reprod Biomed Online. 2007; 14(6): 734–45.

18. Foresta C, Moro E, Ferlin A. Y chromosome microdeletions and alterations of spermatogenesis. Endocr Rev. 2001; 22(2): 226–39.

19. Vogt PH. Azoospermia factor (AZF) in Yq11: towards a molecular understanding of its function for human male fertility and spermatogenesis. Reprod Biomed Online. 2005; 10(1): 81–93.

20. Stahl PJ, Masson P, Mielnik A, et al. A decade of experience emphasizes that testing for Y microdeletions is essential in American men with azoospermia and severe oligozoospermia. Fertil Steril. 2010; 94(5): 1753–6.

21. Philip J, Selvan D, Desmond A. Mumps orchitis in the non-immune postpubertal male: a resurgent threat to male fertility? BJU Int. 2006; 97: 138–41.

22. Masarani M, Wazait H, Dinneen M. Mumps orchitis. J R Soc Med. 2006; 99: 573–5.

23. Osegbe DN. Testicular function after unilateral bacterial epididymo-orchitis. Eur Urol. 1991; 19:204–8.

24. Donat R, McNeill AS, Fitzpatrick DR, et al. The incidence of cystic fibrosis gene mutations in patients with congenital bilateral absence of the vas deferens in Scotland. Br J Urol. 1997; 79: 74–7.

25. Sokol RZ. Infertility in men with cystic fibrosis. Curr Opin Pulm Med. 2001; 7: 421–6.

26. Dörk T, Dworniczak B, Aulehla-Scholz C, et al. Distinct spectrum of CFTR gene mutations in

congenital absence of vas deferens. Hum Genet. 1997; 100: 365–77.

27. Bennetts RJ. The Sperm Cell Production, Maturation, Fertilisation, Regeneration. In: Christopher J. De Jonge CLRB, Eds. Reactive oxygen species: Friend or foe. Cambridge University Press 2006; 170–93.

28. Jones W. The use of antibodies developed by infertile women to identify relevant antigens. Karolinska Symposia on Research Methods in Reproductive Endocrinology Immunological Approach to Fertility Control 1974; Stockholm, Karolinska Institute.

29. Beer AE, Neaves WB. Antigenic status of semen from the viewpoints of the female and male. Fertil Steril 1978; 29(1): 3–22.

30. McLachlan RI, Mallidis C, Ma K, Bhasin S, de Kretser DM. Genetic disorders and spermatogenesis. Reprod Fertil Dev 1998; 10:97–104.

31. Laitinen EM, Vaaralahti K, Tommiska J, Eklund E, Tervaniemi M, Valanne L, Raivio T. Incidence, Phenotypic Features and Molecular Genetics of Kallmann Syndrome in Finland. Orphanet J Rare Dis. 2011; 6: 41.

32. Handelsman, David J, Conway, Ann J, Boylan, Lyn M, Turtle, John R Young's Syndrome. Obstructive Azoospermia and Chronic Sinopulmonary Infections. Obstetrical and Gynecological Survey: June 1984.

33. Terada S, Suzuki N, Uchide K, Ueno H, Akasofu K. Etiology of prune belly syndrome: Evidence of megalocystic origin in an early fetus. *Obstet Gynecol.* 1994; 83: 865–868.

34. Yokota T, Ohno N, Tamura K, Seita M, Toshimori K. Ultrastructure and function of cilia and spermatozoa flagella in patient with Kartagener's syndrome. *Intern Med.* 1993; 32:593–597.

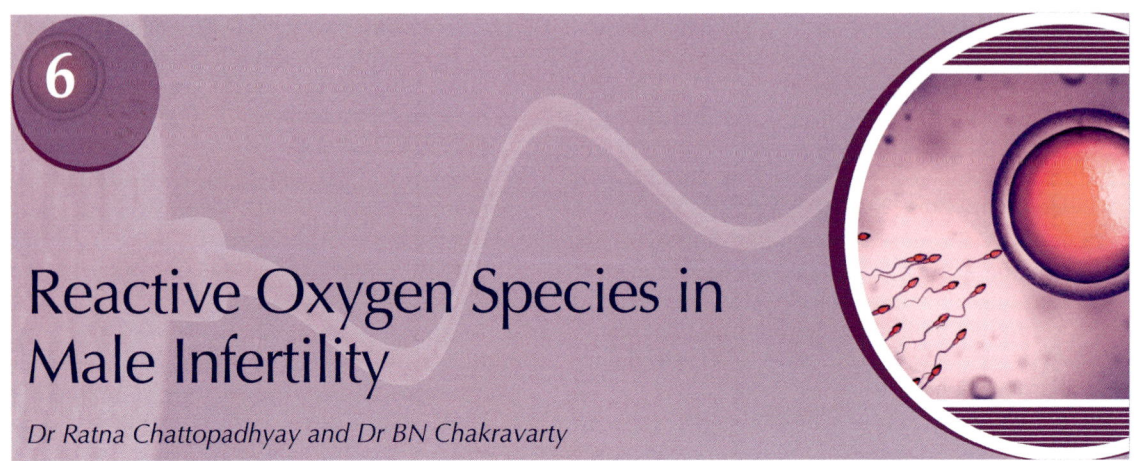

6

Reactive Oxygen Species in Male Infertility

Dr Ratna Chattopadhyay and Dr BN Chakravarty

INTRODUCTION

Semen analysis, undoubtedly, plays a central role in the laboratory diagnosis of male partner infertility. The analysis is expected to provide accurate and clinically useful information. Recent reports indicating worldwide decline of sperm count and increasing incidence of male infertility have aroused public concern.[1] Unfortunately none of the characteristics evaluated during routine semen evaluation gives us accurate data about the complete fertilizing ability of the spermatozoa. Semen parameters are indirect indicators of semen quality and lack specificity and sensitivity. 30% of all patients with normal semen analysis have abnormal sperm function. It is, therefore, obvious that additional sperm function tests are necessary for a better understanding of the problem. Moreover, owing to the complex structure of spermatozoa and considering the fact that a cascade of events occur during fertilisation, it seems reasonable to infer that one single test does not provide complete information on the functional competence of the spermatozoa. One of the factors which may adversely affect physiological function of normal appearing spermatozoa, is reactive oxygen species (ROS). During last two decades, association of ROS with human infertility has created significant interest. In this context, role of ROS in the etiology of male infertility is being increasingly recognised.

REACTIVE OXYGEN SPECIES—WHAT ARE THEY AND HOW DO THEY MODIFY THE FUNCTION OF A NORMAL CELL?

Cells living under aerobic conditions constantly face the oxygen paradox: Oxygen is indispensable for supporting life but its metabolites such as reactive oxygen species (ROS) can modify cell function. ROS includes molecules like hydrogen peroxide, ions like the hypochlorite ion, radicals like the hydroxyl radical and superoxide anion which is both an ion and radical. A radical (also called free radical) is a cluster of atoms one of which contains an unpaired electron in its outermost shell of electrons, e.g. hydrogen-centered radical, sulphur-centered radical, nitrogen-centered radical, etc. The aggressive components in ROS are free radicals. *The most important free radicals in the body, however, are the radical derivatives of oxygen better known as ROS.* Due to a single electron in the outermost shell, ROS are extremely unstable and have a tendency to react with other molecules to attain a stable configuration. The main problem arises when the neighbouring molecules are nucleic acids, fatty acids or lipids because these are the most unstable molecules in the body. The most common ROS that have potential implications in reproductive health include superoxide anion (O_2^-), hydrogen peroxide (H_2O_2), peroxyl radicals (ROO) and very reactive hydroxyl (OH) radicals.

Specific Characteristics of Free Radicals

i. These are atoms or molecules with one or more unpaired electron.

ii. They are highly energetic.

iii. They seek or try to find other electrons with which they want to pair (bind).

iv. In the process they attack healthy cells in order to extract one electron with which they want to bind.

v. In this way, they may modify and damage many different types of biomolecules including proteins, lipids and nucleic acids which are the constituents of healthy cells.

vi. In summary, they damage a healthy cell.

Interestingly, while controlled amount of ROS is necessary for physiological processes such as capacitation, acrosome reaction and acquisition of sperm fertilising ability, excessive generation of ROS is reported to have caused lipid peroxidation of the sperm membrane, affect the integrity of sperm DNA and subsequently cause cell death. Hence, impact of ROS on fertility is a question of degree (amount of ROS) rather than the presence/absence of the pathology (simple presence of ROS). The upper cut off physiological limit of ROS is yet to be critically ascertained. There are many cells in the body which are adversely affected by ROS. Sperm cell is one of them.

Why Sperm Cells are Susceptible to Oxidative Damage?

i. The sperm cell membrane is rich in polyunsaturated fatty acid (PUFA).

ii. Abundance of unsaturated fatty acid is essential for sperm to create membrane fluidity for membrane fusion (plasma membrane with outer acrosomal membrane).

iii. This is essential at the time of sperm entry through zona pellucida at the time of fertilisation.

iv. At this point, membrane fusion followed by dissolution is essential for exocytosis of acrosin (acrosome reaction).

v. Acrosome causes dissolution of zona pellucida after which sperm head can enter into perivitelline space and then penetrate oolemma for entry into ooplasm.

vi. Activated leukocytes contaminating seminal plasma may take the advantage of sperm membrane weakness and cause damage resulting in premature exocytosis of acrosin before sperm head reaches zona pellucida.

vii. Repair mechanism in adult spermatozoa is poor. Sperm cytoplasm contains low level of scavenging enzymes, therefore, sperm cells are unable to repair the injury caused by high ROS.

Therefore, in summary, membrane fusion events are necessary for:

a. Acrosome reaction

b. Sperm oocyte fusion

c. Fertilisation

If membrane fusion and disintegration occur before the sperm head reaches zona pellucida, events of fertilisation do not occur leading to fertilisation failure.

TOXIC EFFECTS OF ROS ON SPERM FUNCTION

1. Lipid peroxidation (LPO): The sperm plasma membrane is remarkably vulnerable to oxidative stress or ROS toxicity, as it is richly endowed with polyunsaturated fatty acids (PUFAs) with six double bonds per molecule which act as an electron sink that makes it highly prone or susceptible to oxidation and other chemical or structural modification.

Lipid peroxidation (LPO) is popularly known as "oxidative deterioration" of PUFA because the overall change reduces sperm plasma membrane fluidity which in turn reduces sperm motility and interferes with membrane fusion events such as acrosome reaction and sperm oocyte fusion at the time of fertilisation.

End product of LPO is malondialdehyde (MDA) which can be estimated in order to evaluate the extent of peroxidative damage.

2. Nuclear DNA damage: DNA and phosphodiester, the backbones of DNA are also susceptible to oxidative damage. Two

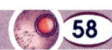

factors such as compact packaging of DNA (protamins) and antioxidants in seminal plasma protect sperm DNA against oxidative insult. But patients with high seminal plasma ROS level having multiple single and double DNA strand breaks have been reported[2] and are the evidence of adverse impact of oxidative stress on sperm integrity.

Exposure of sperm DNA to oxidative stress results in:

   i. DNA base modification

   ii. Formation of base-free sites

   iii. Chromosomal aberration

   iv. DNA cross-linking

   v. Deletions

   vi. Frame shifts

The extent of oxidative damage of DNA can be assessed by a biomarker, 8-hydroxy 2-deoxyguanosine (8-OH-dG).

The assessment can be made by:

   i. HALO sperm assay

   ii. COMET assay

   iii. TUNEL assay

Sperm with DNA fragmentation index (DFI) >15% is considered to be clinically significant and is associated with high risk of fertilisation failure and early embryo death. Details have been described in chapter Sperm Function Test.

3. High ROS may induce apoptosis and thus reduce alive sperm concentration:[3] The level of enzymes, caspases, proteases involved in apoptosis is correlated with ROS levels. They are the causes of oxidative stress with increased apoptosis of adult spermatozoa.

Beneficial Effects of ROS on Sperm Function

Interestingly, controlled generation of ROS appears to be necessary for spermatozoa to acquire fertilising capabilities, which include capacitation, hyperactivation acrosome reaction and sperm oocyte fusion.[4] As a result, several search groups in various assisted reproductive clinics worldwide are working towards the assessment of the threshold level of ROS in sperm cell beyond which conditions may not be favourable for fertilisation. Depletion of essential physiological level of ROS is responsible for "reductive stress" leading to impaired sperm function.[5]

Therefore, subnormal level of ROS may prevent normal sperm function and also elevated normal level may produce oxidative stress and thus may be detrimental for sperm health and function.

ORIGIN OF REACTIVE OXYGEN SPECIES, ANTIOXIDANTS AND OXIDATIVE STRESS IN MALE REPRODUCTIVE TRACT

Origin of reactive oxygen species may be either extrinsic or intrinsic.

Extrinsic origin: Activated leukocytes in seminal plasma can produce enormous amount of ROS. This is known as extrinsic origin of ROS. Extrinsic ROS is a major contributory factor responsible for altered sperm motility, count and morphology. Infected or activated leukocytes can produce 100 fold higher amounts of ROS than non-activated leukocytes.

Intrinsic origin: ROS may also be generated from morphologically abnormal sperm cells or precursor germ cells and this is known as intrinsic origin. DNA damage is strongly correlated with increased intrinsic ROS production. DNA damage in the form of base modification, strand breaks and chromatin cross-linking are commonly observed in oxidative stress.

The cytoplasmic residue of cytoplasmic droplet in immature sperm contains high level of glucose-6-phosphate dehydrogenase which in turn generates NADPH (nicotinamide adenine dineucleotide phosphate). Immature spermatozoa utilize NADPH as a source of electrons to promote generation of ROS.

ROS is generated at two sites of spermatozoa:

   1. Sperm plasma membrane

   2. Mitochondria

Mechanism of mitochondrial ROS generation is still unknown. Any factor affecting redox properties of organelle is a potential inducer of ROS and DNA damage. Mitochondrial inhibitor such as antimycin A, rotenone and excessive quantity of polyunsaturated fatty acids[6] are some factors inducing ROS generation in mitochondria.

Functionally defective spermatozoa may activate mitochondrial ROS generation. Sperm DNA is attacked mainly by mitochondrial ROS.[6–8] Therefore, ROS generated at mitochondrial level is a major contributing factor in male factor infertility. Excessive generation of mitochondrial ROS can be correlated with defective sperm function mainly decreased sperm motility.[7]

The severity of oxidative damage depends not only upon the type and amount of ROS but also on the period of exposure to ROS and other extracellular factors such as temperature, oxygen tension of the surrounding environmental components.

It is known that oxidative stress develops when pro-oxidants outnumber the antioxidants. The balance can be maintained by preventing excess formation of ROS or by scavenging excess ROS by antioxidants. Therefore, antioxidant is an important defense barrier against free radical induced infertility.

Extragenital Sources of Origin of ROS

- Oxidative stress may also be associated with many diseases like cardiovascular disease, diabetes, cancer, brain diseases, etc.
- High amount of alcohol intake has been shown to increase systemic level of oxidative stress.
- A close association exists between cigarette smoking and poor semen quality. Exposure to cigarette smoke generates high level of oxidative stress.
- Men working in heavy metal industries have increased testicular oxidative stress.
- Varicocele has also been involved as a cause of oxidative stress. Alteration of scrotal temperature may cause nuclear DNA damage.
- Oxidative stress is likely to be generated in some of the steps of ART procedure:
  i. Sperm washing
  ii. Incubation.

Sperm Washing

High speed (>1000 rpm/min) rotation during semen preparation may cause breakdown of leukocytes, resulting in production of high level of free radicals. Similarly, abnormal or precursor sperm cells generate high amount of reactive oxygen species. Spermatozoa in semen containing more than one million leukocytes/ml or a large number of morphologically abnormal sperm cells or precursor sperm cells are more prone to develop higher levels of oxidative stress and oxidative damage during sperm preparation.

This can be avoided by density gradient sperm preparation techniques.

Incubation

Altered temperature and chemical composition of media in which sperms are incubated may generate high ROS which is detrimental for sperm health and function.

Antioxidants

Antioxidants are substances which at a low concentration can significantly delay or prevent oxidative damage of an oxidisable substrate.

Though weak, there are antioxidants in seminal plasma to protect against the damaging effects of ROS. These antioxidants are of two types:
  a. Intracellular (within the sperm)
  b. Extracellular (in seminal plasma)

Intracellular Antioxidants

  i. *On sperm membrane*: α-tocoferol, vitamin C, uric acid, tryptophan and taurine.
  ii. *On mitochondria*: Superoxide dismutase (SOD), glutathione, catalase.

Extracellular Antioxidants

These are present in seminal plasma.
  i. Glutathione peroxidase (GPx)
  ii. Superoxide dismutase (SOD)
  iii. Albumin, uric acid, vitamin C

Major Types of Antioxidants

They exist in seminal plasma and act as free radical scavengers. Two types of antioxidants have been detected in seminal plasma: (a) enzymatic and (b) nonenzymatic. Some of the

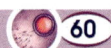
examples of enzymatic and nonenzymatic antioxidants are given below:

- *Enzymatic antioxidants*: SOD (superoxide dismutase), catalase and glutathione peroxidase, glutathione transferase
- *Nonenzymatic antioxidants*: Ascorbate, urate, α-tocopherol, pyruvate, glutathione, taurine, hypotaurine and coenzyme Q10.

Oxidative Stress

Hence, now it is clear that in semen, both ROS generating and ROS scavenging systems exist together. Figure 6.1 illustrates the balance between the ROS generating and ROS scavenging systems in the sample of semen. If the balance is in favour of ROS generating system compared to ROS scavenging system, the resulting condition is known as oxidative stress (OS).

Oxidative stress (OS) is defined as an imbalance between levels of reactive oxygen species (ROS) and total antioxidant capacity (TAC) estimated present in a semen sample.

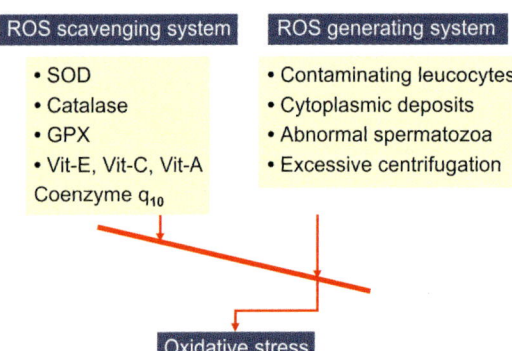

Fig. 6.1: Balance between ROS generating system and scavenging system

Recently, a method based on enhanced chemiluminescence assay has gained popularity in measuring total antioxidant capacity (TAC) in biological fluids.

Assessment of Oxidative Status

As we have seen, oxidative stress is a state of imbalance between ROS production and antioxidant protection, the measurement of ROS level and total antioxidant capacity (TAC) in semen helps in the assessment of oxidative stress level and can be treated by antioxidant supplementation accordingly.

Measurement of ROS

1. Direct assay
2. Indirect assay

Direct Assay

a. Measuring malondialdehyde (MDA) in seminal plasma is the most widely used direct assay as MDA is the end product of sperm plasma membrane lipid peroxidation.[9]

b. Direct assay of intracellular ROS induced oxidative damage can be done by quantification of sperm DNA abnormality. Level of 8-OH-dG is a specific biomarker of oxidative damage to sperm DNA.[10]

Indirect Assay

The most commonly used method of measurement of seminal ROS level is via indirect chemiluminescence assay. It is the less expensive and simpler method of ROS estimation by quantifing redox activities of spermatozoa with the help of an instrument, luminometer using luminol or lucigen as a probe. Indirect assessment of ROS level can also be determined by flow cytometry.

The result is expressed as $\times 10^4$ counted photon per minute per 20×10^6 sperms. Normal ROS level in washed sperm range from 10–100×10^4 counted photon per minute per 10 million sperms.

Upper Cut-off Value

The upper cut-off value of semen samples which correlate well with good semen quality is in order of 75,000–100,000 cpm/10 million cells. The results strongly suggest that excessive generation of ROS causes sperm DNA fragmentation which in turn, may adversely affect the embryo quality and subsequently result in a lowered pregnancy rate. Our study suggests that high ROS has a negative prognostic value with regard to pregnancy outcome in ICSI. In addition to existing WHO guidelines for routine semen parameters, the cut-off value of ROS which has been established to be in range of 75,000–100,000 cpm/10 million cells has the ability to differentiate between good and poor quality semen samples. This 'cut-off' value of ROS is, therefore, expected to provide valuable information to clinicians and assist in predicting semen quality, fertilisation and pregnancy outcome in patients undergoing ART.

Total Antioxidant Capacity

Infertile men compared to fertile men are more likely to have suboptimal level of total antioxidant capacity (TAC) and lower level of individual antioxidants.[11, 12]

Recently, a method based on enhanced chemiluminescence assay has gained popularity in measuring total antioxidant capacity (TAC) in biological fluids.

Imbalance between oxidants and anti-oxidants—oxidative stress (Fig. 6.2).

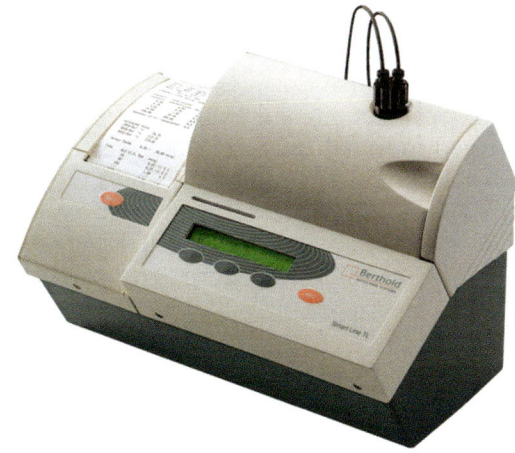

Fig. 6.2: Photograph of a Luminometer—an instrument used for measurement of ROS and total antioxidant capacity (TAC)

ROS-TAC Score

A composite ROS-TAC score is more strongly connected with male infertility rather than ROS or TAC alone.[13]

ROS-TAC score is derived from ROS level in washed sperm and TAC in seminal plasma and considered as a novel assay of oxidative stress. It is superior to ROS or TAC alone in detecting male infertility specially free radical induced male infertility.

The probability of pregnancy is < 10% when the values of ROS-TAC score is < 30 which is the lower limit of normal range. But the probability increases as the score is increased.

Several studies reported that antioxidant supplementation in oxidative stress induced male factor infertility may decrease the level of oxidative stress and may protect the fertilising ability of the new batch of spermatozoa.

Moreover, low cost and low risk of toxicity of antioxidants are gradually making them popular in idiopathic and oxidative stress induced male and female factor infertility.

A combination of lipophilic antioxidants like vitamin E and hydrophilic antioxidants like vitamin C, selenium and zinc have been found to improve semen parameters as observed in some studies.[14]

Management of ROS Toxicity or OS Induced Male Infertility

Abnormal elevation of ROS and subnormal decline of the level of antioxidants in seminal plasma and spermatozoa significantly reduce sperm quantity and quality. The overall effect is abnormal or failed fertilisation and early embryo death. So there is a clear indication for treating abnormal level of ROS in semen sample or abnormal semen profile with unexplained etiology by antioxidants or nutraceuticals. However, up till now treatment procedure has not been rationally standardised by randomised control trial, but plenty of reports are appearing, strongly suggesting the necessity of antioxidants in various areas of ROS toxicity and oxidative stress induced male infertility.

Rational approach of treatment consists of:
  a. Prevention of excess ROS generation
  b. Scavenging of excess ROS already generated
  c. Repair of the oxidative damage in spermatozoa, if possible

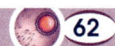

Areas of spermatozoal damage:

1. Sperm plasma membrane
2. Nuclear DNA
3. Mitochondria in mid-piece

} Leading to impaired motility, deficient vitality and fertilisation failure

The treatment procedure can be divided into two groups:

1. Preventive
2. Curative

Preventive

a. By preventing excess formation of ROS— which are commonly associated with systemic diseases or disorders.

   Treatment of the causes of diseases known to generate excessive ROS. For example,

   i. Surgical treatment of varicocele

   A meta analysis on varicocelectomy reported significant benefits in lowering oxidative stress and in spontaneous conception among treated couples versus the control group.[15]

   ii. Control of diabetes

   iii. Eradication of infection of male reproductive tract

b. Reduction of level of ROS through lifestyle modification

   i. Avoidance of cigarette smoking, alcohol consumption, etc.

   ii. Protection from exposure to heavy metals

c. By preventing formation of ROS during sperm washing procedure in ART or IUI cycles

   i. Centrifugation < 1000 rpm/minute for ≤ 5 minutes may reduce ROS formation from trauma of sperm cells and leukocytes.

   ii. Density gradient technique in case of leukocytospermia and asthenozoospermic samples is essential. It significantly reduces the risk of high ROS generation.

   iii. Maintaining optimum temperature, pH and composition of media during incubation after sperm preparation may also prevent ROS formation.

Curative

The basic principles of curative treatment consist of:

a. Removal of excess ROS already generated in seminal plasma or on sperm surface— this may be possible by increasing the level of 'seminal antioxidant scavengers'. Use of antioxidants may help.

b. Stimulating the sperms to be more powerful and energetic to withstand attack by excess ROS through improving health and vitality (metabolism, respiration and locomotion). This may be achieved by addition of 'nutritional factors' or 'mitochondrial energisers'. These molecules are known as 'nutraceuticals'.

Hence the current recommendations for treating excess ROS in male infertility consist of nutraceuticals or antioxidants. Both of them act as 'nutritional factors', 'mitochondrial energisers' and 'free radical scavengers'.

The term 'nutraceutical' indicates a combination of nutritional and pharmaceutical components in a drug which provides health benefits, because dosages used in the combined product exceed those that could be obtained from natural food alone (see chapter on Nutraceuticals in Male Infertility).

Hence the curative treatment of excess ROS which may prevent spermatozoal damage can be broadly classified into three groups.

Classification of Nutraceuticals/Antioxidants

Based on their prime mechanism of action in improving sperm parameters, following classification of nutraceuticals/antioxidants was done:

Nutritional factors	Mitochondrial energisers	Free radical scavengers
Zinc	Coenzyme Q10	Lycopene
L-arginine	L-carnitine	Selenium
Folic acid	Acetyl-L-carnitine	Vitamin E
Vitamin B$_{12}$		Vitamin C
		Glutathione

Published at the 14th International Congress of Endocrinology (ICE) 2010, March 26–30, 2010, Kyoto, Japan.

The areas of sperm likely to be damaged by excess ROS are:

a. Plasma membrane
b. Nuclear DNA
c. Mitochondrial membrane

Except the scavenging role, the functions of nutraceuticals or antioxidants in preventing and repair of a specific spermatozoal defect is still uncertain. Hence, the use of these molecules in the treatment of male subfertility is empirical. But preliminary observations based on published reports indicate that the drugs may be helpful. Extensive research is in progress and vast amount of literature has accumulated in justifying the use of antioxidants and nutraceuticals in ROS induced male subfertility.

A few molecules are quoted below high-lighting the role of specific antioxidants or nutraceuticals which may prevent spermatozoal damage from oxidative stress:

Free Radical Scavengers

Depending upon the range of solubility in lipid and water, the free radical scavengers may be either lipophilic and hydrophilic. The lipophilic antioxidants such as vitamin E, mainly act on sperm plasma membrane. Vitamin E interrupts with lipid peroxidation and enhances the activity of other anti-oxidants and itself helps in scavenging free radicals and improves motility. *Therefore, vitamin E is an important effective antioxidant in treating male factor infertility with elevated ROS.*[16]

Other lipophilic antioxidants like carotenoids such as lycopene, astaxanthin are also used frequently in OS induced male infertility. Three months supplementation of astaxanthin and lycopene significantly improves sperm concentration, motility and pregnancy rate.[17]

Vitamin C is a hydrophilic antioxidant. Fraga, *et al.* (1991)[18], demonstrated a significant relationship between decreased seminal plasma vitamin C level and increased 8-OH-dG. *Vitamin C supplementation can reduce endogenous oxidative DNA damage and thereby decreases the risk of failed fertilisation and genetic defect particularly in patients with low vitamin C level such as smokers. Other hydrophilic antioxidants*

are selenium, zinc, carnitine, N-acetylcysteine (NAC).

Combination of vitamin C and vitamin E acts synergistically to protect against peroxidative attack and DNA damage by high ROS on spermatozoa.[19]

Combined therapy of vitamin E and selenium significantly increases sperm motility and reduces lipid peroxidation markers.[20] Selenium may protect the sperm from high ROS level, moreover, it is essential for normal testicular development, spermatogenesis and helps to maintain the sperm motility and sperm function. *The mode of action of selenium as an antioxidant is still unknown. But selenium is a cofactor of selenoenzymes such as phospholipid hydroperoxide glutathione peroxidase (PHGPX) and sperm capsular selenoprotein glutathione peroxidase which play the role of first line defense against ROS in semen.*

Mitochondrial Energiser (CoQ10)

In humans, each and every cell contains CoQ10 natural molecule, but sperm mitochondria is rich in CoQ10 which acts as an electron carrier to the mitochondrial respiratory chain and is responsible for ATP production, thus providing energy for movement or other energy dependent processes.

Seminal plasma of men with idiopathic male infertility contains significantly low level of CoQ10. Exogenous administration of CoQ10 increases the level and improves sperm kinetic features.[21] At least three months supplementation with CoQ10 ubiquinone significantly improves sperm parameters in idiopathic OATS.[22]

Another important antioxidant, L-carnitine, is present at highest concentration in epididymal fluid. L-carnitine helps in transportation of fatty acid into the mitochondria for generation of ATP.

Nutritional Factors

Folate plays an important role in synthesis of RNA and DNA during spermatogenesis.

L-arginine, administered orally at a dose of 4 mg/day for three months significantly improves sperm count and motility.[23]

Deficiency of vitamin B_{12} has been associated with decreased sperm count and motility and

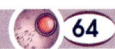

various studies have shown improvement in sperm parameters with methylcobalamine supplementation for at least three months.

A meta analysis of the impact of antioxidant therapy on male infertility was published with a positive conclusion that at least three months supplementation of antioxidants significantly improves pregnancy rate and live birth rate in subfertile couples following ART.[24]

However, further large scale well-designed randomised placebo-controlled trials are necessary to confirm these preliminary observations.

Summary

a. Reactive oxygen species (ROS) is an oxygen metabolite which can adversely modify cell function.

b. ROS may damage different types of biomolecules including proteins, lipids and nucleic acid which are the constituents of healthy cells. There are many cells in the body which are adversely affected by ROS. Sperm cell is one of them. While some amount of ROS is essential for normal sperm function, excess generation of ROS has been reported to be detrimental for sperm integrity and may cause cell death.

c. The susceptibility of sperm cell to ROS attack is primarily due to weak biochemical constituents of sperm cell membrane which is rich in polyunsaturated fatty acid (PUFA).

d. Other sperm cell areas likely to be affected by ROS are sperm head nuclear DNA and mid-piece mitochondrial membrane. The damage affects sperm motility, vitality and reduced fertilising potential.

e. Hence the ultimate adverse effects of ROS on spermatozoa are: (i) Impaired motility, (ii) deficient fertilising potential and (iii) apoptosis—resulting in reduced sperm concentration.

f. The common causes of excess ROS generation in male reproductive tract are: (i) Leukocytospermia, (ii) presence of too many immature or abnormal sperm cells, (iii) varicocele, (iv) high speed sperm washing and (v) altered temperature and chemical composition of media in which the sperms are incubated.

g. Systemic diseases like diabetes, cardio-vascular diseases or cancer may also be responsible for generation of excess ROS. Cigarette smoking and high amount of alcohol consumption have been associated with elevated level of ROS in male reproductive tract.

h. Though weak, there are antioxidants in seminal plasma to protect against the damaging effect of ROS. The antioxidants may be intracellular (within the sperm) or extracellular (in seminal plasma). The balance between the level of pro-oxidants and antioxidant is known as 'oxidative status'

i. If the balance is more in favour of ROS generating system compared to ROS scavenging system, the resulting status is known as 'oxidative stress'. There are methods of measuring the levels of ROS and total antioxidant capacity. The upper 'cut-off value' of ROS in a good quality semen sample has been estimated in the range between 75,000 and 100,000 cpm/10 million cells.

j. Treatment of oxidative stress in male sub-fertility has not yet been standardised. The principles of treatment are: (i) To prevent excess ROS generation, (ii) scavenging excess ROS which has already been generated and (iii) repair of ROS induced spermatozoal damage which is still not possible.

k. Prevention of excess ROS generation after protection of fresh batch of spermatozoa against oxidative stress. This consists of treatment of genital tract infection correction of varicocele if present, treatment of systemic disease or disorders, avoidance of smoking and alcohol and semen preparation for ART procedures with requisite precautions.

l. Curative treatment aims at: (i) Removal of excess ROS already generated through antioxidants and (ii) Supplying nutritional molecules to the sperm to withstand attack by ROS through nutritional factor and mitochondrial energisers'

m. The term 'nutraceutical' indicates combination of nutritional and pharmaceutical components. The advantage of nutraceuticals over simple nutrition is the dosage of drugs used in combined product exceed those which are available in natural food.

n. Depending on their mode of action 'nutraceuticals' or 'antioxidants' have been classified as: (i) Free radicals scavengers, for example, vitamin E (ii) mitochondrial energisers, for example, CoQ10 and (iii) nutritional factors; like L-arginine.

o. Though numerous publications have confirmed positively on the role of antioxidants and nutritional therapy in oxidative stress induced male subfertility, further large scale well-designed trials are necessary to confirm their preliminary observations.

REFERENCES

1. WHO. Report of the meeting on the prevention of infertility at the primary health care level. Geneva: World Health Organization 1984.

2. Denny Sakkas, Juan G. Alvarez. Sperm DNA fragmentation: mechanisms of origin, impact on reproductive outcome, and analysis; Fertility and Sterility; Volume 93, Issue 4, March 2010: 1027–1036.

3. Suresh C. Sikka, Andrology Lab Corner. Role of Oxidative Stress and Antioxidants in Andrology and Assisted Reproductive Technology; Journal of Andrology; Volume 25, Issue 1, 5–18, January-February 2004.

4. Tavilani H, Goodarzi MT, Doosti M, Vaisi-Raygani A, Hassanzadeh T, Salimi S, Joshaghani HR. Relationship between seminal antioxidant enzymes and the phospholipid and fatty acid composition of spermatozoa. Reprod Biomed Online 16(5): 649–656 Cross Ref. 2008.

5. B Lipinski Evidence in support of a concept of reductive stress; British Journal of Nutrition/ Volume 87/Issue 01/January 2002, pp 93–94.

6. Adam J. Koppers, Manohar L. Garg, Robert J. Aitken. Stimulation of mitochondrial reactive oxygen species production by unesterified, unsaturated fatty acids in defective human spermatozoa; Free Radical Biology and Medicine; Volume 48, Issue 1, 1 January 2010, 112–119.

7. Adam J. Koppers, Geoffry N. De Iuliis, Jane M. Finnie, Eileen A. McLaughlin, R. John Aitken. Significance of Mitochondrial Reactive Oxygen Species in the Generation of Oxidative Stress in Spermatozoa; The Journal of Clinical Endocrinology and Metabolism; Volume 93 Issue 8, August 1, 2008.

8. RJ Aitken, GN De Iuliis. On the possible origins of DNA damage in human spermatozoa; Mol. Hum. Reprod. (2010) 16 (1): 3-13.

9. Shang XJ, Li K, Ye ZQ, Chen YG, Yu X, Huang YF. Analysis of lipid peroxidative levels in seminal plasma of infertile men by high-performance liquid chromatography. Arch. Androl. 2004; 50: 411–6.

10. Loft S, Kold-Jensen T, Hjollund NH, et al. Oxidative DNA damage in human sperm influences time to pregnancy. Hum. Reprod. 2003; 18: 1265–72.

11. R. Smith, D Vantman, J Ponce, J Escobar, E Lissi. Andrology: Total antioxidant capacity of human seminal plasma; Hum. Reprod. 1996 11 (8): 1655–1660.

12. Lewis SE, Boyle PM, McKinney KA, Young IS, Thompson W. Total antioxidant capacity of seminal plasma is different in fertile and infertile men.; Fertility and Sterility 1995, 64(4):868-870.

13. Rakesh K. Sharma, Fabio F. Pasqualotto, David R. Nelson, Anthony J, Thomas Jr Ashok Agarwal. The reactive oxygen species—total antioxidant capacity score is a new measure of oxidative stress to predict male infertility; *Hum. Reprod.* (1999) 14 (11): 2801–2807.

14. Parviz Gharagozloo. Treating male infertility secondary to sperm oxidative stress; US Patent 8,377,454, 2013.

15. Joel L. Marmar, Ashok Agarwal, Sushil Prabakaran, Rishi Agarwal, Robert A Short, Susan Benoff, Anthony J. Thomas Jr Reassessing the value of varicocelectomy as a treatment for male subfertility with a new meta-analysis; Fertility and Sterility; Volume 88, Issue 3, September 2007, 639–648.

16. C Ross, A Morriss, M Khairy, Y Khalaf, P Braude, A Coomarasamy, T El-Toukhy. A systematic review of the effect of oral antioxidants on male infertility; Reproductive

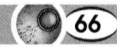

BioMedicine Online; Volume 20, Issue 6, June 2010, Pages 711–723.

17. Narmada P. Gupta, Rajeev Kumar; Lycopene therapy in idiopathic male infertility—a preliminary report; International Urology and Nephrology; 2002, Volume 34, Issue 3, 369–372.

18. C G Fraga, PA Motchnik, MK Shigenaga, HJ Helbock, RA Jacob, BN Ames. Ascorbic acid protects against endogenous oxidative DNA damage in human sperm; Proceedings of the National Academy of Sciences of the United States of America; December 15, 1991, Vol. 88, No. 24.

19. Ermanno Greco, Marcello Iacobelli, Laura Rienzi, Filippo Ubaldi, Susanna Ferrero, Jan Tesarik. Reduction of the Incidence of Sperm DNA Fragmentation by Oral Antioxidant Treatment; Journal of Andrology; Volume 26, Issue 3, 349–353, May-June 2005.

20. Kesker-Ammar, L., Feki Chacroun, N., Rebai, T., Sahnoun, Z., Ghozzi, H., Hammami, S., et al. (2003). Sperm oxidative stress and the effect of an oral vitamin E and selenium supplement on semen quality in infertile men. Archives of Andrology, 49, 83–94.

21. Giancarlo Balercia, Eddi Buldreghini, Arianna Vignini, Luca Tiano, Francesca Paggi, Salvatore Amoroso, Giuseppe Ricciardo-Lamonica, Marco Boscaro, Andrea Lenzi, GianPaolo Littarru; Coenzyme Q_{10} treatment in infertile men with idiopathic asthenozoospermia: A placebo-controlled, double-blind randomized trial; Fertility and Sterility; Volume 91, Issue 5, May 2009, 1785–1792.

22. Mohammad Reza Safarinejad, Shiva Safarinejad, Nayyer Shafiei, Saba Safarinejad. Effects of the Reduced Form of Coenzyme Q_{10} (Ubiquinol) on Semen Parameters in Men with Idiopathic Infertility: a Double-Blind, Placebo Controlled, Randomized Study; The Journal of Urology; Volume 188, Issue 2, August 2012, 526–531.

23. Scibona M, Meschini P, Capparelli S, Pecori C, Rossi P, Menchini Fabris GF. L-arginine and male infertility; Minerva Urologica e Nefrologica = The Italian Journal of Urology and Nephrology 1994, 46(4):251–253.

24. Showell MG, Brown J, Yazdani A, Stankiewicz MT, Hart RJ. Antioxidants for male subfertility (Review); The Cochrane Library; 2011, Issue.

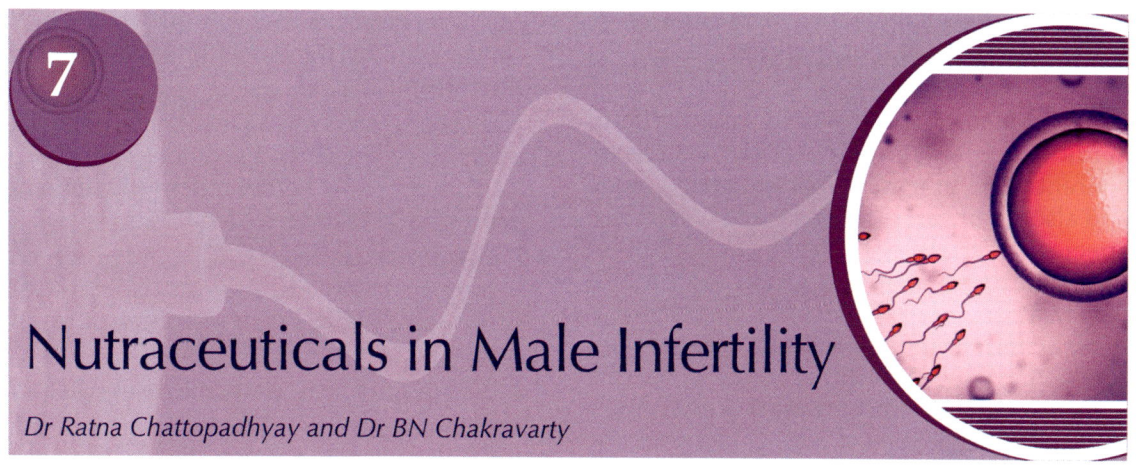

Nutraceuticals in Male Infertility

Dr Ratna Chattopadhyay and Dr BN Chakravarty

INTRODUCTION

Medical management is usually empirical and is often used in idiopathic male infertility. **Nutraceuticals** are diet supplements that provide medical or health benefits, and therefore, used for prevention and/or treatment of diseases in dosages that exceed[1] those that could be obtained from normal foods.

The term 'nutraceutical' is a combination of nutritional and pharmaceutical components and was coined in the late 1980s by Stephen De Felice, MD,[2] Founder and Chairman of the Foundation for Innovation in Medicine.

Hippocrates (460–377 BC) stated "let food be thy medicine and medicine be thy food" referring to the use of plants and their by-products for prevention and treatment of disease.[3]

Nutraceuticals can be **traditional** and **nontraditional**.

Traditional nutraceuticals are simply natural, whole foods with new information about their potential health support qualities.

Many, if not most, fruits, vegetables, grains, fish, dairy and meat products contain several natural components that deliver benefits beyond basic nutrition, such as lycopene in tomatoes, omega-3 fatty acids in salmon or saponins in soy. Even tea and chocolate have been noted in some studies to contain health-promoting attributes.

Nontraditional nutraceuticals, on the other hand, are foods resulting from agricultural breeding or added nutrients and/or ingredients.

The current chapter will focus on nutraceuticals having antioxidant function and their effects on male infertility.

Before discussing nutraceuticals having antioxidant properties, it is essential to have some ideas about reactive oxygen species (ROS) and oxidative stress (OS). Physiologic ROS is essential for certain sperm functions like capacitation and signal transduction events.[4] Whereas high ROS produces oxidative stress and has a negative effect on spermatozoal integrity and fertilising potential.

Nutrition plays a significant role in maintaining male fertility through several mechanisms which are detailed below:

- Involved in the successful maturation of sperm
- Provides nutrition for motility of sperm
- Improvement in sperm count and motility
- Helps in production of sex hormones
- Prevents sperm damage
- Synthesis of RNA, DNA and proteins

ANTIOXIDANTS

The best-studied fertility supplements are the antioxidants, notably vitamins E and C, acetylcysteine and glutathione.

Antioxidants function as ROS scavengers to protect the sperms and other cells against oxidative stress and damage.[5]

Combination therapy with essential fatty acids has been shown to improve sperm concentration in men with low sperm counts and also significantly reduces reactive oxygen species (ROS). Sperm membranes play an important role in sperm ovum fusion and fertilisation. Sperm membranes harbor a higher concentration of polyunsaturated fatty acids (PUFAs) than other human cells. Sperms with the highest concentration of PUFA are thought to have the most normal morphology. ROS can cause instability in membrane permeability through effects on PUFA, as these fatty acids are extremely sensitive to oxidative stress. Indeed, the most protective antiperoxidative mechanism protecting PUFA uses thiol or glutathione-dependent enzymes. For these reasons, ROS scavengers such as glutathione are thought to maintain cell membrane stability. Currently, antioxidant supplements are used empirically in case of low sperm motility and to reduce level of fragmented DNA in sperm.

Based on their prime mechanism of action in improving sperm parameters, the following nutraceuticals have been proposed for improvement of male fertility potential.

- Coenzyme Q10
- L-carnitine
- Lycopene
- Zinc
- Selenium and glutathione
- Methylcobalamine
- Vitamins E and C
- Folic acid
- Arginine

A brief description of each of these nutraceuticals is summarised below (with dietary source of availability and recommended dose):

Coenzyme Q10

- CoQ10 (ubiquinone) is a naturally-occurring compound found in every cell in the body

- In spermatozoa, coenzyme Q10 (CoQ10) is concentrated in the mitochondria located in the mid-piece.
- It acts as an electron carrier in the mitochondrial respiratory chain[6] and provides energy for movement and all other energy-dependent processes in the sperm cell.
- Reduction in levels of CoQ10 are observed in sperm cells and seminal plasma of idiopathic and varicocele-associated asthenozoospermic patients.
- It is found in foods, particularly in fish and meats.

Dietary sources: Cabbage, carrots, whole grains, oily fish (Mackerel, sardines) organ meats (heart, kidney, liver)[7], etc.

The recommended dose range of CoQ10 is 60 mg to 200 mg daily.

L-carnitine

- The main function of L-carnitine in the epididymis is to provide an energy substrate for spermatozoa and it improves sperm motility and maturation.[8]
- L-carnitine is necessary for transport of fatty acids into the mitochondria to produce energy.
- Low levels of L-carnitine reduces fatty acid concentrations within the mitochondria, leading to decreased sperm motility.
- Significantly high levels of free L-carnitine is observed in the seminal plasma of fertile men compared to infertile men.
- The level of free L-carnitine in the semen has positive correlation with sperm concentration, sperm motility and vitality of sperm cells.
- Moreover, L-carnitine functions as anti-oxidant providing protection against ROS.[9]
- Carnitine supplementation improves sperm concentration, motility, morphology, vitality and total oxidative capacity.

Dietary sources: Fish, poultry, red meat, dairy products, etc.

The recommended dose range of L-carnitine is 1 to 3 gm daily.

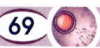

Lycopene

- Lycopene is a non-provitamin vitamin A carotenoid antioxidant which is a red pigment synthesized by plants.
- It plays an important role in cell growth regulation, gap junction communication, gene expression, modulation of immune responses and protection of lipid peroxidation.[11]

The general mechanism by which lycopene works is by preventing oxidative damage to sperms, which includes:

- Damage to the cell membrane
- DNA molecules (DNA oxidation is reduced by 75%)
- Lipids (lipid peroxidation is reduced by 80%)
- Proteins
- DNA fragmentation (COMET assay) is reduced by 40%.

Dietary sources: Tomato, red fruits like watermelons, guava, etc.

Lycopene has been demonstrated to be the most potent antioxidant with the ranking: lycopene >α-tocopherol >α-carotene > lutein.

The recommended dose range of lycopene is 4,000 mcg to 22.6 mg.

Zinc

- It is implicated in the genetic expression of steroid hormone receptors and has anti-apoptotic and antioxidant properties.
- It is a micronutrient which serves as a cofactor for more than 80 enzymes involved in DNA transcription and protein synthesis.[12]
- Low level of zinc is associated with decreased testosterone levels and sperm count.
- Levels are generally lower in men with diminished sperm count and testosterone level and with compromised function of immune system.[13]
- Zinc is known to improve sexual potency, sperm count and concentration, motility and morphology by improving testosterone concentration.

Dietary sources: Seeds (pumpkin, sunflower, sesame), wheat, meat, etc.

The recommended dose range of zinc is 24 mg to 500 mg daily.

Selenium

- Selenium is an essential trace element as well as important antioxidant.
- It is a component of glutathione peroxidase which involves reduction of antioxidant enzymes.[14]
- Deficiency of selenium can lead to instability of the mid-piece, resulting in defective motility.
- However, it can be toxic, if consumed in excess.

Dietary sources: Cereal, eggs, nuts, meat, seafood, etc.

Glutathione

- Glutathione is one of the most important endogenous antioxidants and plays an important role in reduction of exogenous antioxidant.
- Glutathione supplementation in infertile male improves sperm motility and along with vitamin E and vitamin C, glutathione supplementation improves sperm count and reduces DNA fragmentation.

Dietary sources: Fruits, vegetables, meat, etc.

Methylcobalamin

- Vitamin B_{12} is important in cellular replication, especially for the synthesis of RNA and DNA, and deficiency states have been associated with decreased sperm count and motility.
- Various studies have shown that methyl-cobalamin improves the sperm parameters.
- However, studies show that methyl-cobalamin is effective in only just over 20% of infertile men.

Dietary sources: Fish, meat, poultry, dairy products, etc.

Vitamins E and C

- In small studies, vitamin E (tocopherol) has been shown to improve sperm function and

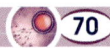
IVF success rates. Ascorbic acid (vitamin C) has been reported to protect sperm DNA from the damage induced by exogenous oxidative stress *in vitro*. Other studies have also shown that higher levels of sperm DNA fragmentation, a marker of oxidative stress and possibly reduced fertility, are associated with lower levels of seminal ascorbic acid.

- Combination therapy significantly reduces DNA fragmentation rate.[15]
- Oral supplementation with vitamin E significantly decreases the malondialdehyde concentration and improves the sperm motility.
- Although *in vitro* studies have proved the efficacy of vitamin E, human studies are lacking.

Dietary sources of vitamin C: Fruits (citrus, papaya, strawberry) vegetables, etc.

Dietary sources of vitamin E: Fruits, vegetables, cereals, vegetable oil, dairy, poultry, meat, etc.

Folic Acid

Folic acid is an important micronutrient that has been documented for its effects on preventing neural tube defects in the developing embryo. Folate also plays a role in RNA and DNA synthesis during spermatogenesis and has antioxidant properties.[16] While older studies have shown no benefit for folic acid supplementation on the semen quality of infertile men, newer studies suggest that there may be benefit, especially for tobacco users. Most recently, when combined with zinc, folate supplementation was shown to increase sperm concentration in infertile men in a blinded, randomized, controlled trial.

Dietary sources: Dark green leafy vegetables, avocado, beans, Brewer's yeast, etc.

Arginine

- Arginine is thought to be essential for sperm motility.
- According to a study by Schachter, *et al.* arginine significantly improved sperm count and motility after intake of 4 gm/day for three months.[17]
- A recent study conducted in Italy also showed that arginine is effective in male infertility.

- However, the dosage of arginine is higher compared to other micronutrients.

Dietary sources: Barley, brown rice, chocolate, coconut, cereal, etc.

Conclusion

Currently, nutraceuticals are marketed extensively and are some of the popular drugs used by the infertility specialist prior to or during ART though there is lack of enough proven scientific data about the composition and dosing regimen.

The lack of uniformity in public studies makes direct comparison difficult.

Small size, short study period, lack of dose standardisation and absence of double blinding are some of the deficiencies in the published reports.

Confusion about the composition, dose, and period of treatment has not yet been cleared and precise conclusion regarding their effects on male subfertility are yet to be ascertained. But Cochrane review[18] in 2011 demonstrated an improvement in pregnancy and child birth rate following nutraceutical therapy.

However, it is possible that nutraceutical supplementation containing traditional antioxidants will help in protecting sperm from ROS already produced.

REFERENCES

1. Brower V. Nutraceuticals poised for a healthy slice of the healthcare market? Net Biotechnol 1998; 16: 728–31.
2. Kalra EK. Nutraceutical-definition and introduction. AAPS Pharmsci 2003; 5(3): 1–2.
3. Bagchi D. Nutraceuticals and functional foods regulations in United States and around the world. Toxicology 2006: 5(3) 1–2.
4. de Lamirande E, Lamothe G. Reactive oxygen induced reactive oxygen formation during human sperm capacitation. Free Radic Biol Med 2009'c 46: 502–10.
5. Ross C, Morriss A, Khairy M, et al. A systemic review of the effect of oral antioxidants on male infertility.
6. Hidaka T, Fuijii K, Funahashi I, et al. Safely assessment of co-enzymes Q10 (CoQ10), Biofact 2008; 32: 199–208.

7. Pravst I, Zomitek J. Coenzyme Q 10 contents in food and fartification strategies. Crit Rev Food sci Nutr 2010; 50: 269–80.

8. Palemo S, Bottazzi C, Cost M, et al. Metabolic effects of L carnitine on pre-pubertal rat Sertoli cells. horm Metab Res 2000; 32: 887–90.

9. Vicari E, Lavigera S, Calogero A. Antioxidant treatment with carnitines is effective in infertile patients with prostatovesiculoepididymitis and elevated seminal leukocyte concentrations after treatment with nonsteroidal anti-inflammatory compounds Fertil Steril 2002; 6: 1203–8.

10. Zhou X, Liu F, Zhai S. Effect of L carnitine and/or L-acetyl carnitine in nutrition treatment for male infertility, a systematic review. Asia Pac J clin Nutr 2007; 16: 383–90.

11. Rao AV, Min MR, Rao LG. Lycopene Adv Food Nutr Res 2006; 51: 99–164.

12. Ebisch IM, Thomas CM, Peters NH, et al. The importance of Folate, zinc and antioxidants in the pathogenesis and prevention of sub-fertility. Hum Reprod Update 2007; 13: 163–79.

13. Prasad AS. Zinc in human health, Effect of zinc on immune cells. Mol Med 2008; 14: 353–7.

14. Brown KM, Arthur JR. Selenium , Selenoprotein and human health: a review. Public Health nutr 2001; 4: 593–9.

15. Greco E, lacobeli M, Reinzi L, et al. Reduction of the incidence of sperm DNA fragmentation by oral antioxidant treatment. J Androl 2005; 26: 349–53.

16. Ebisch IM, Thomas CM, Peters WH, et al. The importance of folate, zinc and antioxidants in the pathogenesis and prevention of subfertility. Hum Reprod Update 2007; 79: 829–43.

17. Schibona M, Mseschini P, Cappavells, et al. L-arginine and male infertility. Minerva Urol Nefrol 1994: 46 (4) 251–3.

18. Showell MG, Brown J, Tazdani A, et al. Anti-oxidants for male infertility. Cochrane Databese Syst Rev 2011; (1): CD007411.

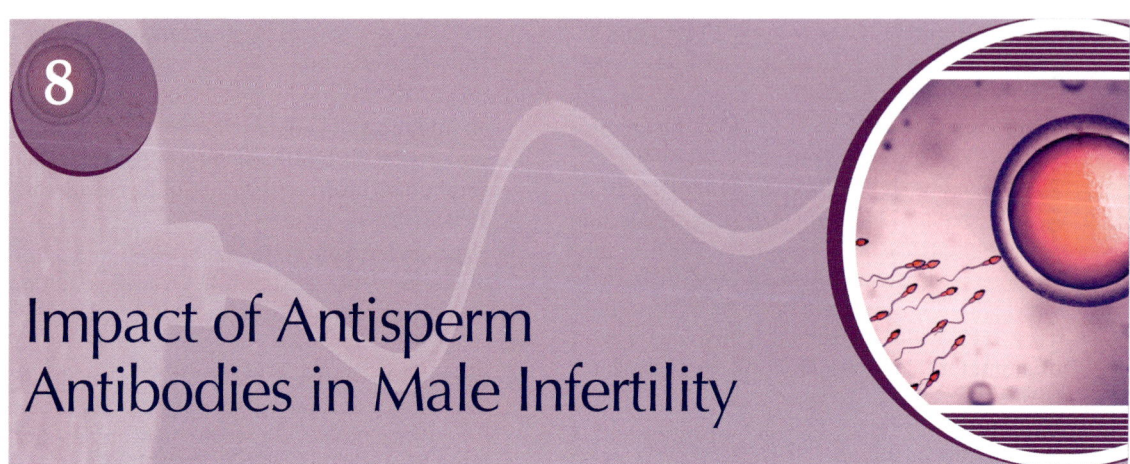

Impact of Antisperm Antibodies in Male Infertility

There are plenty of evidence to suggest that antisperm antibodies (ASAs) may have significant role in immune-related human infertility. These antibodies are directed to various sperm antigens and implicated in sperm dysfunction. Couples with unexplained infertility are more likely to have antisperm antibodies. At least 40% of all infertile couples have problem with sperm and about 10% of infertile men have ASA *versus* 2% of normal fertile men.[4]

Major histocompatibility complex (MHC) antigen family on sperm surface is most likely to be involved in reproductive immune system. These antigens are probably absent on human germ cell.[1, 2] Some antigens like PH20 and RSA-1 in animals are regulators of spermatozoa, enzyme receptor, capacitation and sperm zona interaction. One of these antigens, fertilisation antigen-1 (FA-1) is a glycoprotein and regulator of sperm-oocyte interaction in humans. Antibody against this antigen inhibits fertilisation at sperm-zona level without reducing sperm motility.[3, 4]

There are about 30 types of antigens found in seminal plasma and on spermatozoa, of which 6 are sperm-specific. In response to these antigens, two types of antibodies develop.

a. Autoimmunity: In this variety, male partner himself develops antibodies in response to his own antigens. This happens following testicular trauma, infection or following vasectomy (at least 2 years after vas ligation). The disruption of blood-testis barrier (formed in the seminiferous tubules by tight apical junction of adjacent Sertoli cells) or epithelial barriers, an immunosuppression defect or genital tract trauma are the primary mechanisms responsible for leakage of sperm antigens and formation of ASA. The antigens on developing spermatozoa pass into general circulation through testicular connective tissue—and are processed by reticulo-endothelial system. Antibodies produced by reticuloendothelial (RE) system pass back into the seminiferous tubules and affect the developing spermatozoa. This is known as autoimmune reaction. ASAs are found in three locations: in the serum, seminal plasma, and sperm surface (sperm-bound). Among these, sperm-bound are the most critically relevant antibodies.

b. Isoimmunity: Isoimmunity or antibody formation against spermatozoa occurs following deposition of spermatozoa in the female genital tract. 7 to 17% of infertile women can produce antisperm antibodies in their cervical fluids.[5, 6]

Mechanism of Production of Antibodies in Male Partner

Testis is an immunologically privileged site. The germ cells and spermatozoa within the testis harbor antigen considered "foreign" by the immune system; still no immunoresponse is generated because these cells are well protected in the testis and separated from the circulatory system by a blood-testis barrier. Components of the barrier may include cells, immunosuppressive molecules and undefined genetic contribution. All these factors contribute to a sanctuary state of immunological tolerance within the seminiferous tubules. In humans, Sertoli cell is the most important morphological barrier to immunity in the testis. In between Sertoli cells, there are specialised epithelial cells called occlusive junction or popularly known as tight junction. It has been reported[7,8] that the tight junction of efferent tubules contains some gaps; these gaps allow small, but constant leakage of sperm antigen to the systemic circulation which results in desensitisation of the immunosystem. But when the barrier is disrupted there is leakage of large dosage of antigen which initiates a pathologic immunoresponse which means formation of 'antisperm antibody'.

Formation of antisperm antibody to sperm is a consequence of:

  i. Breaches in blood-testis barrier
  ii. Overwhelming inoculation of sperm antigen
  iii. A defect in active immunosuppression

Conditions responsible for antisperm antibody formation:

  a. *Physical injury*: Trauma, torsion, biopsy, coitus
  b. *Infections*: Orchitis, epididymis, prostatitis
  c. *Obstruction*: Absence of vas deferens, vasectomy, testicular
  d. *Thermal injury*: Varicocele, cryptorchidism
  e. *Genetic*: Human lymphocyte antigen.

Mechanism of Production of Antibodies in Female Partner (Isoimmunity)

After semen is deposited in the vagina following intercourse, sperms are phagocytosed by macrophages and carried to reticuloendothelial cells in the body like spleen and lymphoid tissues. The sperm antigens are processed in these tissues and three types of antibodies develop. The significant antibodies are IgG and IgA. IgM is a very insignificant antibody and is rarely found in female serum. IgG and IgA are relatively more significant and are involved in immobilising the sperm. They are found on the sperm surface and in the cervical mucous. These are known as sperm specific and local antibodies respectively.

Types, Clinical Significance and Source of Origin of Antisperm Antibodies

Three types of antibodies are produced, e.g. IgG, IgA and IgM, of these IgG and IgA are the most significant antisperm antibodies. IgG which is both locally derived and transuded from serum, and IgA which is thought to be purely locally produced (on the sperm surface) are the most frequently implicated in the pathogenesis of human immune infertility.[9]

  A. *Local antibodies*:
    a. Sperm surface antibodies
    b. Seminal plasma antibodies
    c. Cervical mucous antibodies (IgG and IgA).
  B. *Humoral antibodies (IgG, IgA and IgM—in serum)*; of these three types of antibodies IgM is rarely found in the serum of female partner.
  C. *Systemic antibodies*: This is rarely encountered—may sometimes lead to anaphylactic shock. Clinical examples— severe cramping of the uterus after pushing raw unprepared semen in IUI treatment.

Indications, Materials and Methods of Testing Antisperm Antibodies

At present there is no single assay which may be considered as a global indicator for assessment of immunological subfertility. In order to understand immunological defect as cause of unexplained infertility, a combination test in some cases may be helpful.

Mixed antiglobulin reaction (MAR) or immunobead test combined with sperm agglutination in serum or seminal plasma are the best methods for assessment of ASA-mediated subfertility.

In general, antisperm antibody (ASA) testing is not performed routinely. This is

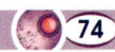

because no prospective study has demonstrated decreased fecundity in ASA positive couples compared to those who are ASA negative.

But circumstantial evidence suggest that ASA can sometimes alter sperm function. Hence test for ASA should be performed when this is indicated.

The indications for ASA testing are

A. Semen analysis reveals:
    a. Abnormal clumping
    b. Agglutination
    c. Unexplained decreased motility
B. History of genital tract trauma or infection
C. Abnormal PCT

Though PCT is not done as a routine in infertility workup, there are specific indications for PCT
These are:

a. Semen hyperviscosity
b. Increased or decreased semen volume with good sperm density
c. Unexplained infertility

Hence it is apparent, that under some situations in infertility workup there are indications for performing antisperm antibody test.

Which ASA test is of practical significance?

As has already been described before, anti-sperm antibodies can be produced systemically or locally. It has also been pointed out that circulating ASA (humoral antibodies) is not a sufficient proof of immunologic infertility. But sperm surface ASA may indicate a cause of infertility (auto-antibodies may indicate a cause of immunologic infertility). Local antibodies as in cervical mucous or in uterine fluid (isoimmunity) may also contribute as etiological factors of immunological infertility.

Materials for testing antisperm antibodies

a. Serum
b. Seminal plasma
c. Cervical mucous
d. Reproductive tract fluid (uterine, cervical, tubal, follicular fluid)
e. Surface of spermatozoa.

Methods of testing for ASA—these are only screening tests and not specific.

Before ART was introduced (1978) these tests were performed extensively in infertility practice. But since IVF was introduced sperm washing technique has become a routine procedure to wash out the surface antibodies on sperm surface. Also to overcome the cervical mucous antibodies IUI is being practiced.

Hence the tests which are being mentioned below are not practiced routinely nowadays, and they are only of historical interest.

A. Agglutination test:
    • Kibrick's test (gelatin agglutination test, GAT)
    • Franklin and Duke's test (Tube's slide agglutination test)
    • Friberg's test (tray agglutination test, TAT)
B. Immobilisation test:
    • Isojima test

Brief description of agglutination test
Principles

a. The donor sperm is treated with media (Ham's F10) and serum albumin.
b. The test sample (seminal plasma, cervical mucous or serum) is also treated with media (Ham's F10) and serum albumin.
c. The two (a and b) are mixed together and kept at room temperature for about half an hour.
d. Observation and conclusion—the test is positive when large agglutination forms with donors' spermatozoa.

Brief description of Immobilisation test

Isojima test: The principle is the same as in agglutination test. Donor spermatozoa become immotile in presence of a complement. This is considered to be less sensitive than agglutination test.

Detection of sperm surface antibodies

This is more specific than detection of antibodies in serum, seminal plasma or cervical mucous. Two types of tests were performed, but currently not popular because of introduction

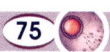

of sperm washing technique in ART practice. The two tests commonly used were:

a. Mixed antiglobulin reaction test (MAR test)

b. Immunobead test

Mixed antiglobulin reaction test (MAR test):[10]

The steps are:

a. MAR is similar to Coomb's test

b. Three ingredients are essential
   i. Semen sample (test)
   ii. Sensitised group O Rh (+ve) human RBC
   iii. Rabbit or goat monospecific anti-G antiserum

c. These ingredients are mixed together— incubated for 10 min and observed under light microscope.

d. Agglutination is seen as mixed clumps of spermatozoa and red cells with a 'shaky' movement.

e. Test is positive when more than 50% agglutination is present.

Immunobead test

Materials: Immunobead reagent consists of polyacrylamide beads 5–10 μm in diameter coated with antihuman immunoglobulins of either IgA, IgG or IgM class.

These beads are available in lyophilised form and can be reconstituted by adding 10 ml of sterile Tyrode's or Ham's F10 solution.

Procedure and conclusion: One drop of immunobead reagent mixed with one drop of semen sample is placed on a slide covered by cover slip. This is incubated on a moist petridish for 10 min at room temperature.

The test is positive when 20% or more spermatozoa show positive binding.

The diagnosis of immunological infertility requires two conditions to be satisfied:[9]

a. Fifty percent or more of the motile spermatozoa (progressive and non-progressive) have attached beads. It should be noted, however, that particle binding restricted to the tail tip is not associated with impaired fertility and can be present in fertile men.

b. Sperm-bound antibodies interfere with sperm function; this is usually demonstrated by using functional tests such as the sperm–mucous penetration test, zona binding assays and the acrosome reaction

At present, flow-cytometry seems to be a promising technique to assess exact amount of IgG and IgA on individual spermatozoa.[11]

In routine infertility practice, these tests are seldom performed. Commonly performed and also clinically informative tests are:

a. Sperm cervical mucous contact test (SCMCT)

b. Sperm cervical mucous penetration test (SCMPT)

Figure 8.1 illustrates agglutination of sperm head and tail in cervical mucous.

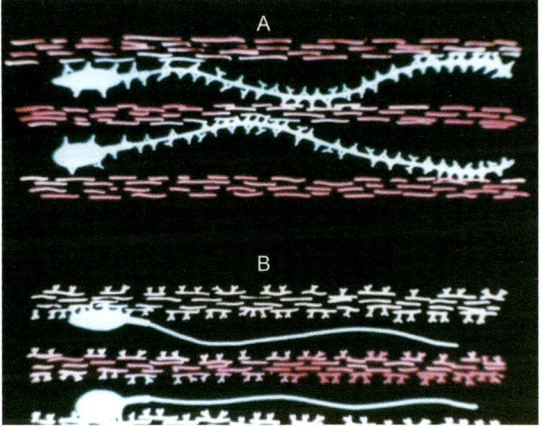

Fig. 8.1: Agglutination of sperm and tail in cervical mucous

Treatment of Antisperm Antibody Positive Cases

Treatment options previously practised and now abandoned

a. **Short-term use of condom:** Idea was to avoid exposure of the female partner from antigenic stimulus of seminal plasma, thereby avoiding production of antibodies. During the short period while the female partner was free from antisperm antibody, chances of pregnancy were expected to increase following either timed intercourse or IUI.

b. **Corticosteroid:** Idea was to achieve immunosuppression. However, the results were not encouraging. Moreover,

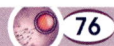

corticosteroid may be detrimental for the health of female partner.

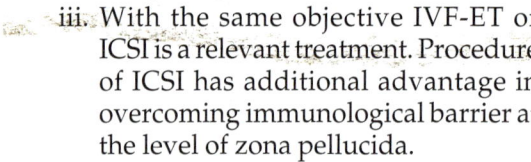

Currently practised therapeutic approaches are

a. IUI with second part of split ejaculate or second masturbated sample of semen: The background of this approach is as follows:

  i. There is fixed daily production rate of ASA. Therefore, level of antibody will be lower in the second part of split ejaculate or second masturbated sample of semen.

  ii. For IUI, the semen is to be collected in a special container containing washing buffer or media, from which the sperm may be collected. This will be retrieved after washing and used for IUI. The buffer or media is expected to washout the sperm surface antigens adequately.

  iii. With the same objective IVF-ET or ICSI is a relevant treatment. Procedure of ICSI has additional advantage in overcoming immunological barrier at the level of zona pellucida.

However, in many cases antisperm antibodies may not be the only factor causing infertility, and therefore, a search for other causative factors should also be performed.

Conclusion

Though sperm immunology provides us with useful information about latent subfertility or unexplained infertility still ideas are vague about the exact role of antisperm antibodies (IgG, IgA) in the etiopathogenesis of human infertility. This is because of the following reasons:

1. Even with highest level of ASA (particularly IgA) viable pregnancies have been reported. What level of ASA causes subfertility is not known.

2. A multicentric study by WHO on antibodies to reproductive antigens could not find any clinical relevance and no significant difference was observed between fertile and infertile groups.

3. Clear distinction between IgG and IgA is difficult to make because most infertile men with ASA have a mixture of these two immunoglobulin classes on their spermatozoa.

REFERENCES

1. Anderson DJ, Narayan P, DeWolf WC. Major histocompatibility antigens are not detectable on postmeiotic human testicular germ cells, J Immunol 133: 1962, 1984.

2. Hass GG Jr, Nahhas F. Failure to identify HLA, ABC and DR antigens on human sperm, Am J Reprod Immunol Microbiol 10: 39, 1986.

3. Abdel-Latif A, Mathur S, Rust PF. Cytotoxic sperm antibodies inhibit sperm preparation of zona-free hamster eggs, Fertil Steril 45: 542, 1986.

4. Bronson RA, Cooper JW, Rosenfeld DL. Autoimmunity to spermatozoa: effect on sperm penetration of cervical mucus as reflected by post-coital testing, Fertil Steril 41: 609, 1984.

5. Jones W. The use of antibodies developed by infertile women to identify relevant antigens. Karolinska Symposia on Research Methods in Reproductive Endocrinology Immunological Approach to Fertility Control 1974; Stockholm, Karolinska Institute.

6. Beer AE, Neaves WB. Antigenic status of semen from the viewpoints of the female and male. Fertil Steril 1978; 29(1): 3–22.

7. Anderson DJ, Hill JA. Cell-mediated immunity in infertility, Am J Reprod Immunol Microbiol 17: 22, 1988.

8. Suzuki FF, Nagano T. Regional differentiation of cell junctions in the excurrent duct epithelium of the rat testis as revealed by freeze-fracture, Anat Rec 191: 503, 1978.

9. Turek PJ. Male infertility. In: Tanagho E MJ. Smith's General Urology. 17th ed: McGraw-Hill 2008; 684–716.

10. Bronson RA. Antisperm antibodies: a critical evaluation and clinical guidelines. J Reprod Immunol 1999; 45(2): 159–83.

11. Ke RW, Dockter ME, Majumdar G, Buster JE, Carson SA. Flow cytometry provides rapid and highly accurate detection of antisperm antibodies; Fertility and Sterility 1995, 63(4): 902–906.

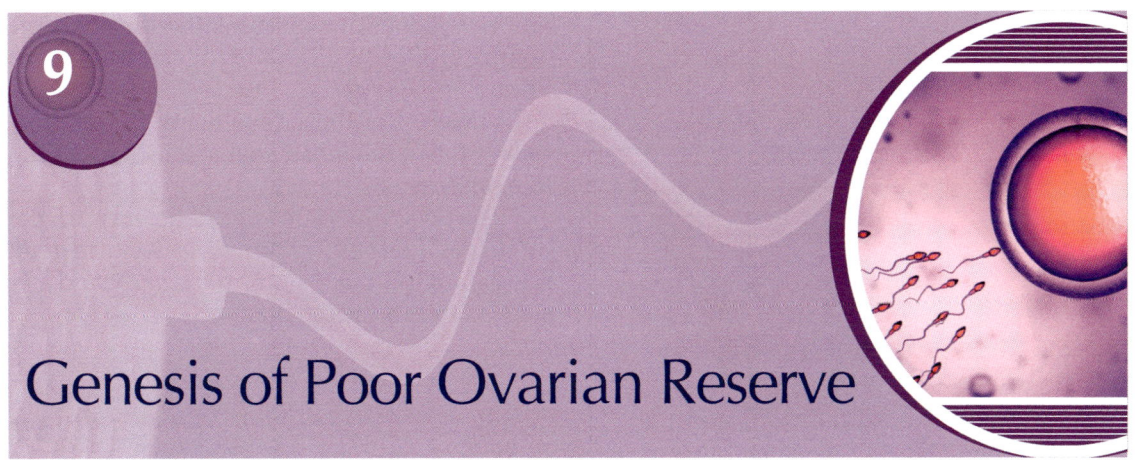

Genesis of Poor Ovarian Reserve

INTRODUCTION

Ovarian reserve is a term that is used to determine the capacity of the ovary to provide eggs that are capable of fertilisation, resulting in a healthy and successful pregnancy. With advanced maternal age the number of eggs that can be successfully recruited for a possible pregnancy declines, constituting a major factor in the inverse correlation between age and female fertility and poor reproductive potential. Folliculogenesis, the developmental progression of an ovarian follicle from the primordial to the preovulatory state, is a key reproductive event in the female.[1] The process begins before birth and continues throughout reproductive life. Generally, the lifetime quota of follicles in the female is established at birth,[2, 3] although recent evidence suggests the existence of proliferative germ cells capable of oocyte/follicle production in the postnatal mammalian ovary.[4] The number of primordial follicles, which constitute the ovarian reserve at birth, the rate of replenishment during postnatal life[4], and the rate at which follicles are recruited dictate the functional ovarian life span of an individual.[2–7]

When the total number of follicles is less than normal at birth or there is increased rate of atresia before menopause, the ovaries will contain less number of follicles during childbearing age leading to a clinical con-dition of 'poor ovarian reserve'. In addition, even if the follicular stock is normal, but sensitivity of follicular receptors to circulating gonadotropin is deficient, a similar state of low ovarian reserve will be the consequence. Also, suboptimal bioactivity of pituitary gonadotropin (which is found in elderly women) may also be responsible for poor ovarian reserve. The later two conditions are not due to low follicular stock, but in spite of follicular stock being normal, the functioning potential of a follicle in stimulated cycle is either deficient, or functionally asynchronous even if numerically adequate. Asynchronous follicles mean that different follicles in a maturing follicular cohort respond differently to endogenous or exogenous gonadotropin stimulation. Some behave normally to become fully mature while others remain erratic and remain semi-mature.

Hence the broad etiological factors of poor ovarian reserve are:
- i. Low follicular stock
- ii. Accelerated atresia of the existing number of follicles
- iii. Low follicular response to endogeneous or exogeneous gonadotropins
- iv. Low bioactive FSH

These factors have been diagrammatically represented in Fig. 9.1.

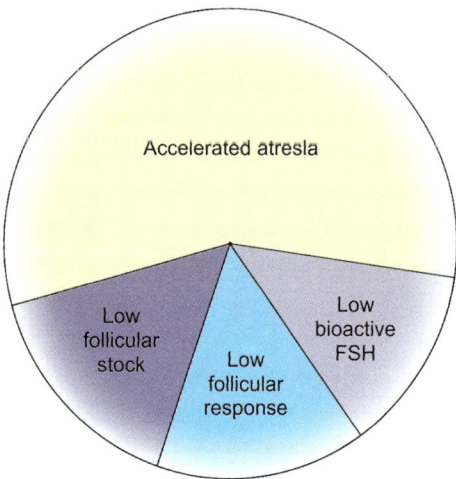

Fig. 9.1: Broad etiological factors

Initial Inadequate Stock of Follicles

Considering normal physiology, the germ cells (oocytes) originating from hind gut and yolk sac of embryos at 6–7 weeks intra-uterine life migrate to genital ridge where they multiply by mitotic division. By 12 weeks, the number of germ cells (oocyte) becomes 6–7 million. This process is activated by fetal thymus. Hence hypoplasia or aplasia of the fetal thymus may lead to ovarian insufficiency. This is one way by which low follicular stock might exist from the initial stages of fetal development in the intrauterine life.

There is another mechanism by which the follicular stock may be deficient from the very beginning of intrauterine life. This also depends on defect in the earlier stages of follicular development. As has already been stated, by 12 weeks of gestation the number of follicles becomes 6–7 million and remains in "resting pool". At an interval of 70–80 days, cohort of follicles is selected from 'resting pool' (primordial follicle); they grow and run for maturity and eventually become atretic. Before gonadotropins are available, growth and development of follicles depend on a variety of factors locally produced and regulated; important ones are—TGF-β superfamily of proteins, activins, inhibins, AMH, etc.

After puberty, the cohort of follicles recruited, during the last 20 days of 80 days cycle (late luteal phase of previous cycle) few

becomes gonadotropin-sensitive through the action of GH, IGF-1, androgens and other unknown factors.

Deficiency of these sensitising factors may reduce the number of effective follicles, leading to ovarian insufficiency.

Figure 9.2 illustrates the deficiency of the different factors responsible for reduced number of follicular stock in the early and late stages of intrauterine life.

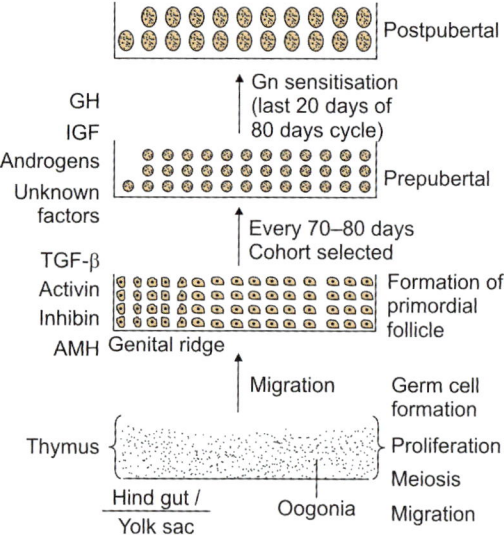

Fig. 9.2: Stage of follicular development and gradual migration

Accelerated Atresia

The second important cause of follicular depletion is accelerated follicular atresia.

Though follicular growth and atresia (apoptosis) are physiological processes in folliculogenesis, accelerated atresia reduces the available number of follicles for utilisation.

Etiology of Accelerated Atresia

The broad etiological factors are:

    a. Immunologic

    b. Infective

    c. Metabolic

    d. Iatrogenic

    e. Chromosomal/Genetic

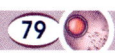

Immunological Causes

Approximately 4% of women with premature ovarian insufficiency (POI or POF) have autoimmune disease.

Autoimmune polyglandular syndrome (APS) both type I and type II are also associated with ovarian failure. But more significant associations of this syndrome are Addison's disease, IDDM, hypoparathyroidism, etc.

Type I APS presents in childhood with typical features of hypoparathyroidism often associated with adrenal insufficiency (60–80%) and POF (60%); the cause is mutation of a gene located on chromosome-21. Type II APS has an adult onset and is characterised by adrenal insufficiency (100%) and thyroid autoimmunity (70%) and type I diabetes (50%). 25% of women with this disorder have amenorrhoea, and 10% have POF/POI (premature ovarian insufficiency).

The strong association between autoimmune adrenal and ovarian failure justifies screening for antiadrenal antibodies in all women with POF. Patients with positive antiadrenal antibodies should be further evaluated to exclude asymptomatic adrenal insufficiency by measuring morning sample of serum cortisol level.

Isolated autoimmune ovarian failure is commonly associated with histologic picture of lymphocytic oophoritis. Common association is hypothyroidism. Circulating antibodies against ovarian antigen may be found in these women. However, the antibodies are more pronounced in ovarian vessels than in general circulation because the antibodies are mixed up with other antibodies found in these women with autoimmune polyglandular syndrome (APS). Hence it is difficult to identify ovarian antibodies separately for the diagnosis of autoimmune ovarian failure.

Apart from syndromes described above, ovarian insufficiency has also been reported in association with myasthenia gravis, SLE, rheumatoid arthritis and Crohn's disease.

Infective Causes

Mumps oophoritis has been associated as one of the causes of follicular destruction leading to low ovarian reserve. However, mumps oophoritis is a less frequent cause of gamete depletion in female compared to mumps orchitis in male (2% in females against 25% in male).

Caseous and fibrocaseous lesion of the ovary in tubercular infection is a significant cause of premature follicular depletion. In genital tubercular infection, in general, even when the ovaries are not involved directly there may be follicular depletion because of toxins liberated from *Mycobacterium tuberculosis* (MTB). POI has also been encountered in latent female genital tuberculosis.

Cytomegalovirus and nonspecific salpingo-oophoritis have also been implicated in the genesis of POI (premature ovarian insufficiency).

Metabolic

Galactose toxicity has been reported as an important cause of premature ovarian insufficiency (galactosaemic ovarian insufficiency). This is due to deficiency of an enzyme—galactose-I-phosphate uridyl transferase.

The damage is caused at the time of oocyte migration from yolk sac to genital ridge. This has been supported by our observation published earlier.[8]

Iatrogenic

Surgical trauma or repeated assault on the ovary at the time of laparoscopy may reduce the number of follicles in the ovary as in recurrent surgery for chocolate cyst (endometriomas). Similarly, ovarian drilling with or without use of diathermy may reduce the number of follicles in the ovary.

Unilateral oophorectomy reduces the number of follicles to be recruited in each ovarian cycle (70–80 days), which run for maturity; because the number of follicles to be recruited in each ovarian cycle depends on the number of follicles existing in resting pool.

Chemotherapy is one of the significant causes of ovarian follicular depletion. Majority of the cytotoxic treatments cause ovarian failure in about 50% women. Alkylating agents and cyclophosphamide specifically cause gonadal damage. Women with haematological malignancies receiving total body irradiation experience irreversible ovarian failure.

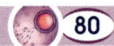
Lastly, cigarette smoking has an inverse relationship with age of menopause.

Chromosomal/Genetic Defect

This is a significant cause of ovarian failure. The defects are broadly classified as:

a. Chromosomal

b. Genetic

Chromosomal Defect

Chromosomal defect may be either autosomal or sex chromosomal

Both sex chromosomal and autosomal defects can be subclassified as:

a. Numerical

b. Structural.

Both X chromosomes must be present and active in oocytes to avoid the accelerated loss of follicles. The findings of a normal karyotype in patients with ovarian failure, commonly observed in clinical practice, is most perplexing, suggesting subtle reasons for loss of activity probably due to specific gene alteration. It is essential that specific genes confined to a portion of X chromosome are necessary for normal ovarian function.

The common ovarian anomalies associated with aneuploidy, namely Turner (45XO) has complete depletion of ovarian follicles before birth and they present with primary amenorrhoea at puberty. Mosaic Turner (46XX/45XO) and super females (47XXX) may present with low follicular reserve and premature ovarian insufficiency.

Structural anomalies leading to poor ovarian reserve or even total absence of follicles and primary amenorrhoea have been observed in women with X isochromosome, ring chromosome and part of X chromosome translocated to an autosome. Different types of sex chromosomal and autosomal anomalies (structural and numerical) associated with poor ovarian reserve or premature ovarian failure are illustrated in Figs 9.3 and 9.4.

Genetic Defect

Multiple genes on sex chromosomes and autosomes are involved in regulating female fertility and reproductive life span.

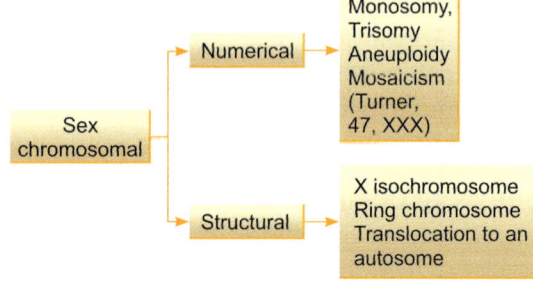

Two X chromosomes and an intact gene located on autosome Xq13 are essential for normal oocyte meiosis. Impairment of the gene results in meiotic arrest and oocyte depletion.

Fig. 9.3: Sex chromosomal anomalies

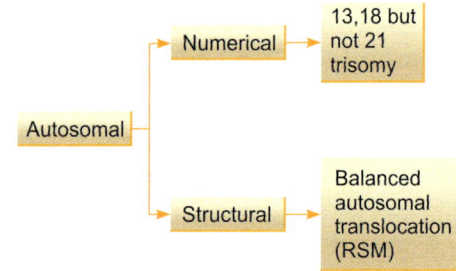

Fig. 9.4: Autosomal anomalies

From that point of view, genes on X chromosomes are more vital than genes on autosomes. Multiple genes on X chromosome regulate different aspects of female fertility and reproductive life span. In this respect, genes on short arm rather than on long arm of X chromosomes are more commonly involved for normal ovarian function.

Examples of a few genetic defects associated with ovarian failure

a. FMR-1 gene—this gene is located on Xq27.3, which is absent or mutated. Women with this type of chromosome and genetic defect are known as "X fragile syndrome". The complete mutation of gene leads to mental retardation with primary amenorrhoea, whereas partial mutation is responsible for ovarian insufficiency.

b. Genes located on Xq13 are involved in reactivation of inactive X during oocyte maturation. When this gene is defective, there may be maturation arrest and oocyte depletion.

c. BPES syndrome (blepharophimosis, ptosis and epicanthus inversus syndrome)— the features of this syndrome are characterised by drooping, tethered eyelids and ovarian insufficiency. The defect is in autosome 3q2. An example of BPES syndrome is presented in Fig. 9.5 which was published by our team.

Genetic defect in women has been worked out to some extent by our team in collaboration with CCMB, Hyderabad. A brief report of this work has been published in 2005.[9]

Dysfunction of Follicles

In a few women, follicular number may be normal, but their functions are abnormal, resulting in features of ovarian insufficiency.

The etiological factors of this subnormal function with normal follicular stock are:

a. FSH receptor defect.

b. Bioactive gonadotropins deficiency.

FSH Receptor Defect

In these cases, both the number of existing follicles and quality and quantity of gonadotropins secreted by the pituitary are normal. But the receptors located on the surface of the follicles which are supposed to receive gonadotropins to make the follicles work are defective. A most common clinical example is Savage syndrome (resistant ovary syndrome).

FSH receptors are more often partially functional. The more severe form with total receptor dysfunction presents with primary amenorrhoea and absent secondary characteristics. The follicles are normal in number, but FSH is elevated.

Complete loss of FSH receptors results in small ovaries, but this is rarely found in Savage syndrome. Surprisingly men with FSH receptor mutation have variable suppression of sperm count and few of them may be fertile. Isolated LH receptor defect is rarely found in men and women. When found in women, they present with primary amenorrhoea with typical picture of primary ovarian failure.

Summary

Low ovarian reserve or premature ovarian insufficiency (POI) indicates either low follicular stock or inadequate functioning of follicles even if the number of follicles is adequate. Depleted stock may be due to deficient number of follicles existing from intrauterine life or accelerated destruction of follicles resulting from a variety of etiological factors.

Some of the congenital causes of deficient number in the resting follicular pool may be due to defect in either embryonic thymic activity or intrinsic oocyte quality. Follicular depletion due to accelerated atresia may be attributed to immunologic intolerance (autoimmune ovarian failure), viral infections (mumps), metabolic, iatrogenic, chromosomal and genetic defects.

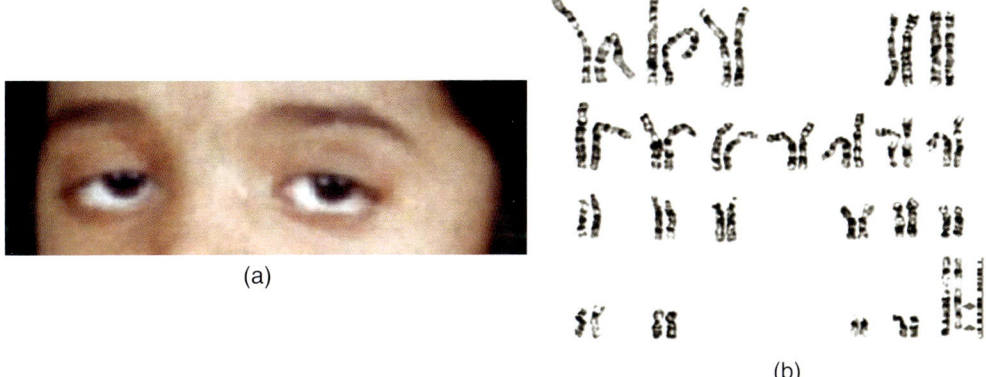

(a)

(b)

Figs 9.5a and b: (a) Photograph of the patient with BPES showing peculiar ocular deformities, (b) GTG-Banded results showing two break points on one of the X chromosomes

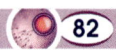

Apart from depletion of follicular number, follicular dysfunction may also be a significant cause of poor ovarian response. Dysfunction is primarily due to receptor defect in the follicular wall or may be because of deficiency of synthesis and release of normal amount of bioactive pituitary gonadotropin.

REFERENCES

1. Adashi EY The ovarian follicular apparatus. In: Adashi EY, Rock JA, Rosenwaks Z, eds. Reproductive endocrinology, surgery and technology. New York: Lippincott-Raven 1995; 17–40.

2. Zuckerman S. The number of oocytes in the mature ovary. Recent Prog Horm Res 1951; 6: 63–109.

3. Block E. Quantitative morphological investigation of the follicular system in women. Variations at different ages. Acta Anat 1952; 14: 108–123.

4. Johnson J, Canning J, Kaneko T, Pru JK, Tilly JL. Germline stem cells and follicular renewal in the postnatal mammalian ovary. Nature 2004; 428: 145–150.

5. Faddy MJ. Follicle dynamics during ovarian ageing. Mol Cell Endocrinol 2000; 163: 43–48.

6. Richardson SJ, Senikas V, Nelson JF. Follicular depletion during the menopausal transition: Evidence for accelerated loss and ultimate exhaustion. J Clin Endocrinol Metab 1987; 65: 1231–1237.

7. Gougeon A, Ecochard R, Thalabard JC. Age-related changes of the population of human ovarian follicles: increase in the disappearance rate of non-growing and early-growing follicles in aging women. Biol Reprod 1994; 50: 653–663.

8. S Bandopadhyay, J Chakraborti, S Banerjee, A K Pal, D Bhattacharyya, S K Gosh, B N Chakravarty and S N Kabir; Parental exposure to high galactose adversely affects initial gonadal pool of germ cells in rats; Human Reproduction 2003, Vol. 18, no. 2, 276–283.

9. Mutation screening of coding region of growth differentiation factor of gene in Indian women with ovarian failure—Menopause 2005.

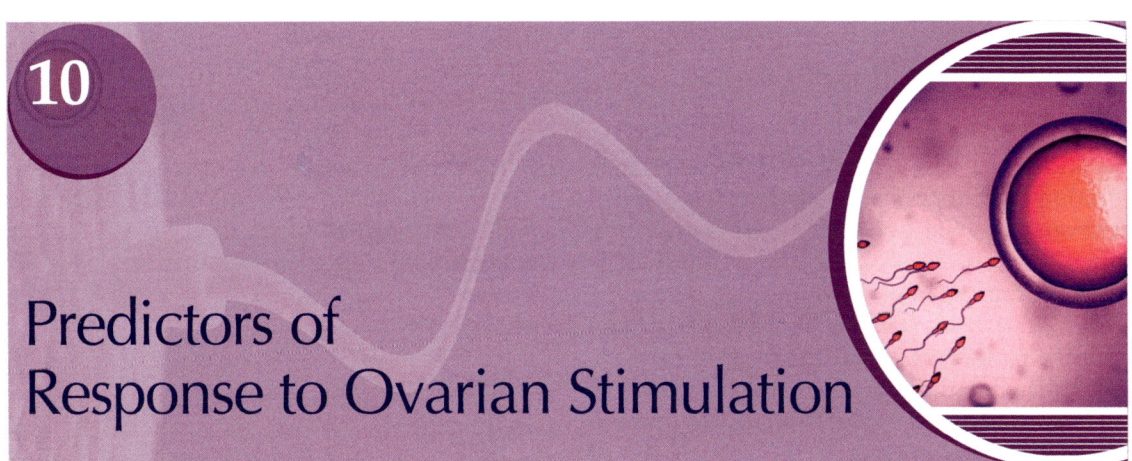

10

Predictors of Response to Ovarian Stimulation

INTRODUCTION

The aim of ovarian stimulation in IVF is the recruitment of multiple follicles in an effort to compensate for the inefficiencies of embryo culture, embryo selection for transfer and subsequent implantation.[1] But excessive response to ovarian stimulation generates many oocytes that may lead to a compromised oocyte quality[2-4] and hence chances of pregnancy may decrease.[5] An excessive response may also typically introduce the risk of ovarian hyperstimulation syndrome (OHSS), a potentially life-threatening condition.[6] Poor response to ovarian stimulation usually indicates a reduction in follicular response resulting in a reduced number of retrieved oocytes and a lower cumulative pregnancy rate.

It is hence important to anticipate the response to ovarian stimulation and individualise the regimen for each patient.

This chapter deals with different 'markers' which may identify the specific regime of ovarian stimulation for an individual patient. A single 'marker' may not be specific or sensitive enough for prediction of ovarian response. Therefore, identification of more than one marker will have a better predictive value. This chapter highlights the conventional 'markers' in some details with a brief description of additional markers which may help positively the conventional markers for prediction of 'ovarian reserve'.

Conventional Markers

The following are the conventional markers which have been used to predict ovarian reserve:

a. Age

b. Basal FSH

c. Basal oestradiol

d. Basal inhibin level

e. Basal antral follicle count (AFC)

f. Measurement of mean ovarian volume

g. Clomiphene citrate challenge test (CCCT), exogenous FSH ovarian reserve test (EFORT), and GnRH-agonist stimulation test (GAST) are dynamic methods that have been used in the past to assess ovarian reserve.[7]

Additional Markers

a. Anti-müllerian hormone: Anti-müllerian hormone is currently believed to be the most informative serum marker and should be considered as an important predictor of ovarian reserve. It is more informative than basal FSH and can be assessed at any point in the cycle as its estimation does not depend on feedback mechanism of hypothalamic-pituitary-ovarian axis.

b. Basal plasma androgen measurement.

c. Insulin resistance (IR) assessment.

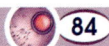

The efficacy of these tests are detailed in the following paragraphs:

AGE

Secondary to the physiological decline in the ovarian follicle pool with ageing, the ovarian response to FSH decreases with advancing age.[8] Though chronologic and reproductive ageing progress in parallel, the rate of decline varies in different individuals. In some women quantitative and qualitative declines are dissimilar, and therefore, fertility potential does not always depend on the available number of eggs in elderly women. The prevalence of poor ovarian response usually increases with age, and in women over 40 years of age it is > 50%.[9]

BASAL FSH MEASUREMENT

An elevated day 3 FSH level ranging from ≥ 7 mIU/ml to ≥ 15 mIU/ml has been proposed as an additional criterion[10–13] along with advanced patient age ≥ 40 years[13] for prediction of poor ovarian reserve. Single measurement in one cycle may not be assuring specially in borderline cases. Single measurement may not be confirmative, but will be predictive of follicular sensitivity to gonadotropin stimulation (Fig. 10.1). At least two estimations in consecutive cycles are essential. Basal FSH measurement (D1/D2/D3) will be more diagnostic when combined with either antral follicle count (AFC) or with AMH.

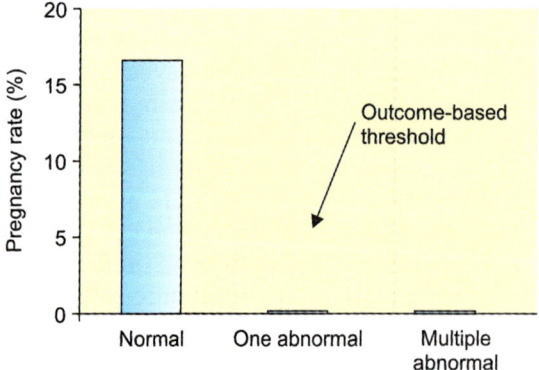

Fig. 10.1: FSH as a predictor of poor ovarian reserve

BASELINE E2 LEVEL

High baseline E2 with normal FSH is not predictive of correct ovarian reserve. Because high baseline E2 may mask abnormal FSH level in patient with occult diminishing ovarian reserve. In general, basal oestradiol level compared to basal FSH level is not a dependable predictor of diminishing ovarian reserve.

INHIBIN-B

Inhibin-B is a granulosa cell product from antral follicles which directly suppress pituitary FSH. Therefore, decline of inhibin level is the first sign of failing ovarian function and hence it should be a valid marker for declining ovarian reserve. Unfortunately, in few women decline of basal inhibin is not always parallel to rise of basal FSH. This is because basal FSH is also partly dependant on basal E2 level. Hence inhibin-B is also not a totally dependable marker. It reflects the ovarian function in assisted reproduction, but is less reliable in prediction of outcome.[14]

OVARIAN VOLUME

Following the rapid increase in the use of transvaginal sonography, the measurement of ovarian volume has become quick, accurate and cost-effective. Ovarian volume measurement has become a potentially useful tool in the screening, diagnosis and monitoring of the treatment of conditions such as polycystic ovarian syndrome and ovarian carcinoma, and in the prediction of superovulation during IVF.[15] Ovarian volume is not dependent on age. An ovarian volume of < 3 ml is predictive of a poor response to ovulation induction by HMG for IVF, very suggestive of reduced ovarian reserve.[16]

CLOMIPHENE CITRATE CHALLENGE TEST (CCCT)

A few women with incipient ovarian failure may have a 'normal' screening basal FSH level (false negative test result). They may be exposed by repeat screening for basal FSH in consecutive cycles or by CCCT. CCCT

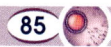

values are independent of patient's age. CCCT values consist of:

- Estimation of baseline FSH (D1/D2/D3)
- Administration of clomiphene citrate (50 mg twice daily from D3 to D7)
- Estimation of FSH (D10): Interpretation and conclusion: Higher level of D10 FSH compared to baseline FSH suggests a poor ovarian reserve. This is because of absence of rise of oestradiol, and therefore, absence of negative feedback on FSH secretion. On the other hand, if D10 FSH is less than or equal to baseline FSH, the conclusion will be in favour of adequate ovarian reserve.

BASAL ANTRAL FOLLICLE COUNT (AFC)

The AFC comprises the number of 2–5 or 2–9 mm diameter follicles measured in the ovaries at the start of the menstrual cycle[17] and is highly correlated to the number of oocytes retrieved at pick up.[18, 19]

To do these tests it is essential to use software application, namely the 'inversion mode' to 3D ultrasonography machine which may enhance the specificity of counting the entire number of antral follicles within the ovaries.[20] Apart from count and volume, assessment of ovarian vascularity is of additional predictive value.

The predictive criteria are—6 to 10 follicles (2–9 mm in diameter); they may be considered as normal responders. More than 20 such follicles in each ovary indicate risk of OHSS. Around 10 follicles in each ovary is an evidence of borderline PCOS, whereas less than 6 follicles indicate poor response.

Diagnosis of borderline number of antral follicles is difficult with conventional ultrasound machine and 3D machine is more reliable than 2D.

ANTI-MÜLLERIAN HORMONE (AMH)

AMH has been implicated as the most valuable marker of ovarian reserve as serum concentrations correlate highly with baseline AFC and the number of oocytes retrieved at aspiration.[21–26]

Predictive Value of AMH

Like inhibin-B, AMH is also synthesised and released by the granulosa cells of the ovary. Unlike other biomarkers like FSH and inhibin-B, estimation of anti-müllerian hormone can be performed on any day of menstrual cycle. Predictive value of AMH for poor or hyperresponse is parallel or even better than procedures like FSH, E2 or inhibin-B. This may be because level of serum FSH, E2 and inhibin-B depends on individual 'feedback' mechanism, whereas production of AMH does not depend on 'feedback' mechanism.

AMH performs two broad functions in folliculogenesis and ovulation—(a) preservation of follicle (follicular reserve) and (b) monofollicular ovulation. These functions are due to (i) in the first phase of migration, AMH controls recruitment of too many follicles from 'resting' pool to 'active' pool to prevent unnecessary apoptosis and (ii) in second phase, AMH decreases responsiveness of gonadotropin-sensitive follicles to FSH—preventing multifollicular dominance and helping monofollicular ovulation from that follicle in which gonadotropin sensitivity is maximum (Figs 10.2 and 10.3).

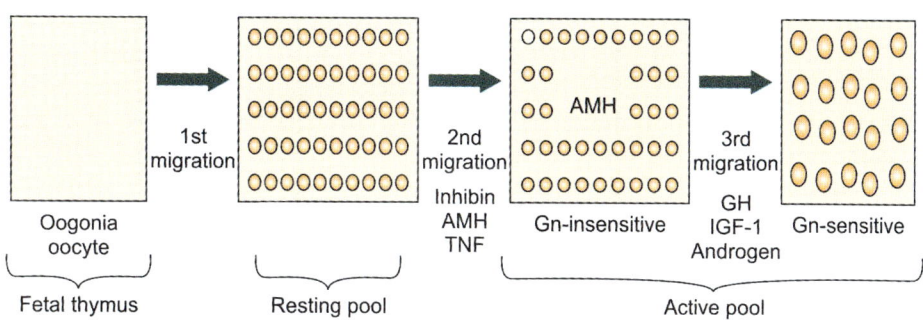

Fig. 10.2: Phases of follicular migration

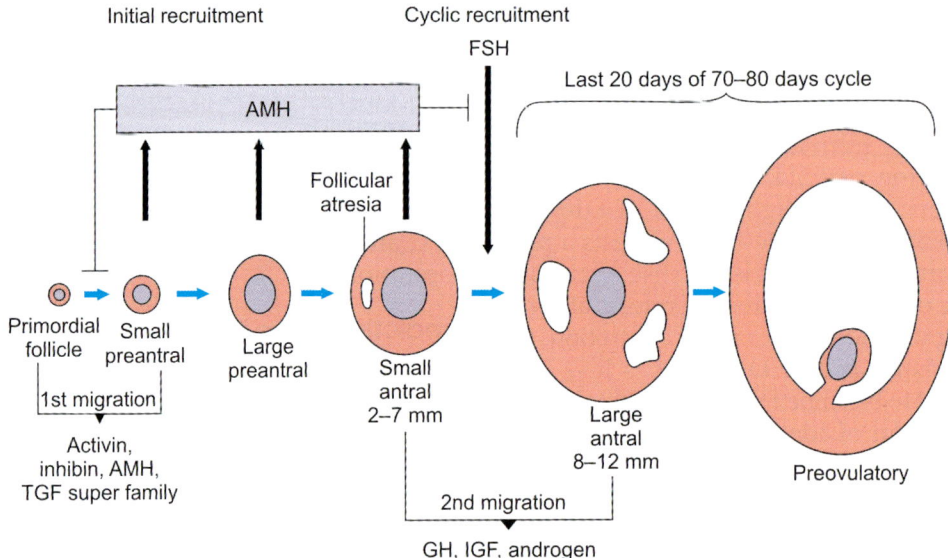

Fig. 10.3: AMH in follicular preservation and monofollicular ovulation

Cut-off Value of AMH

There is a wide variation between lower and upper range of AMH (0.19 to 9.13 ng/ml). Accepted cut-off value is < 0.2 ng/ml—range of poor responder. Value > 4 ng/ml is the range of hyper-responders, usually found in PCOS women.

COMPARATIVE EVALUATION OF SPECIFICITY AND SENSITIVITY OF AMH VS AFC

AMH has a higher predictive value for 'qualitative' assessment of good or bad oocytes, whereas AFC offers better 'quantitative' prognostication (number of oocytes) of ovarian reserve.

AMH is a cycle independent test,[27–30] so any measurement in the period before starting the ART cycle will be at the disposition of the clinician, making the test an ideal tool.

For the AFC, standardisation needs to be dealt with by the physician[31], implying choices on ultrasound equipment, dedicated personnel and a systematic visualisation and counting process. As the intra- and intercycle stabilities for the AFC may be comparable to that for AMH[32], the unlimited availability of this test makes it the preferable one for the short-term.

BLOOD PLASMA ANDROGEN MEASUREMENT

This test has been currently recommended specially in PCOS women. Androgen production is closely linked to ovarian response to gonadotropin stimulation.

A recent study attempted to establish a correlation between AFC with baseline and stimulated serum androgen levels (testosterone, androstenedione, 17-OHP and DHEA).

Stimulation was given by 0.1 mg Decapeptyl on d2, d3 (like GnRH agonist stimulation Test, GAST). This was preceded and followed (24 hours after injection) by blood sampling for 4 different types of androgens mentioned earlier. Levels of different serum androgens, both pre- and post-GnRH injection were correlated with the number of antral follicles categorised into 3 groups, namely category 1—less than 10 follicles, category 2—10 to 20 follicles and category 3—more than 20 follicles.

Significant correlation was observed between pre- and poststimulated 17-OHP only and number of follicles observed. Similar correlation was not observed with any of the other types of androgens (testosterone, ADD and DHEA).

Poststimulated compared to prestimulated 'low 17 OHP' in the presence of large number of antral follicles indicate deficiency

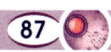

of endogenous LH because 17-OHP production is regulated through LH which stimulates theca cells to produce androgens. Hence these patients are marked as 'poor responders'. Perhaps they benefit by addition of LH in the stimulation protocol.

On the other hand, when poststimulated 17-OHP is very high, possibility of high LH may be presumed. This may add to the risk of OHSS. In these situations, stimulation protocol requires careful adjustment and vigilant monitoring.[33]

Screening for Insulin Resistance (IR)

About 50 to 80% of PCOS women have insulin resistance. The clinical and biochemical markers of insulin resistance are briefly described as follows:

Clinical Evaluation of an Insulin-resistant Patient

A. Endocrine parameters

There are three specific endocrine features which are typical of hyperinsulinemic PCOS women. These are:

- Increased levels of testosterone
- Low sex hormone binding globulin
- Impaired LH/FSH ratio is found in non-insulin resistant PCOS women; but a normal ratio has been observed in the insulin resistant group. Several other studies have also stressed that high BMI and insulin resistance are not associated with an increase in LH levels or LH/FSH ratio.

B. Confirmation of diagnosis of insulin resistance (IR)

- Ratio between fasting insulin and fasting glucose
- Insulin challenge test
- Approaches for assessing insulin sensitivity and resistance *in vivo*.

a. Fasting insulin and fasting glucose ratio

If the ratio is more than 4.5, then the individual is insulin-resistant. On the other hand, if it is less than 4.5, the individual is insulin-sensitive. This is the practical definition for insulin resistance.

75 gm of glucose is to be administered to non-diabetic PCOS patients and non-diabetic control. Mean glucose and insulin are estimated at time zero and every hour for 2 hours following glucose administration. Fasting insulin levels in response to glucose administration are found to be significantly higher in one group of PCOS patients than in the other healthy, normally ovulating female subjects, thus defining two distinct groups: insulin resistance (IR) and non-IR.

b. Insulin challenge test

Insulin plays a vital role in glucose metabolism and homeostasis and a resistance to it precedes onset of type 2 diabetes by a few years—may be decades. Hence, role of insulin is generally considered as an important factor in the pathogenesis of the disease. Insulin challenge test helps to evaluate the glucose response to insulin. Usually the subjects are assessed in the first week of their menstrual cycle. After a baseline sample has been drawn, insulin is injected IV in a bolus dose of 0.1 unit/kg body weight. Blood samples are obtained at 2, 6, 10, 12 and 15 minutes for the assessment and evaluation of fall in glucose in PCOS as well as in non-PCOS subjects (control) (Fig. 10.4).

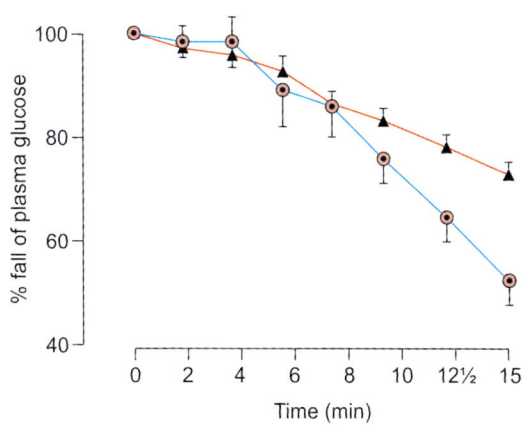

Fig. 10.4: The percentage fall of plasma glucose in PCOS subjects (dark triangles) and non-PCOS controls (open circles), after 0.1 u/kg soluble insulin given IV at 0 min

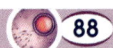
c. Approaches for insulin sensitivity and resistance *in vivo*

The direct evidence of insulin resistance is very difficult to elicit because of the complicated steps and expense. The procedures are more of academic importance and can be used only for research purpose. The procedures are: (a) Hyperinsulinemic euglycemic glucose clamp and (b) homeostatic measurement assessment of insulin resistance (HOMA-IR). However, latter one is more patient friendly and can be used in clinics (Table 10.1).

Impact of Insulin Resistance or Obesity on Ovarian Response

Both IR and obesity have adverse impact either alone or in combination on ovarian response to COS. Both may lead to either explosive or poor ovarian response. Therefore, pre-IVF weight reduction or use of insulin sensitisers either before or along with gonadotropin stimulation are essential for optimal ovarian response.

Accuracy of Prediction of Poor Ovarian Reserve

It has been suggested[34] that through statistical analysis (AUC-ROC) there are three markers

Table 10.1: GIR, glucose infusion rate; M-glucose disposal rate; IST, insulin suppression test; SI, insulin sensitivity index; HOMA-IR, homeostasis model assessment of insulin resistance

Method	Measurement of insulin sensitivity
Hyperinsulinemic euglycemic glucose clamp	Steady state GIR = $M \times SI_{Clamp} = M/(G \times \Delta I)$, where M is normalized for G (steady state blood glucose concentration) and ΔI (difference between fasting and steady state plasma insulin concentrations)
HOMA-IR	HOMA-IR = {[fasting insulin (mU/ml)] × fasting glucose (mmol/l)}/22.5

which can be reliably accepted as 'predictors' of response to controlled ovarian stimulation. These markers are—FSH, AMH and AFC (value of AUC being 0.70) (Fig. 10.5).

Conclusion

An ideal marker should have the potential to predict both qualitative as well as quantitative response to ovarian stimulation. From statistical

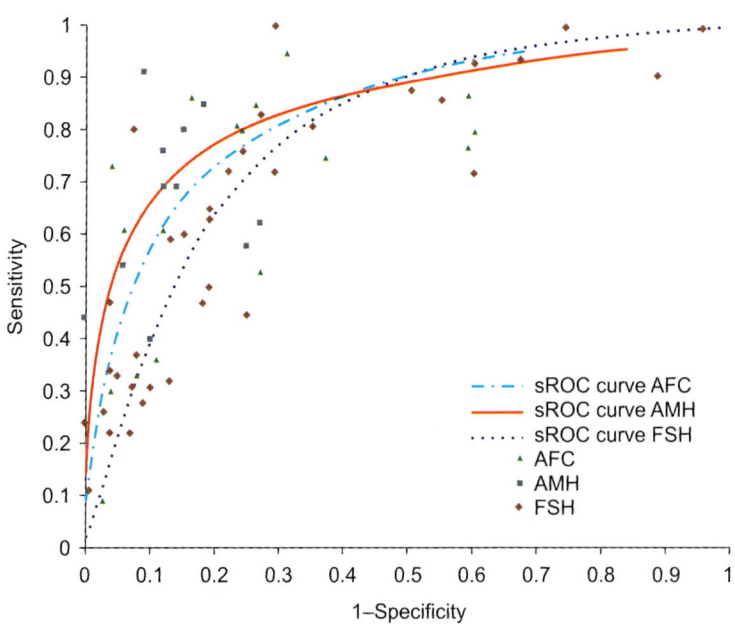

Fig. 10.5: Accuracy of poor response prediction

evaluation, it has now been generally accepted that three markers FSH and AMH and AFC either alone or in combination can reliably predict the response to controlled ovarian stimulation.

REFERENCES

1. Macklon NS, Stouffer RL, Giuduce LC, Fauser BC. The science behind 25 years of ovarian stimulation for in vitro fertilisation. Endocr Rev 2006; 27: 170–207.

2. Baart EB, Martini E, Eijkemans MJ, Van OD, Beckers NG, Verhoeff A, Macklon NS, Fauser BC. Milder ovarian stimulation for *in vitro* fertilisation reduces aneuploidy in the human preimplantation embryo: A randomized controlled trial. Hum Reprod 2007; 22: 980–988.

3. Heijnen EM, Eijkemans MJ, de Klerk C, Polinder S, Beckers NG, Klinkert ER, Broekmans FJ, Passchier J, Te Velde ER, Macklon NS, Fauser BC. A mild treatment strategy for *in vitro* fertilisation: A randomised non-inferiority trial. Lancet 2007; 369: 743–749.

4. Verberg MF, Macklon NS, Nargund G, Frydman R, Devroey P, Broekmans FJ, Fauser BC. Mild ovarian stimulation for IVF. Hum Reprod Update 2009; 15: 13–29.

5. Van der Gaast MH, Eijkemans MJ, van der Net JB, de Boer EJ, Burger CW, van Leeuwen FE, Fauser BC, Macklon NS. Optimum number of oocytes for a successful first IVF treatment cycle. Reprod Biomed Online 2006; 13: 476–480.

6. Fauser BC, Diedrich K, Devroey P. Predictors of ovarian response: Progress towards individualized treatment in ovulation induction and ovarian stimulation. Hum Reprod Update 2008; 14: 1–14.

7. Erdhem M, Erdhem E, Gursoy R, Biberoglu K. Comparison of basal and clomiphene citrate induced FSH and inhibin B, ovarian volume and antral follicle counts as ovarian reserve tests and predictors of poor ovarian response in IVF. J Assist Reprod Genet 2004; 21: 37–45.

8. Goverde AJ, McDonnell J, Schats R, Vermeiden JP, Homburg R, Lambalk CB. Ovarian response to standard gonadotrophin stimulation for IVF is decreased not only in older but also in younger women in couples with idiopathic and male subfertility. Hum Reprod 2005; 20: 1573–1577.

9. A.P. Ferraretti, A. La Marca, B.C.J.M. Fauser, B. Tarlatzis, G. Nargund, and L. Gianaroli. ESHRE consensus on the definition of 'poor response' to ovarian stimulation for in vitro fertilisation. Human Reproduction, Vol.26, No. 7; 1616–1624, 2011.

10. Droesch K, Muasher SJ, Brzyski RG, Jones GS, Simonetti S, Liu HC, Rosenwaks Z. Value of suppression with a gonadotropin releasing hormone agonist prior to gonadotropin stimulation for *in vitro* fertilisation. Fertil Steril 1989; 51: 292–297.

11. Feldberg D, Farhi J, Ashkenazi J, Dicker D, Shalev J, Ben-Rafael Z. Minidose gonadotropin releasing hormone agonist is the treatment of choice in poor responders with high FSH levels. Fertil Steril 1994; 62: 343–346.

12. Faber BM, Mayer J, Cox B, Jones D, Toner JP, Oehninger S, Muasher SJ. Cessation of gonadotropin-releasing hormone agonist therapy combined with high-dose gonadotropin stimulation yields favorable pregnancy results in low responders. Fertil Steril 1998; 69: 826–830.

13. Karande V, Gleicher N. A rational approach to the management of low responders in IVF. Hum Reprod 1999; 14: 1744–1749.

14. Hall JE, Welt CK, Cramer DW. Inhibin A and inhibin B reflect ovarian function in assisted reproduction but are less useful at predicting outcome. Hum Reprod 1999; 14: 409–415.

15. Lass A and Brinsden P. The role of ovarian volume in reproductive medicine. Hum Reprod Update 1999; 5,256 ± 266.

16. Lass A, Skull J, McVeigh E, Margara R and Winston RML (1997b). Measurement of ovarian volume by transvaginal sonography before ovulation induction with human menopausal gonadotrophin for *in vitro* fertilisation can predict poor response. Hum Reprod 12,294 ± 297.

17. de Carvalho BR, Rosa e Silva AC, Rosa E Silva JC, dos Reis RM, Ferriani RA, Silva de Sa MF. Ovarian reserve evaluation: State of the art. J Assist Reprod Genet 2008; 25: 311–322.

18. Kwee J, Schats R, McDonnell J, Themmen A, de Jong F, Lambalk C. Evaluation of anti-müllerian hormone as a test for the prediction of ovarian reserve. Fertil Steril 2008; 90: 737–743.

19. Broer SL, Mol BW, Hendriks D, Broekmans FJ. The role of anti-mullerian hormone in prdiction of outcome after IVF: Comparison with the antral follicle count. Fertil Steril 2009; 91: 705–714.

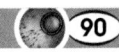

20. A. Nazzaro, A. Salerno, M. Rubino, N. I. Leccia, P. Fusco; Embryo implantation rate is related to endometrial and subendometrial vascularization measured by 3D ultrasound and power Doppler angiography; Ultrasound in Obstetrics and Gynecology; Volume 32, Issue 3; 266–267, August 2008.

21. van Rooij IA, Broekmans FJ, te Velde ER, Fauser BC, Bancsi LF, Jong FH, Themmen AP. Serum anti-müllerian hormone levels: A novel measure of ovarian reserve. Hum Reprod 2002; 17: 3065–3071.

22. Eldar-Geva T, Ben Chetrit A, Spitz IM, Rabinowitz R, Markowitz E, Mimoni T, Gal M, Zylber-Haran E, Margalioth EJ. Dynamic assays of inhibin B, anti-müllerian hormone and estradiol following FSH stimulation and ovarian ultrasonography as predictors of IVF outcome. Hum Reprod 2005; 20: 3178–3183.

23. Tremellen KP, Kolo M, Gilmore A, Lekamge DN. Anti-mullerian hormone as a marker of ovarian reserve. Aust N Z J Obstet Gynaecol 2005; 45: 20–24.

24. Nakhuda GS, Chu MC, Wang JG, Sauer MV, Lobo RA. Elevated serum mullerian-inhibiting substance may be a marker for ovarian hyper-stimulation syndrome in normal women undergoing in vitro fertilisation. Fertil Steril 2006; 85: 1541–1543.

25. Nakhuda GS, Sauer MV, Wang JG, Ferin M, Lobo RA. Mullerian inhibiting substance is an accurate marker of ovarian response in women of advanced reproductive age undergoing IVF. Reprod Biomed Online 2007; 14: 450–454.

26. Riggs RM, Duran EH, Baker MW, Kimble TD, Hobeika E, Yin L, Matos-Bodden L, Leader B, Stadtmauer L. Assessment of ovarian reserve with anti-müllerian hormone: A comparison of the predictive value of anti-müllerian hormone, follicle-stimulating hormone, inhibin B, and age. Am J Obstet Gynecol 2008; 199: 202–208.

27. Cook CL, Siow Y, Taylor S, Fallat ME. Serum müllerian-inhibiting substance levels during normal menstrual cycles. Fertil Steril 2000; 73:859–861.

28. Hehenkamp WJ, Looman CW, Themmen AP, de Jong FH, te Velde ER, Broekmans FJ. Anti-müllerian hormone levels in the spontaneous menstrual cycle do not show substantial fluctuation. J Clin Endocrinol Metab 2006; 91: 4057–4063.

29. La Marca A, Stabile G, Artenisio AC, Volpe A. Serum anti-müllerian hormone throughout the human menstrual cycle. Hum Reprod 2006; 21: 3103–3107.

30. Tsepelidis S, Devreker F, Demeestere I, Flahaut A, Gervy C, Englert Y. Stable serum levels of anti-müllerian hormone during the menstrual cycle: A prospective study in normo-ovulatory women. Hum Reprod 2007; 22: 1837–1840.

31. Broekmans FJ, de ZD, Howles CM, Gougeon A, Trew G, Olivennes F. The antral follicle count: Practical recommendations for better standardization. Fertil Steril 2009. Epub ahead of print July 7.

32. van Disseldorp J, Lambalk CB, Kwee J, Looman CW, Eijkemans MJ, Fauser BC, Broekmans FJ. Comparison of inter- and intra-cycle variability of anti-müllerian hormone and antral follicle counts. Hum Reprod 2010; 25:221–227.

33. Cedrin I. Durnerin, K. Erb, R. Fleming, H. Hillier, S.G. Hillier, C.M. Howles, J. N. Hugues, A. Lass, H. Lyall, P. Rasmussen, J. Thong, I. Traynor, L. Westergaard and R. Yates. Effects of recombinant LH treatment on folliculogenesis and responsiveness to FSH stimulation. Hum Reprod 2008; 23–2; 421–426.

34. Broekmans FJ, Kwee J, Hendriks DJ, Mol BW, Lambalk CB. A systematic review of tests predicting ovarian reserve and IVF outcome. Hum Reprod Update 2006; 12:685–718.

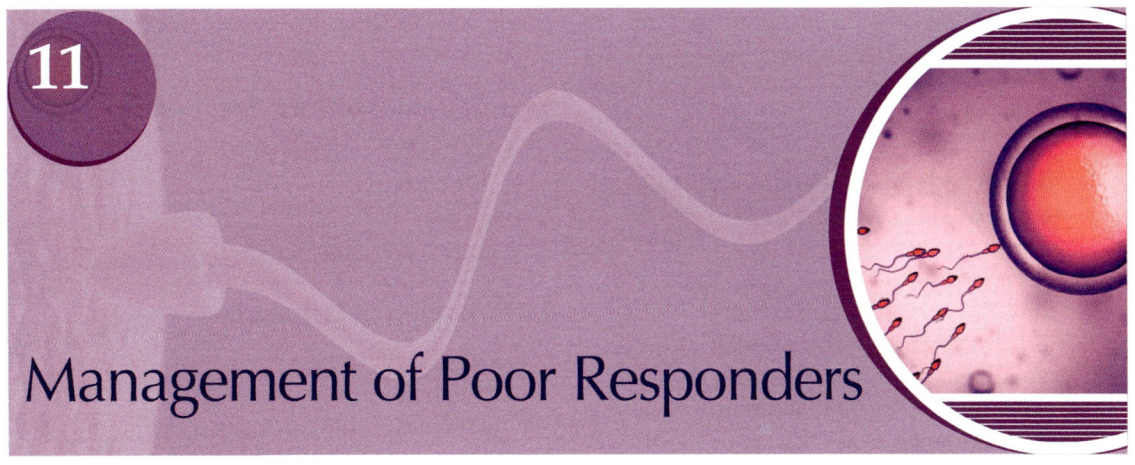

11

Management of Poor Responders

INTRODUCTION

The genesis and predictive markers of poor ovarian reserve have already been outlined. Age is one of the very important factors which is responsible for poor follicular response in controlled ovarian stimulation. This may be due to age related follicular apoptosis and increase in gynaecological disorders. Increase in ovulatory disorders is also a contributory factor which may have its adverse impact on hypothalamic pituitary ovarian axis. A compromised uterine vascular supply is an additional cause of reduced chance of implantation.

Spontaneous pregnancy and viable delivery after the age of 45 years is 0.2% of total deliveries. 80% of them are grand multipara.[1] IVF may, however, improve the chances of conception in these women. Deliveries have been reported, after the age of 45 years, if more than 5 oocytes were retrieved in the treatment cycle. However, even in younger women ovarian response to conventional stimulation protocol is often unsatisfactory.

Definition of Poor Responders

There is lack of uniformity in the definition of 'poor ovarian response'. Various definitions include: (i) Peak E2 levels between less than 300 pg/ml and less than 500 pg/ml; (ii) low number of dominant/codominant follicles and/or number of eggs retrieved from less than 3 to less than 6 dominant follicles observed on hCG day or less than 3 to less than 5 eggs retrieved after OPU; (iii) D3 FSH less than 12 mIU/ml and (iv) female partner age > 40 years, and many others.

However, European Society for Human Reproduction and Embryology (ESHRE), a working group on poor ovarian reserve (POR), met at Bologna, Italy, and has formulated a consensus definition of POR as follows:

At least two of the three following features should be present:

   i. Advanced maternal age or any other risk factor(s) of POR

  ii. History of previous POR with retrieval of less than 3 eggs following a conventional stimulation protocol

 iii. An abnormal ovarian reserve test, e.g. antral follicle count—less than 6; or anti-müllerian hormone—0.5 to 1.1 ng/ml.

In addition, following points require special consideration while defining a patient with 'poor ovarian reserve'.

  a. Two episodes of POR after conventional ovarian stimulation are sufficient to define a patient as having POR, even in young women with normal 'ovarian reserve'.

  b. By definition, the term POR means 'poor ovarian response', and therefore, one stimulated cycle is essential to confirm that the ovarian response is 'poor'. But

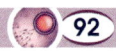

patients over 40 years of age and an 'abnormal ovarian reserve' test in young women, may be classified as poor responders. Both these factors predict reduced ovarian reserve and can be considered as surrogate of 'ovarian stimulation cycle'. However, these women should be precisely defined as expected PORs.

c. 'Risk factors' as mentioned in 'Bologna definition' indicate maternal age more than 40 years and in addition, include all the known genetic and acquired conditions which are associated with reduced number of resting follicles.

d. POR is considered when a cycle is cancelled because of less than 3 dominant follicles or in previous cycle less than 3 eggs were collected following a stimulation protocol using at least 150 units of gonadotropin. However, collection of less than 4 eggs with 'soft' stimulation protocol is not to be considered as poor response.

e. Each criterion (risk factor in previous cycle and ovarian reserve test) individually is not used for defining POR. At least two criteria should be present before the term POR is used.

Management

Management of poor ovarian responders is difficult. At the moment, no uniform effective agent has been established.[2] In fact a positive impact of different protocols reviewed in literature for the treatment of 'poor ovarian responders' is negligible. Still before referring them to 'egg donation' programme, which may be unacceptable and unaffordable to many patients, it is worthwhile attempting therapeutic options which are less interventional and may be of benefit at least to some of the poorly responding women.

Principles of Therapeutic Approaches

a. Modification of the existing protocol
b. Pharmacological manipulation of endocrine profile in both follicular and luteal phases of the treatment cycle with innovative protocols

c. Oocyte donation
d. Surrogacy.

Management of Poor Responders

a. Cycle cancellation
b. Low pregnancy rate
c. Cost.

Poor response may be ovarian or endometrial.

Modification of Existing Protocols

Modification involves:

a. Modification of starting dose of gonadotropin
b. Modification of long agonist downregulation
c. Modification of short agonist downregulation
d. Modification of antagonist protocol

Starting dose of gonadotropin: Three modifications have been attempted:

i. Persistently high dose: This schedule has been introduced with the idea that perhaps follicles may be more susceptible at a higher than conventional dose. The dose of gonadotropin between 300 and 450 IU has been tried. However, the dose beyond 450 IU is not very effective. Hence the recommended highest dose of gonadotropin for poor responders has been suggested to be between 300 and 450 IU.[3]

ii. Initially low, but subsequently high (step up): Initial recommended dose is 225–300 IU with maximum increment up to 450 IU. This schedule has been recommended in many studies, but does not work well because follicles are recruited in early and not in late follicular phase. Dominant and codominant follicles are already selected by D5 and not beyond that. Hence late increment of gonadotropin does not help in recruitment of more number of codominant follicles.[4]

iii. Initially high and then low (step down): This is preferable and more effective with short flare protocol because the gonadotropin is not downregulated and the follicular receptors have been sensitised

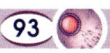

by endogenous gonadotropin. This helps in recruitment of a large number of codominant follicles. And the response persists to even lower doses of gonadotropin after D5 or D6.[5]

Modification of the Long GnRH Agonist Protocol

Brief Outline of Conventional 'Long' GnRH Agonist Protocol

GnRH agonist (Leuprolide, Buserelin, Triptorelin, etc.) in a dose of 400–500 µg is started on D21 (mid-luteal phase of preceding menstrual cycle) and is continued for 15 days thereafter or till D1 or D2 of the next menstrual cycle, whichever is earlier. On this day, LH, E2 and progesterone are estimated for confirmation of downregulation. If the values of estimation are satisfactory (i.e. downregulation confirmed), then dose of GnRH analogue is reduced to 200 µg daily and stimulation with gonadotropin (rFSH or HMG) in appropriate dose is started.

However, sometimes GnRH in conventional 'long downregulation' protocol may 'oversuppress' ovarian response to exogenous gonadotropin even in normofollicular women in following ways:

i. Altered biologic effect of endogenous gonadotropin
ii. Direct effect on gonadotropin receptors (oversuppression—hypersensitive receptors for GnRH) on the ovarian follicle

These factors can cause oversuppression of FSH receptors on the developing follicles, and therefore, there may be interference with follicular recruitment during ovarian stimulation.

To avoid these undesirable responses, two modified protocols of downregulation have been suggested:
a. Mini-dose downregulation
b. Stop protocol downregulation.

Mini-dose Long GnRH-a Downregulation

It is known that to suppress gonadotropin effect on ovarian follicle, a minimum dose of 15 µg of triptorelin is essential. In IVF triptorelin is used at a dosage of 100 µgm which is enough. Hence in poorly responding patients to minimize oversuppression of the ovary, a 'mini-dose' GnRH-a protocol is recommended. The actual protocol consists of—(a) 200 µg GnRH-a (Leuprolide acetate) instead of 500 µg from D21 of the previous menstrual cycle and (b) in addition, progesterone is sometimes added from D21 till the start of stimulation of gonadotropin to inhibit production of endogenous FSH. Endogenous FSH secretion during the phase of initial flare up of downregulation may have two adverse effects on stimulation—(i) recruitment of asynchronously maturing follicles (this is common in poor responders) and (ii) cyst formation during the early phase of stimulation. Progesterone in the luteal phase may avoid these two undesired effects of GnRH-a adverse problems.[6] After downregulation has been achieved, dose of GnRH-a is further reduced to 100 µgm/day (Fig. 11.1).

Stop Protocol Long GnRH-a Downregulation

In this protocol, GnRH analogue downregulation is started on D21 and continued till downregulation has been achieved. The

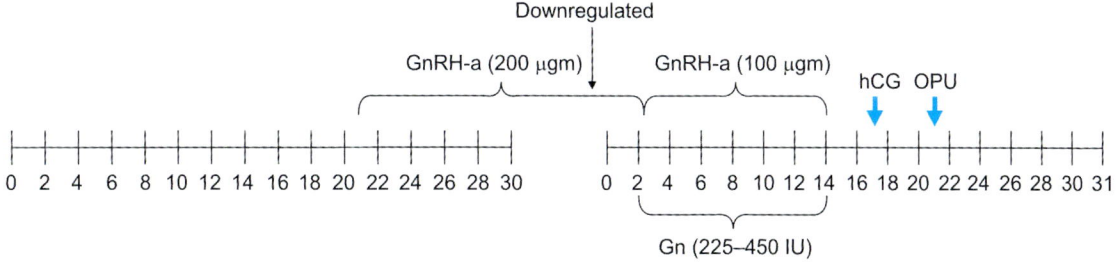

Fig. 11.1: Protocol-I (reducing chances of 'over' downregulation with GnRH)

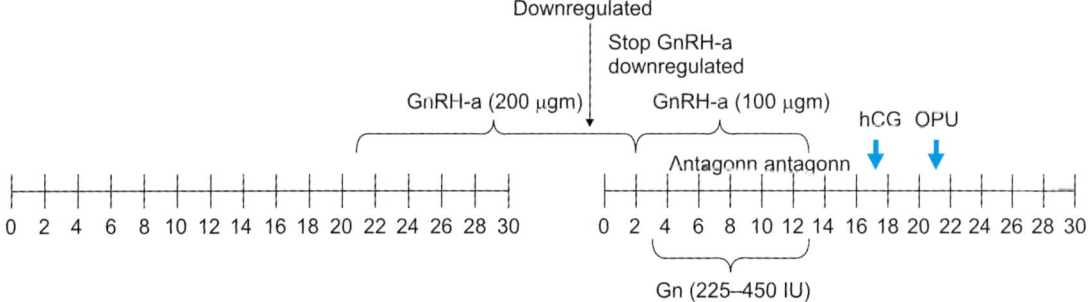

Fig. 11.2: Protocol-II (no GnRH after downregulation, antagonist SOS)

starting dose of GnRH-a is usually reduced as in the previous protocol. Once stimulation is started, no further analogue is continued. However, in the later phase of the stimulation after the dominant follicle(s) achieves a diameter of 14 mm, sometimes GnRH antagonist may have to be added for 2 or 3 days to prevent premature LH surge. This protocol produces better result than the previous one.[7,8]

Modification of 'Short Flare'

Brief Outline of Conventional 'Short Flare' Protocol

The protocol consists of suppression of both FSH and LH with the use of GnRH agonist starting from early follicular phase (D1/D2). Immediately thereafter from D3 or D4 gonadotropin stimulation is started. The advantage of initiation of analogue before gonadotropin is due to 'upregulation' effect of analogue, there is 'flare' of endogenous FSH in early follicular phase. This early flare augments the action of exogenous gonadotropin on the follicles which are already sensitised by endogenous gonadotropin. Therefore,

exogenous gonadotropin effect may be more pronounced than in long protocol. However, flare effect continues up to D5 only and thereafter, the receptors of LH is down-regulated. Hence patients are protected from premature LH surge up to the end of the stimulation phase.

But there are disadvantages as well. Flare involves elevation of LH level also. Elevated LH in early follicular phase stimulates production of thecal androgen and progesterone. The result is that oocytes grow in androgen-rich environment. This leads to poor quality oocytes which is responsible for deficient fertilisation and poor pregnancy rate. Conventionally used "short flare' protocol is represented in Fig. 11.3.

Modification of Flare Protocol to Avoid the Disadvantage

The problems of disadvantage of 'LH-flare' in early follicular phase can be solved in two ways (suitable for poor responders)—(a) pre treatment with OC pills or with progesterone used in the luteal phase and (b) reduction of

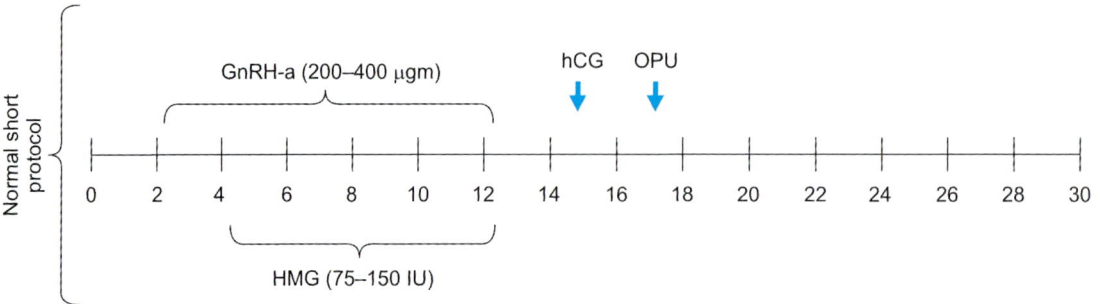

Fig. 11.3: Short flare protocol (conventionally used protocol)

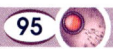

dose of GnRH agonist in flare protocol and microdose flare protocol.

a. OC pill or luteal progesterone prior to flare protocol: The advantages are: (a) Elevated progesterone and oestrogen specially in the luteal phase can effectively suppress gonadotropin (LH) in next early follicular phase (avoiding adverse impact of high LH, and therefore, progesterone and androgen), and (b) sensitisation of oestrogen receptors at the follicular and endometrial level, thereby increasing sensitivity of follicle to FSH and offering a better chance for development of good endometrial receptivity. This positive effect is brought about by oestrogen in OC pill. Though theoretically sound, effectivity of this protocol is yet to be proved by case control study.[9, 10]

b. Microdose (low dose) flare protocol: This is a similar approach to the mini-dose protocol of long downregulation. The protocol consists of 100–200 µg of leuprolide with gonadotropin from D2. This regime of downregulation may theoretically prevent premature LH surge, but reported studies did not reveal specific advantages over long protocol using mini-dose GnRH analogue (Fig. 11.4).[11]

GnRH ANTAGONIST PROTOCOL

General Considerations

Mechanism of Action

The drug competitively blocks GnRH receptors in the pituitary gland, thereby causing immediate dose-related suppression of gonadotropin release. Within 6 hours gonadotropin levels, particularly LH, is significantly reduced.

Advantages Over Agonist Protocol

Antagonist is generally administered later in the follicular phase; thereby it avoids suppression of endogenous FSH during the phase of early follicular recruitment (unlike long protocol). Follicles, therefore, get the benefit of exposure to endogenous FSH before pituitary is suppressed by downregulation. Another advantage of antagonist is that there is no flare up of gonadotropin in the early follicular phase leading to cyst formation, as sometimes found in association with short agonist (flare) protocol. In addition, there is less risk of ovarian hyperstimulation following antagonist downregulation. The treatment period is also relatively shorter and unlike long protocol posttreatment menopausal side effect is reduced.

Antagonist and Poor Responders

Literature survey through retrospective and prospective studies reveals that there is no significant difference in pregnancy and cancellation rate when results were compared between:

a. Antagonist *vs* long protocol
b. Antagonist *vs* short protocol
c. Antagonist *vs* microflare protocol
d. OC pill/progesterone pretreatment (D18 to D25 *vs* no OC pill pretreatment in antagonist protocol)

However, with alternative approaches, GnRH antagonist has proved itself to be an useful drug specifically for poor responders. The situations in which GnRH antagonist may be useful in poor responders are:

a. Restricting use of GnRH antagonist where baseline FSH is less than 8 mIU/ml

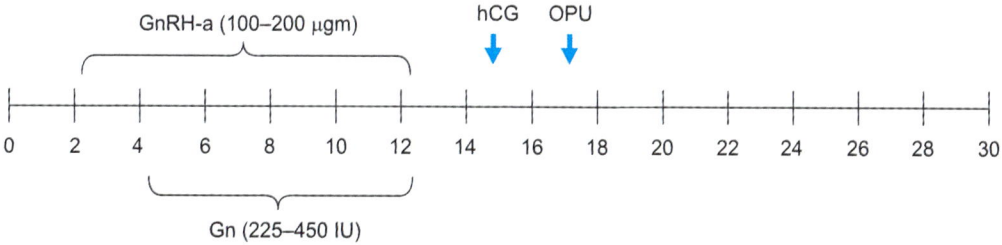

Fig. 11.4: Microdose GnRH-a (flare) protocol

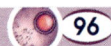
b. In most of the poor responders, follicular phase is short; antagonist has been used to make follicular phase longer.

c. To suppress ill-effect of LH in GnRH flare used for poor responders, GnRH antagonist has been used with improved success rate.

Antagonist protocol suggested to increase the length of follicular phase in poor responders:

In majority of poor responders, the follicular phase is shorter. As a result of short follicular phase, the recruitment of follicles becomes deficient. Antagonist protocol may help to increase the length of follicular phase in two ways:

i. Antagonist Preceding and Following Gonadotropin Stimulation Protocol

The protocol was suggested by Frankfurter, et.al.[12] Patient receives two doses of 3 mg cetrorelix, the first on cycle between D5 and D8 and second 4 days later. Along with cetrorelix, medroxyprogesterone acetate (MPA) is given at a dose of 10 mgm daily till

ovarian suppression is achieved. MPA is then discontinued to allow vaginal bleeding. A combination of recombinant FSH (225 IU SC twice a day) and recombinant hCG (2.5 mg SC 4 times a day) are administered. hCG acts as a surrogate for LH, alternatively rLH (75 IU) can be used. When the mean follicular diameter reaches 14 mm, GnRH antagonist (cetrorelix) is reinitiated till ovulation triggered by hCG. This protocol helped in improved oocyte-embryo yield and an improved implantation and clinical pregnancy rate. The conventional antagonist (flexible protocol) and the modified antagonist protocol approach as described above have been illustrated in the following two diagrams (Figs 11.5 and 11.6).[12]

ii. Combined GnRH Agonist (Flare) with Antagonist Protocol[13]

This simplified approach also helps to increase length of follicular phase. This protocol consists of combination of microdose GnRH flare + GnRH antagonist (flexible dose schedule). The idea is to suppress the elevated LH level

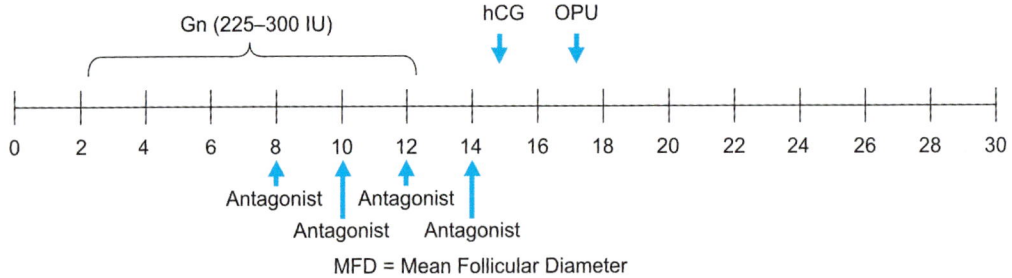

Fig. 11.5: Conventional Gn/antagonist protocol

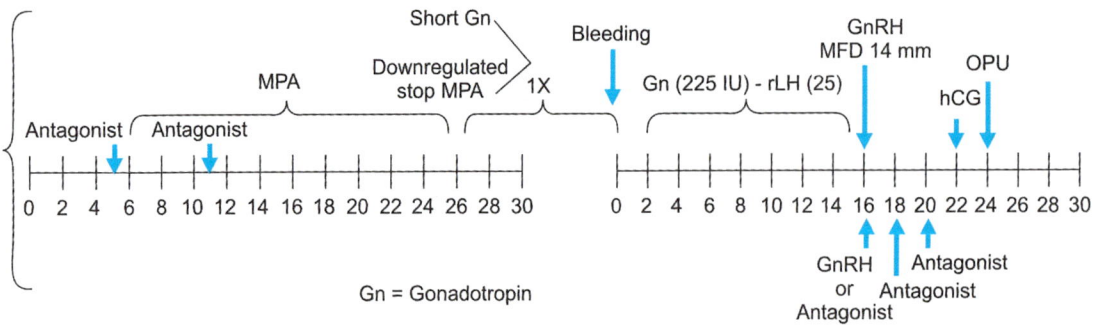

Fig. 11.6: Modified antagonist approach (to increase follicular phase length)

induced by GnRH flare by an antagonist in addition to the beneficial effect of FSH release with GnRH flare. The actual protocol consists of: (a) Administration of buserelin (100 µg SC) from D1 to D3, (b) high dose (225–300 IU) of gonadotropin from D3 till the lead follicle achieves a diameter of 14 mm and (c) GnRH antagonist (0.25mg daily) is initiated till the day of hCG trigger.

The entire protocol is illustrated in Fig. 11.7.

ENDOCRINOLOGICAL MANIPULATION IN FOLLICULAR AND LUTEAL PHASES IN POOR RESPONDERS

There are certain endocrine problems in poor responders which may be intelligently modified by manipulating or supplementing endocrine mechanism in the follicular and luteal phases of the treatment cycle. These manipulations consist of:

a. Calculating the starting dose of gonadotropin for ovarian stimulation
b. LH requirement in the stimulation regime
c. Supplementation of growth hormone (GH) for ovarian stimulation
d. Androgen supplementation
e. Manipulating 'short follicular' into a 'long follicular' phase for recruitment of more codominant follicles (follicular phase is usually shorter in poor responders)
f. To avoid recruitment of asynchronously developing follicles
g. Natural or modified natural cycles often used in poor responders

Patients from (a) to (d)—require follicular phase endocrine manipulation; (e) and (f)—these groups require luteal phase endocrine

adjustment; (g)—requires both follicular and luteal phase endocrine maneuvering.

Calculation of Starting Dose of FSH in Poor Responders

It is known that there may be genetic variations in receptor sensitivity to FSH stimulation. These variations are more common in poor responders and elderly patients. Attempt is being made to calculate starting dose of FSH in poor responders and elderly patients. Calculation may be made by dose calculator using basal FSH, BMI, age and number of follicles < 11 mm on baseline screening.

Requirement of LH in Poor Responders

Of the two gonadotropins synthesised and released by pituitary, FSH is involved in folliculogenesis while LH performs the function of steroidogenesis which is essential for synchronous cytoplasmic and nuclear maturation. The exact quantity of LH essential for such maturation is still controversial. It has now been generally agreed that the minimum requirement of LH is less than 1% follicular LH occupancy. However, low and high levels of LH are equally ineffective. Fluctuating rather than exact level is not desirable. Fluctuating level is commonly found in women with PCOS and poor responders. Serum LH levels by immunoassay do not exactly indicate bioavailability of LH. Optimum serum level of LH for steroidogenesis essential for follicular growth is exactly not known. However, in the early follicular phase, the requisite level should be 1 to 3 mIU/ml. This is the therapeutic window.[14–16] 'Therapeutic window' is essential for optimum steroidogenesis, but more importantly within this 'therapeutic window' there should not be too

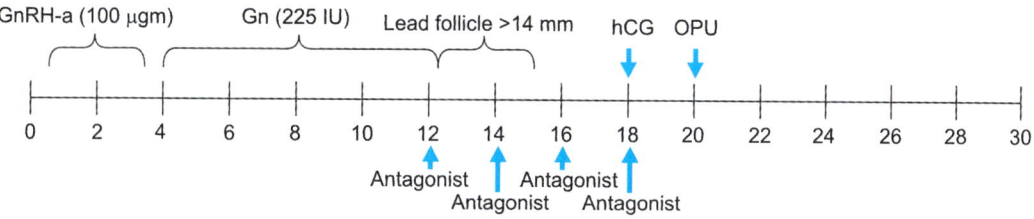

Fig. 11.7: Combined GnRH-a (flare) + GnRH antagonist protocol (to increase follicular phase length)

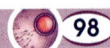

many fluctuations. This is found in women with PCOS and low ovarian reserve.

Preferable LH preparation for poor responders may be either rLH or uHMG. Obviously rLH is preferable because uHMG contains hCG which is surrogate for LH and other undesirable contaminants.

What is 'Ceiling' Level of LH?

Level below which effects of LH is beneficial and above that the effect is detrimental. Cut-off value of ceiling level is 10 miu/ml. The base line (d1, d2, d3) optimum physiological level of LH should be 1–3 miu/ml. Below 1 miu/ml E_2 synthesis is not optimum, and therefore, oocyte maturation and follicular development are not adequate. Above the level of 3 mIU/ml oocyte maturation and follicular development become difficult because of undesirable adverse impact of excess androsterone (ADD) generated by excess LH.

Beneficial Functions of Intrafollicular E2 Induced by LH-mediated Conversion of Thecal Androgen

a. Synchronous nuclear and cytoplasmic maturation of oocytes
b. LH-mediated E2 also helps in increased endometrial receptivity, thereby helping implantation, and hence an increased pregnancy.

When to Start LH in Poor Responders?

a. In hypogonadotropic women, LH should be initiated from the beginning of the stimulation. This is specifically applicable in women with hypogonadotropic hypogonadism. Currently, recombinant combination is available in the name of "Pergoveris" (Serono—rFSH/rLH—2:1 ratio). For cost factor HMG may also be used and the results have been claimed to be equally satisfactory.[17]
b. In poor responders or in elderly women, LH (rLH or HMG) should be initiated in the later phase of stimulation (D5–D6). The theoretical rationality of this approach is based on the fact that LH receptors in the dominant or codominant follicle(s)

appear in the mid-follicular phase induced by FSH in the early follicular phase.

Benefits of LH Supplementation in Poor Responders

In ART treatment protocol, there are 3 groups of patients who respond poorly to the conventional stimulation protocol.

a. Elderly women
b. Over downregulated patients
c. Women with so called "ovarian resistance" have normal basal follicle count and are normogonadotropic. But due to follicular receptor defect (genetic) or due to less availability of bioactive LH in the endrogenously released gonadotropin, the follicles do not respond adequately to the conventional dose of exogenous gonadotropin. They require additional LH stimulation for adequate ovarian response.

Also with advancing age endogenous FSH and LH increase; but testosterone decreases. LH supplementation in these women helps testosterone synthesis from theca cell—more E2.

Moreover, a number of functional LH receptors in the follicle with advancing age decreases. Biologically active endogenously produced LH in poor responders is also less.

These are the reasons for which addition of exogenous LH in the stimulation protocol may help to improve the outcome of IVF treatment, specially in elderly women.

LH supplementation in agonist and antagonist protocol (in poor responders).

Published reports indicate that this is beneficial in agonist protocol, but in antagonist cycles the outcome of LH addition in poor responders is still controversial. Further studies are necessary to come to a conclusion.

Specific groups of patients of poor responders where LH supplementation may help, consist of—(a) elderly patients and (b) normogonadotropic patients, but with ovarian resistance. These groups of patients may have either receptor defect or low level of circulating endogenous bioactive LH.

The time of addition of LH to FSH in hypogonadotropic women is from the start of stimulation, and in normogonadotropic poor responders, from D6 to D7 of stimulation.

ROLE OF ANDROGENS IN POOR RESPONDERS

It is now well-established that androgen has a definite role in women poorly responding to conventional stimulation protocol. This is because androgens help in follicular growth in two ways:

a. Before follicles become sensitive to gonadotropin (small antral stage 0.15–2 mm), androgen induces FSH receptors in follicles.

b. After follicles become sensitive to gonadotropin ($\geq$ 2 mm to large antral stage), androgen enhances FSH action on developing follicles.

Necessity of Androgen Supplementation in Poor Responders

With advancing age, ovarian androgen secretion declines. In impending menopause, FSH rises; so also oestrogens, but ovarian androgens do not increase. Hence aromatised androgen induced E2 diminishes. Therefore, in these women, addition of androgen may increase oestradiol level which in synergy with exogenous FSH, help follicular growth and development.

In addition, in poor ovarian reserve even in young women, boosting with androgen may help both recruitment and growth of follicles.

How to Supplement Androgens?

This can be done in three ways:

a. **In downregulated cycles, rLH 5 to 7 days before starting rFSH stimulation:** Pretreatment with rLH down regulated cycle before rFSH is started. This schedule provides better results than in patients who do not receive rLH pretreatment.[18]

b. **Testosterone and DHT supplementation before gonadotropin stimulation:** In this procedure, transdermal testosterone (20 µg/kg body weight daily) supplementation is provided 5–15 days prior to FSH supplementation.[19]

There is another method of testosterone supplementation in poor responders which is currently very popular. This consists of DHEA (80 mg/day) administered for two months prior to ovarian stimulation.[20] Androgen supplementation augments the effect of gonadotropin stimulation via IGF-1.

c. **Blocking intraovarian conversion of androgen to oestrogen by aromatase inhibitors:** In this procedure, letrozole is administered for 5 days along with gonadotropin at the beginning of the stimulation protocol. It has been observed that in the follicular fluid the level of testosterone and ADD were increased compared to those observed in women who did not receive letrozole in their gonadotropin stimulation protocol.[21]

Growth Hormones in Poor Responders

It is known that IGF and IGF-binding protein (IGFBP) families are actively involved for follicular growth. Growth hormone is directly responsible for stimulating IGF-1 activity. Therefore, growth hormone is suggested to improve follicular growth.[22] But no significant data is available to support the role of growth hormone in improving follicular responsiveness to gonadotropin. However, further studies are essential for defining the dose of growth hormone and finding out the select population who may benefit from growth hormone co-treatment;[23] because growth hormone is extremely expensive.

OC PILL PRETREATMENT

It has been reported that use of OC pill in the previous cycle may increase pregnancy rates especially in poor responders.[24] This is because OC pill has a positive role in improving oestrogen receptor sensitisation induced by oestrogen component of the pill. In addition, OC pill also has a suppression effect of pituitary LH when used in combination with GnRH agonist. Biljan, et al. 1998,[25] reported superior pregnancy rate with GnRH + OC pill suppression compared to GnRH suppression alone. It has also been observed that OC pill

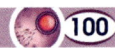
pretreatment may induce alteration of local ovarian growth factors along with changes at the endometrial level which may account for improved pregnancy rate associated with OC pill pretreatment.

Though there is a general feeling that OC pill pretreatment might be of assistance for ovarian response in poor responders, specially in 'flare up' regimens, but till now sufficient data is not available to confirm this approach.

LUTEAL PHASE MANIPULATION

What is the Basis for Luteal Phase Manipulation in Poor Responders?

It has been observed very frequently that in poor responders the size of antral follicle recruited is heterogeneous in size. This may be due to early exposure of FSH-sensitive follicles to gradient of FSH concentration during the preceding luteal phase. This leads to asynchronous development of follicles during the late luteal phase which continues to develop in the similar asynchronous manner during the early follicular phase of the treatment cycle. Ovarian stimulation leads to asynchronous growth and development of the follicle, ultimately ending in poor IVF outcome.

Luteal FSH suppression, therefore, may prevent premature exposure of FSH sensitive follicle to endogenously produced pituitary FSH. Thereby it prevents discordant follicular development. And at the same time this may allow synchronous coordinated follicle size development after exogenous gonadotropin stimulation.

The suppression of exogenous pituitary gonadotropin may be achieved either with administration of luteal phase oestrogen or with GnRH antagonist. The protocol is as follows:

a. Oestradiol valerate (4 mg daily) from cycle D21 till stimulation of D3 (status of downregulation to be monitored by LH) or alternatively

b. On D25, single dose of 3 mg cetrorelix.

These protocols prevent follicular size discrepancy of early antral follicle through suppression of luteal phase elevation of FSH, because some of the follicles in cohort may have receptors which are more sensitive to FSH than others in the same cohort.

There is an alternate protocol which is slightly different and known as GnRH agonist antagonist conversion with oestrogen priming (AACEP). This has also been used in poor responders with prior IVF failures. This is, however, a bit more complicated protocol and is not commonly used.

The AACEP protocol emphasises on improving oestrogenic dominance in the stimulated ovary and at the same time prevents ill-effects of LH flare and androgen, which are commonly seen in GnRH-a flare and antagonist protocol. The actual protocol consists of OC pill and GnRH analogue overlapping last 5 days of the pill until the onset of menses (previous cycle). From cycle D2, low dose GnRH antagonist (0.125 mg/day) and oestradiol valerate (2 mg) are given IM, followed by oestrogen suppository until a dominant follicle is detected. Ovarian stimulation consisted of use of high dose FSH/HMG (450–600 IU/day).[26]

Appearance of dominant follicle indicated administration of hCG followed by OPU. The entire protocol has been presented in Fig. 11.8.

This combination protocol is also known as oestrogen-priming protocol. Oestrogen-priming in low responders ensures oestrogen dominance in stimulated ovaries and counteracts ill-effects of LH and androgens, associated with GnRH flare and antagonist protocols. Similar benefit was achieved by a simplified protocol (Letrozole-antagonist) suggested by Elassar et al., 2011.[27]

Letrozole antagonist protocol consists of:

Letrozole (5 mg) from D2 – 5 days

↓

Gonadotropin (rFSH/HMG) from D5 till dominant follicle (18 mm)

↓

Flexible protocol antagonist (0.25 mg) at 14 mm follicle diameter

↓

hCG

Both these protocols are acceptable alternatives in poor responder groups.

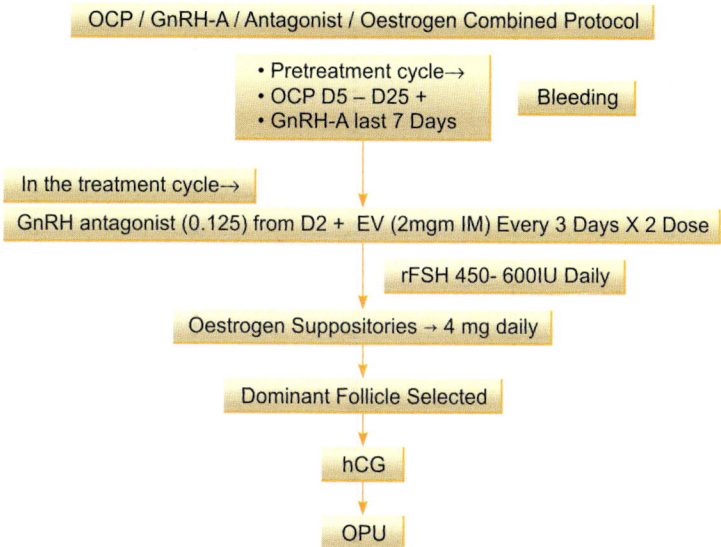

Fig. 11.8: Asynchronous follicular maturation—correction starts in preceding menstrual cycle

NATURAL CYCLE (NC) OR MODIFIED NATURAL CYCLE (MNC) IN POOR RESPONDERS

The rationality of use of this protocol is that the approaches are less invasive and less expensive. There are sporadic reports which indicate that the success rates are not inferior to those expensive protocols conventionally used for 'poor responders'.

Protocols for Modified Natural Cycle (MNC)

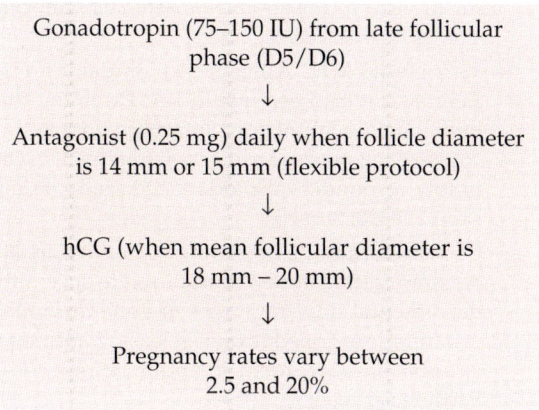

The disadvantages of these protocols are: (a) High cancellation rate, (b) negative oocyte retrieval rate, (c) high rate of dropouts and (d) unacceptably low pregnancy rates.

MNC has not been very popular because following questions are yet to be answered

a. In MNC, best time of hCG administration and time interval between hCG and OPU has not been exactly defined. Early triggering with hCG (around 16 mm size) has been preferred.[28] Some have advocated use of GnRH agonist for ovulation triggering.[29]

b. Are oocyte and embryo quality better in natural cycle? The popular belief is that it is better but it has never been confirmed by RCT.

c. How many attempts are to be made?—3 to 5 maximum.[30]

d. What is the dose of gonadotropin?—usually 100 to 225 IU has been suggested, but the optimal dose with GnRH antagonist administration has not been adequately determined.[31]

e. There is no definite information about the benefits and drawbacks of either cleavage and blastocyst stage transfer.

f. Should LH be included in gonadotropin regimen?—it is preferable to add LH in poorly responding elderly women.[32] The specific benefits of use of LH in these women have already been discussed in previous paragraphs of this chapter.

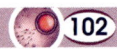

Currently, there is hardly any convincing evidence to prove that these interventions can improve results in poor responders in general IVF cycle; but may have some positive impact in women ≥ 38 years of age and in those who had 2 or 3 cycles previous IVF attempt failures.

ADDITIONAL INTERVENTIONS IN POOR RESPONDERS

This is particularly useful in protocols where there is disparity between follicular growth/endometrial development/E_2 levels.

a. **Low dose aspirin:** The mode of action of aspirin in poor responders may be brought about in two ways: (i) Inhibition of vasoconstricting prostaglandins (Thromboxane-A2) and (ii) augmenting vasodilating prostaglandins (prostacycline).

b **PGD (preimplantation genetic diagnosis):** This is an invasive method for diagnosis of embryo quality. Moreover, the method does not guarantee the quality of embryo with certainty for assessment of embryo quality. Research is ongoing for finding out non-invasive markers like follicular fluid biochemical constituents, cumulus cell gene expression profile and metabolomics and proteomics in spent media by spectroscopic examination.

c. **Assisted hatching with chemical material like Tyrode's solution:** May improve fertilisation rate in selected cases like advanced maternal age or more than three previous IVF attempts. However, currently evidence is insufficient to recommend hatching in poor responders.[33]

PRACTICAL POINTS TO REMEMBER FOR IMPROVEMENT OF RESULTS IN POOR RESPONDERS

For improvement of result in these groups of women it is crucial to acquire maximum clinical expertise and experience. In addition, the following points are to be noted:

a. Higher dose of gonadotropin (maximum 300–450 IU)

b. Long GnRH agonist protocol; still preferable with following modifications:
  i. Preceding luteal phase progesterone with GnRH agonist (to prevent recruitment of asynchronous follicles)
  ii. Mini-dose GnRH agonist
  iii. Stop protocol GnRH agonist

c. OC pretreatment followed by short agonist or microflare protocol

d. Failure to respond to long or short GnRH protocol; before cancelation one should try either stop protocol or antagonist protocol or modified natural cycle protocol.

e. Addition of LH is must in final stage of stimulation (D5/D6 onwards).

f. Androgen supplementation or pretreatment with DHEA or addition of rLH in elderly women is theoretically preferable but they require further studies.

REFERENCES

1. Laufer N, Simon A, Samueloff A, et al. Successful spontaneous pregnancies in women older than 45 years. Fertil Steril 2004; 81: 1328–32

2. Shahine LK, Milki AA, Westphal LM, Baker VL, Behr B, Lathi RB. Day 2 versus day 3 embryo transfer in poor responders: A prospective randomized trial. Fertil Steril 2011; 95: 330–2

3. Hofmann GE, Toner JP, Muasher sJ, Jones GS. Highdose follicle-stimulating hormone (FSH) ovarian stimulation in low-responder patients for in vitro fertilisation. J In vitro Fert Embryo Transf 1989; 6: 285–9.

4. Van Hooff MH, Alberda AT, Huisman GJ, Zeilmaker GH, Leerentveld RA. Doubling the human menopausal gonadotrophin dose in the course of an *in vitro* fertilisation treatment cycle in low responders: a randomized study. Hum Prod 1993; 8: 369–73.

5. Cedrin-Durnerin I, Bstanding B, Herve F, et. al. A comparative study of high fixed-dose and decremental dose regimens of gonadotropins in a minidose gonadotropin-releasing hormone agonist flare protocol for poor responders. Fertil Steril 2000; 73: 1055–6.

6. Feldberg D, Farhi J, Ashkenazi J, et al. Minidose gonadotropin-releasing hormone agonist is the treatment of choice in poor responders with high follicle-stimulating hormone levels. Fertil Steril 1994; 62: 343–6.

7. Corson SI, Batzer FR, Gocial B, et al. Leuprolide acetate-prepared *in vitro* fertilisation-gamete intra-fallopian transfer cycles: efficacy versus controls and cost analysis. Fertil Steril 1992; 57: 601–5.

8. Fujii S, Sagara M, Kudo H, et al. A prospective randomized comparison between long and discontinuous long protocols of gonadotropin-releasing hormone agonist for *in vitro* fertilisation. Fertil Steril 1997; 67: 1166–8.

9. Cedrin-Durnerin I, Bulwa S. Herve F, et al. The hormonal flare-up following gonadotrophin-releasing hormone agonist administration is influenced by a progestogen pretreatment. Hum Reprod 1996; 11: 1859–63.

10. al-Mizyen E, Sabatini L, Lower AM, et al. Does pre-treatment with progestogen or oral contraceptive pills in low responders followed by the GnRHa flare protocol improve the outcome of IVFR-ET? J Assist Reprod Genet 2000; 17: 140–6.

11. Deaton JL, Bauguess P, Huffman CS, Miller KA. Pituitary response to early follicular-phase minidose gonadotropin releasing hormone agonist (GnRHa) therapy: evidence for a second flare. J Assist Reprod Genet 1996; 13: 390–4.

12. Frankfirter D, Dayal M, Dubey A, Peak D, Gindoff P. Novel follicular-phase gonadotropin-releasing hormone antagonist stimulation protocol for *in vitro* fertilisation in the poor responder. Fertil Steril 2007; 88: 1442–5.

13. Orvieto R, Kruchkovich J, Rabinson J, al. Ultrashort gonadotropin-releasing hormone agonist combined with flexible multidose gonadotropin-releasing hormone antagonist for poor responders in *in vitro* fertilisation/embryo transfer programs. Fertile Steril 2008; 90: 228–30.

14. Howles CM. Role of LH, FSH in ovarian function. Mol Cell Endocrinol 2000; 161: 25–30.

15. Chappel SC, Howles C. Reevaluation of the roles of luteinizing hormone and follicle-stimulating hormone in the ovulatory process. Hum Reprod 1991; 6: 1206–12.

16. Hiller SG. Current concept of the roles of follicle stimulating hormone and luteinizing hormone in folliculogenesis. Hum Reprod 1994; 9: 188–91.

17. Caglar GS, Asmakopoulos B, Nikolettos N, Diedrich K, Al-Hasani S. Recombinant LH in ovarian stimulation. Reprod Biomed Online 2005; 10: 774–85.

18. Durnerin CI, Erb K, Fleming R, et al. Effects of recombinant LH treatment on folliculogenesis and responsiveness to FSH stimulation. Hum Reprod 2008; 23: 421–6.

19. Massin N, Cedrin-Durnerin I, Coussieu C, et al. Effects of transdermal testosterone application on the ovarian response to FSH in poor responders undergoing assisted reproduction technique-a prospective, randomized, double-blind study. Hum Reprod 2006; 21: 1204–11.

20. Casson PR, Lindsay MS, Pisarska MD, Carson SA, Buster JE. Dehydroepiandrosterone supplementation augments ovarian stimulation in poor responders: a case series. Hum Reprod 2000; 15: 2129–32.

21. Mitwally MF, Casper RF. Aromatase inhibition improves ovarian response to follicle-stimulating hormone in poor responders, Fertil Steril 2002; 77: 776–80.

22. Adashi EY, Resnick CE, Hurwitz A, et al. Insulin-like growth factors: the ovarian connection. Hum Reprod 1991; 6: 1213-19.

23. De Ziegler D, Streuli I, Meldrum DR, Chapron C. The value of growth hormone supplements in ART for poor ovarian responders. Fertil Steril 2011; 96: 1069–76.

24. Gonen Y, Jacobson W, Casper RF. Gonadotropin suppression with oral contraceptives before *in vitro* fertilisation. Fertil Steril 1990; 53: 282–7

25. Biljan MM, Mahutte NG, Dean N, et al. Effects of pre-treatment with an oral contraceptive on the time required to achieve pituitary suppression with gonadotropin releasing hormone analogues and on subsequent implantation and pregnancy rates. Fertil Steril, 1998; 70: 1063–9.

26. Fisch ZD, Keskintepe L, Sher G. Gonadotropin releasing hormone agonist/antagonist conversion with oestrogen priming in low responders with prior *in vitro* fertilisation failure. Fertil Steril, 2008; 89: 342–7.

27. Elassar A, Engmann L, Nulsen Benadiva C. Letrozole and gonadotropin versus Luteal estradiol and gonadotropin-releasing hormone antagonist protocol in women with a prior low response to ovarian stimulation. Fertil Steril 2011; 95: 2330–4 .

28. Ellenbogen A, Gidoni Y, Atamna R, et al. Last chance before egg donation: Modified natural cycle *in vitro* fertilisation in poor responder patients; the role of follicle diameter on the day of hCG administration in order to improve results. Fertil Steril 2009; 92: S162.

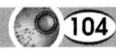

29. Segawa T, Yelian Y, Kato K, et al. Natural cycle IVF is an excellent treatment option for women with advanced age. Fertil Steril 2009; 92: S54.

30. Schimberni M, Morgia F, Colabianchi J, et al. Natural cycle *in vitro* fertilisation in poor responder patients: A survey of 500 consecutive cycles. Fertil Steril 2009; 92: 12907–301.

31. Elizur SE, Aslan D, Shulman A, et al. Modified natural cycle using GnRH antagonist can be an optional treatment in poor responders undergoing IVF. J Assist Reprod Genet 2005; 22: 75–9.

32. Hill MJ, Levens ED, l Levy G, et al. The use of recombinant luteinizing hormone in patients undergoing assisted reproductive techniques with advanced reproductive age: A systematic review and meta-analysis. Fertility and sterility 2012; 97:1108–14 e1.

33. Bider D, Livshits A, Yonish M, Yemini Z, Mashiach Dor J, Assisted Hatching by zona drilling of human embryos in women of advanced age. Hum Reprod, 1997; 12: 317–20.

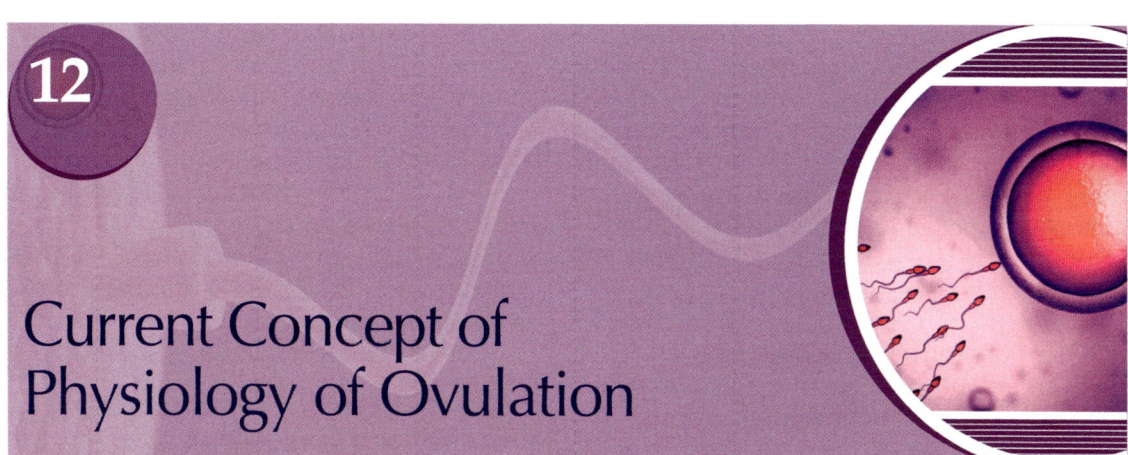

12

Current Concept of Physiology of Ovulation

INTRODUCTION

Folliculogenesis followed by ovulation is one of the basic events in female reproduction. Over the years, the concept of tightly regulated endocrine control and biophysical changes in follicular growth and development leading to either ovulation or atresia has changed considerably. The current concept of these changes are discussed in this communication under the following broad headings:

This chapter focuses on:

- Folliculogenesis—follicular growth and atresia—emergence of dominant follicle

- Role of AMH—regulation of follicular recruitment, preservation of follicle and monofollicular development

- Dominant role of E2 in endocrine control of ovulation—how and why?

- Difference in ovulatory and menstrual cycle—are they same?

- Events in ovulatory cycle—endocrine and biophysical

- Events in non-ovulation

Physiology of Folliculogenesis—Follicular Growth, Ovulation and Atresia

At around 6–8 weeks of gestation, germ cells originating from hind gut and yolk sac migrate to genital ridge. They multiply by mitotic division and stimulate the mesoderm to form granulosa cells. A single layer of flat cells surrounds each germ cell (oocyte) leading to origin of primordial follicles. These primordial follicles contain immature oocytes surrounded by flat, squamous granulosa cells (the support cells) that are segregated from the oocyte's environment by the basal lamina. They are quiescent, showing little to no biological activity. By 12 weeks of intrauterine life they become 6–7 million in number and remain in a 'resting' pool.

Follicles containing oocytes arrested in the stage of meiosis I constitute the ovarian follicular reserve which provides a woman with reproductive potential for her entire lifetime. The number of follicles occupying the follicular reserve is estimated to be 7 million at 20 weeks gestation.[1]

At an interval of 70–80 days, a cohort of these follicles is selected from the resting pool (primordial follicles); they grow and run for maturity and eventually become atretic. This is the first phase of follicular migration within 'resting' to 'active' pool.

So from the resting phase the follicles become active at an interval of 70–80 days. This dynamic process of follicular development and atresia starts from intrauterine life and the follicular reserve is reduced to 2 million at birth and 300,000 at puberty. Depletion of the ovarian follicular reserve continues throughout a

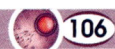

woman's lifetime,[1–5] irrespective of ovulation or anovulation, pregnancy and intake of OC pills.

The dynamicity of the follicular growth and atresia depends on a variety of factors locally produced and regulated— the important ones are TGF-β (transforming growth factor-β), super family of proteins, activins, inhibins, AMH, etc. These factors play an important role before gonadotropin is available, i.e. before puberty.

After puberty, some follicles in the 'active pool' are recruited to become gonadotropin-sensitive.[2, 6–8] Migration from gonadotropin-insensitive to gonadotropin-sensitive pool occurs during the last 20 days of 70 to 80 days cycle. This is the 2nd 'migration' during follicular maturation and occurs in between small antral and large antral stages of follicular growth (Fig. 12.2). The gonadotropin-sensitive follicles continue to grow and others become atretic.

The gonadotropin sensitivity is perhaps brought about by growth hormone, IGF1, androgen and some other unknown growth factors. The privileged follicles which become gonadotropin-sensitive are predetermined by some intrinsic factors within the follicles or within the germ cells, i.e. oocytes. These intrinsic factors are not clearly known.

Each one of these gonadotropin sensitive follicles compete for maturation under the influence of pituitary gonadotropin and one may be successful for final ovulation whereas the others become atretic.

In summary, there are two stages of follicular recruitment from the development of primordial follicle (resting pool) till ovulation. These are:

a. Recruitment from the resting pool— 70–80 days cycle—they run for maturity but cannot reach final stages of maturation and eventually become atretic. The factors regulating recruitment, though not exactly known, may be TGF-β super family of proteins, activins, inhibins, AMH, etc. This is the first stage of follicular migration.

b. Recruitment from the cohort running for maturity—gonadotropin sensitive during last 20 days of the 80 days cycle.[9]

The factors responsible for recruitment are growth hormone, IGF1, androgen and some other unknown growth factors. This is the 2nd stage of follicular migration.

The number of follicles to be primarily recruited each cycle, which eventually undergo atresia, depends on the number of follicles existing in the resting pool. Therefore, atresia is maximum in the intrauterine life. For the same reason, after unilateral oophorectomy recruitment rate certainly diminishes.

Stages of Follicular Recruitment, Growth, Maturation and Ovulation

The process involves recruitment from resting pool, growth and maturation through different stages (with or without gonadotropin influence), dominant follicle selection, ovulation and atresia. Details have been elaborated in Figs 12.1 and 12.2 and their legends.

Anti-müllerian Hormone (AMH)—Influence on Follicular Recruitment, Preservation and Monofollicular Development

AMH is expressed by granulosa cells of the ovary during the reproductive years. It has a role in folliculogenesis and follicular preservation.[10] Unlike E2, it is not controlled by gonadotropin. AMH has got antagonistic and regulating effect on FSH, E2 and aromatase in follicular microenvironment. AMH performs two functions: (a) Controls formation of primary follicles and their preservation by inhibiting unnecessary and excessive recruitment of follicles at two stages of migration (from primordial to small and large preantral, and from small to large antral follicles), and (b) AMH also indirectly helps in monofollicular development. Monofollicular development is achieved by decreasing responsiveness of gonadotropin-sensitive follicles to FSH so that instead of many follicles developing simultaneously, only one may reach the stage of dominance, because all preantral and small antral follicles produce AMH (*see* Fig. 12.2). As they reach large antral stage, AMH, through FSH inhibition in each follicle, reduces their further growth. But during the last 20 days of 80 days cycle, when some of the follicles

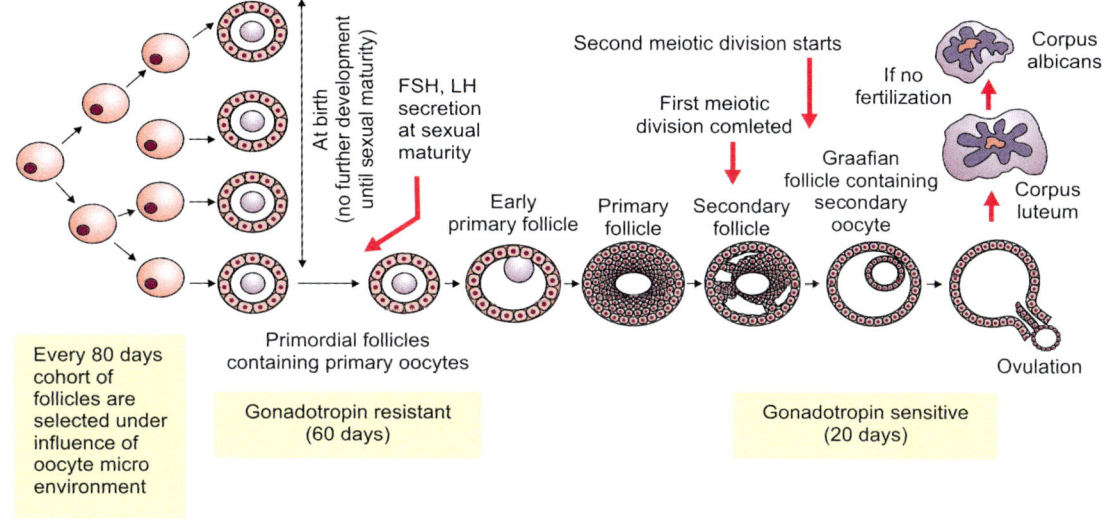

Fig. 12.1: Folliculogenesis, emergence of dominant follicle and ovulation

In intrauterine life and following birth, but before sexual maturity is reached, the follicles remain gonadotropin-insensitive. But every 80 days a cohort of follicles is selected under the influence of oocyte microenvironment, namely activin, inhibin, AMH and transforming growth factors, etc. They grow and run for maturity, but in the absence of gonadotropin, they are not able to reach full maturity and finally become atretic.

Just before puberty, some of these follicles become gonadotropin-sensitive during the last 20 days of the 80 days cycle. The factors responsible to make follicles gonadotropin-sensitive are growth hormone, IGF1, androgens and some unknown factors. How some follicles become gonadotropin-sensitive and others are denied of the privilege is not known. The gonadotropin-sensitive follicles run for maturity and one or two become dominant and others become atretic.

The privileged follicle which enjoys the maximum gonadotropin stimulation becomes the dominant follicle. Under the influence of LH surge the oocyte undergoes the first meiotic division and eventually the follicle ruptures leading to ovulation. The ruptured follicle undergoes a dramatic transformation into the corpus luteum, a steroidogenic cluster of cells that maintains the endometrium of the uterus by secreting large amount of progesterone and minor amounts of estrogen. This is ultimately converted to corpus albicans in the absence of pregnancy.

become FSH-sensitive, the production of AMH is suppressed by rising level of FSH. Still AMH does not allow many follicles to grow rapidly and prevents them to become dominant.

But one large follicle has more dominant FSH receptors. As it grows it produces less AMH, enabling this follicle to grow faster. Rest of the follicles cannot grow because of weak follicle FSH receptors and dominant AMH control, thereby resulting in monofollicular development and hence resulting in mono-follicular ovulation.

Follicles exist in the ovaries in two functional states: (a) In resting pool (primordial, primary) and (b) active pool (preantral → preovulatory). After puberty, the active pool becomes subdivided into two subgroups: (a) gonadotropin-insensitive and (b) gonadotropin-sensitive. The value of AMH which is estimated during child-bearing period represents amount of AMH being synthesised by the follicles in the gonadotropin-insensitive pool. This is because follicles of gonadotropin-sensitive pool are unable to synthesise adequate AMH.

Estimation of serum AMH (female, 25–40 years 0.19–9.13 ng/ml—normal range; range is variable in different estimations; *see* Chapter 20, Vol 2) level on any day of menstrual cycle indicates the follicular sensitivity to gonadotropin. Though there is a wide difference between upper and lower limits of normal range of AMH, for all practical purposes,

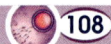
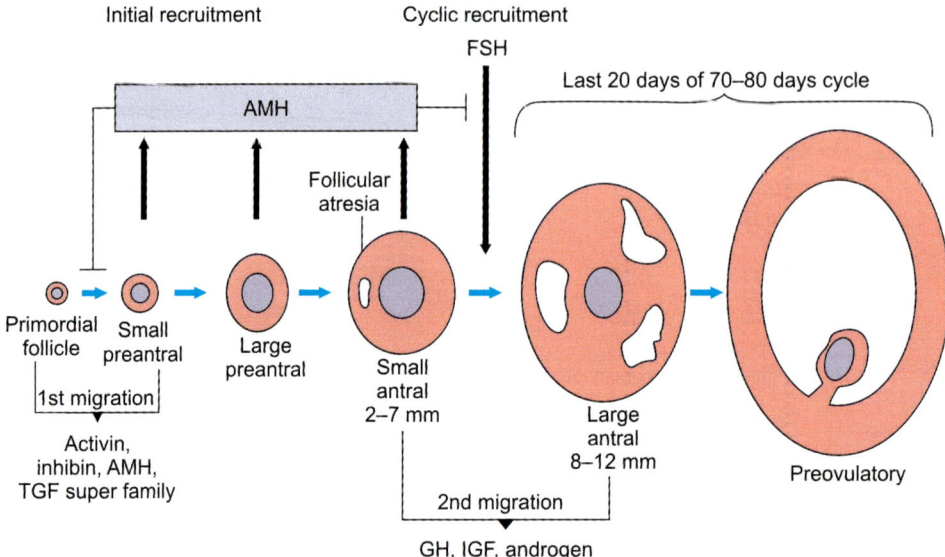

AMH in follicular preservation and monofollicular ovulation

Fig. 12.2: AMH control of folliculogenesis

The diagram represents stages of folliculogenesis starting from primordial follicle (resting pool)—small preantral, large preantral, small antral, large antral—preovulatory—finally ending in ovulation. Preantral (small and large) and small antral follicles produce AMH. AMH is produced by granulosa cells and production is not dependent on FSH or does not have any feedback mechanism. The function of AMH is to prevent undesirable follicular migration at two stages of follicular development. The first stage of migration occurs from primordial (resting pool) to preantral (active pool) stage every 70 to 80 days. The process continues from intrauterine life till menopause. During this period of 70 to 80 days, follicles run for maturity and finally undergo apoptosis. The number recruited in the first stage of migration depends on the number existing in the resting pool. Ordinarily 200 to 300 follicles are recruited every 80 days from 'resting' to 'active' pool.

The second phase of migration occurs when small antral follicles pass into the large antral follicles. At this stage some of the follicles become FSH-sensitive. FSH-sensitivity of follicles starts around the age of puberty and continues throughout the reproductive period. This occurs during the last 20 days of 80 days follicular maturation cycle. A cohort of follicles (30–40 in number) amongst many follicles recruited in 80 days cycle become gonadotropin-sensitive in the late luteal phase of a menstrual cycle. When gonadotropin starts rising, one of the gonadotropin-sensitive follicles become dominant which is destined to ovulate. Others become atretic. The exact controlling factor of migration is not known. But it appears that, the first phase of migration is brought about by inhibin, activin, AMH and TGF super family. The second phase of migration is brought about by growth hormone, IGF-1 androgen, etc. This is the reason for using growth hormone and androgen in poorly responding women in IVF stimulation cycles. Growth hormone and androgen may make some of the gonadotropin-insensitive to sensitive follicles and recruit them to become codominant follicles in the stimulation cycle.

AMH is produced by preantral (small and large) and small antral follicles which prevent excessive migration at both the stages. AMH also helps in monofollicular development by inhibiting FSH activity in codominant follicle (see previous section of this chapter).

the lower normal limit has been accepted as 1 ng/ml. Granulosa cells of polycystic ovaries produce more AMH than granulosa cells of non-polycystic ovaries. Higher values of AMH can be used as 'markers' for diagnosis of PCOS.

Endocrine Control of Ovulation

So long it was known that hypothalamus and pituitary are the controlling factors for endocrine feedback mechanism in the process of ovulatory menstrual cycle. But recently it has been suggested that ovary (oestrogen) plays a 'dominant' role in ovulatory orchestra. Neither the pituitary nor the hypothalamus has the primary role to play.

How and Why Does E2 Play the Dominant Role?

It is now clear that cyclicity of ovulation and menstruation depends on the following factors:

a. Oestrogen must decline in late luteal phase allowing FSH to rise for recruitment of fresh batch of follicles which run for maturity and ovulation during the next menstrual cycle.

b. Oestrogen must also rise in the mid-menstrual phase of the next menstrual cycle for rupture of dominant graffian follicle allowing ovulation to occur.

c. Androgens within the follicle must be aromatised to oestrogen, allowing events in follicular phase to occur for the follicles to grow and finally rupture leading to ovulation.

Hence estrogen must rise and must decline once in the menstrual cycle for ovulation to occur. Decline of oestrogen allows low FSH to rise in the late luteal phase of the previous menstrual cycle. Static oestrogen level (as in PCOS) throughout the menstrual cycle prevents ovulation.

Specific Endocrine Mechanism Involved in the Process of Ovulation

As has already been stated, E2 generated from granulosa cell, and through aromatisation of thecal androgen under the influence of rising FSH gradually increases and reaches a peak in mid-follicular phase (100–150 pg/per mature follicle). It remains in plateau at that level for 48 hours. During this period, at any point of time there may be LH surge, and this leads to ovulation. Inadequate amount of oestradiol peak leads to attenuated LH surge leading to either ineffective ovulation (ovum not competent to be fertilised) or to a clinical situation of luteinised unruptured follicle (LUF).

Control of E2 synthesis and release is initially by FSH and subsequently entirely by LH (LH receptor has already developed in dominant follicles).

In early follicular phase, synthesis of E2 is not entirely dependent on FSH. Some amount of LH also has a role to play. Because LH generates androgen from the thecal cell and this is aromatised to estrogen. FSH induces production of enzyme aromatase by granulosa cell. Estrogen in synergy with FSH induces follicular growth and maturation. Hence some amount of LH (not very high, otherwise follicular environment will be androgenised) is essential for production of estrogen which is absolutely essential for follicular growth and development. Excess androgen under the influence of elevated LH is converted to dihydrotestosterone (DHT) which prevents aromatase formation and consequently turns follicular environment more androgenised rather than oestrogenised.

The endrocrine regulation and control of ovulatory menstrual cycle is diagrammatically represented in Figs 12.3a and b.

Other Endocrine Factors in the Mechanism of Ovulation

With intact hypothalamic-pituitary-ovarian axis—the key role in the mechanism of ovulation is played by oestradiol produced by the dominant follicles.

Dominant follicle selection depends on FSH. But FSH action on follicle is modulated by 'growth factor (IGF-1)' generated by autocrine/paracrine mechanism in the follicle itself, under the influence of growth hormone (GH).

Hence ovulatory mechanism has a dual tropic hormone axis support, namely:

• Somatotropic axis support—GH, IGF-1, SHBG, IGFBP

• Gonadotropin axis support—FSH, LH, E2, inhibin, activin.

Therefore, growth hormone has a significant role in the process of folliculogenesis.

Role of Androgens in the Process of Folliculogenesis and Ovulation

In the earlier stages of folliculogenesis, androgens are essential to recruit follicles from the 'preantral' pool and make them gonadotropin-sensitive. Therefore, poorly

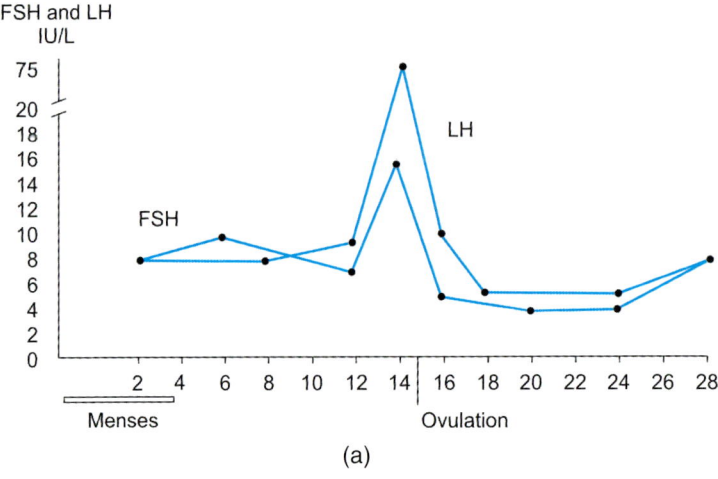

(a)

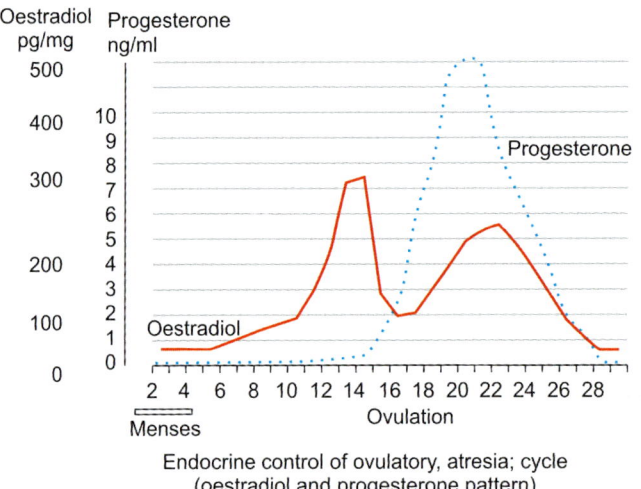

Endocrine control of ovulatory, atresia; cycle
(oestradiol and progesterone pattern)

(b)

Figs 12.3a and b: The endrocrine regulation and control of ovulatory menstrual cycle is diagrammatically represented

responding women in COH protocol are sometimes treated with androgens to make them gonadotropin-sensitive.

In the maturing follicles, androgen receptors are present in the granulosa cells. LH-mediated thecal androgens are aromatised to estrogen within the follicle in the early follicular phase. This helps in making the intrafollicular micro-environment into an oestrogenised milieu, in which the oocytes can mature well. However, when androgens are at a higher level they are converted to 5α reduced androgens which inhibit aromatase activity. Follicular micro-environment is androgenised instead of

being oestrogenised. This may prevent oocyte development and maturity. Therefore, high level of LH (>threshold level) in the early follicular phase is detrimental for folliculogenesis and oocyte maturity.

Ovulatory and Menstrual Cycle—are they Same?

There is a difference in physiological and biophysical changes in menstrual and ovulatory cycles. Hence strictly speaking there should be different definitions for these two important physiological events in a woman's reproductive years.

Menstrual cycle: Menstrual cycle begins on day 1 of bleeding of the preceding cycle and ends on day 1 of the subsequent cycle.

Ovulatory cycle: Ovulatory cycle begins in the late luteal phase (around D21 of a regular menstrual cycle) of the preceding menstrual cycle and ends in mid-menstrual phase (D14–D16 of a regular menstrual cycle) of the subsequent cycles.

Menstrual cycle has got four distinct phases as:

 a. Bleeding phase
 b. Follicular phase
 c. Ovulatory phase
 d. Luteal phase

Similarly, ovulatory cycle also has four distinct phases as:

 a. **Late luteal phase:** This begins from D21 of the previous menstrual cycle and continues up to early follicular phase of the subsequent menstrual cycle. During this period E2 declines and FSH starts rising allowing recruitment of fresh batch of follicles which run for maturity during the next menstrual cycle.

 The events in late luteal phase are diagrammatically represented in Fig. 12.4.

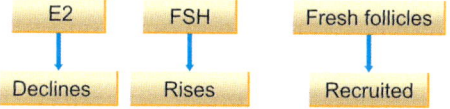

Fig. 12.4: Events in late luteal phase

 b. **Menstrual and early follicular phase:** This phase starts from D1–D4 of the subsequent menstrual cycle and continues up to mid-follicular phase. During this period follicular recruitment continues— the follicles grow and try to become mature. Under the influence of rising FSH four important events occur during this period: (a) Multiplication of granulosa cell and growth of follicle, (b) synthesis of aromatase enzyme in the follicle, (c) induction of LH receptors in addition to FSH receptors within the follicle and (d) synthesis and production of oestradiol

through aromatase conversion of LH-mediated thecal androgen. FSH in synergy with E2 leads to further follicular growth.

Endocrinologic and biophysical events in early follicular phase are represented in Fig. 12.5.

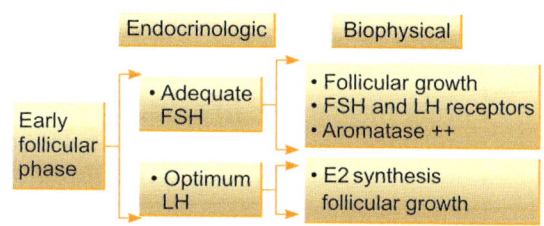

Fig. 12.5: Endocrinologic and biophysical events in early follicular phase

 c. **Mid-follicular phase:** Period around D4–D5 of the subsequent menstrual cycles. During this period, of all the follicles running for maturity one becomes dominant and others become atretic. The mechanism by which a follicle becomes dominant and others become atretic is not very clear. However, it is known that the dominant follicle is privileged to have more FSH receptors than the non-dominant follicles, and therefore the non-dominant follicles under the influence of rising LH become atretic. But the privileged "dominant" follicle having more FSH receptors continues to grow initially under the influence of FSH and subsequently under the control of LH, because by this time the dominant follicle has produced adequate LH receptors also. Endocrinology and biophysical events in mid-follicular phase are represented in Fig. 12.6.

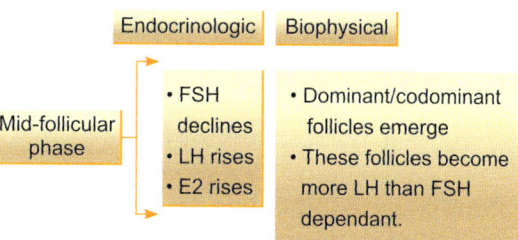

Fig. 12.6: Mid-follicular phase events

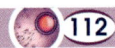

d. Late follicular phase: Starts from D6–D7 of the subsequent menstrual cycle and continues till ovulation (around D13–D14 of the subsequent menstrual cycle). During this period the dominant follicle is under control of LH and not FSH. The follicle can function under the influence of LH because enough LH receptors have been generated during the early follicular phase. Three important events occur during this period: (i) Luteinisation of granulosa cell—they form the large luteal cell of the future corpus luteum, (ii) first meiotic division of the maturing oocyte and release of first polar body in perivitelline space. Oocyte maturation during the intrauterine life, gets arrested at the stage of prophase by oocyte maturation inhibitory factor (OMIF). The inhibitory action of OMIF is suppressed by progesterone induced by rising LH in the follicular fluid just around ovulation and (iii) Ovulation—during this period E2 has reached its peak (around 150 pg/per mature follicle) and remains in plateau for about 48 hours. This exerts a negative feedback effect on pituitary synthesis of FSH and positive feedback effect on release of LH. A bolus of LH is released from the pituitary and this is known as 'LH surge'. This event leads to "ovulation" of the dominant follicle (Fig. 12.7).

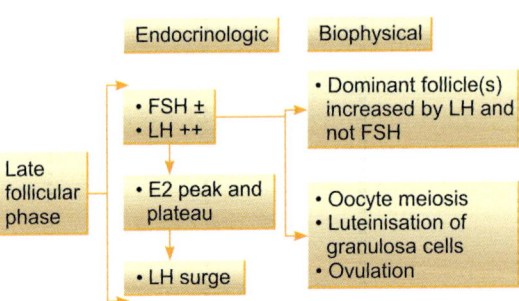

Fig. 12.7: Late follicular events

Summary of the important points in selection of dominant follicle(s) and events leading to ovulation:

Important points to note for selection of dominant follicle:

a. Local interaction of oestrogen and FSH within the privileged follicle.
b. Negative feedback of oestrogen on pituitary secretion of FSH—withdrawal of FSH effect on less developed follicle → atresia of remaining follicles.

Normal and Abnormal Events in the Periovulatory Period

- Shift of control of dominant follicle from FSH to LH in the mid-follicular phase
- Rising level of LH in late follicular phase causes follicular atresia other than the dominant follicle. Otherwise multiple pregnancy would have been more frequent.
- Multiple pregnancy is common after induction of ovulation.
- LH surge occurs after oestradiol reaches a peak (100–150 pg/follicle) and then remains in plateau for 48 hours. "Surge" actually occurs any time during this plateau period.
- There may be unscheduled LH surge, if E2 level is prematurely elevated, when the granulosa cells are not yet mature → premature luteinisation and 'progeric' egg → unsuitable for fertilisation
- Also premature luteinisation of granulosa cells results in defective corpus luteum formation
- Duration of LH surge is about 27 hours; this period is essential for first meiotic division of the oocyte to occur. LH surge has a crescendo, peak and descendo. Peak level of LH should be 75 to 90 ng/ml.
- Attenuated LH surge may lead to ovulation, but a dysmature egg is liberated which is unsuitable for fertilisation.
- LH induced progesterone (not more than 1.8 ng/ml) within the follicle inhibits the influence of OMIF (oocyte maturation inhibitory factor) which releases the first polar body of the oocyte and makes it fertilisable.
- Actual process of ovulation is induced by thinning of perifollicular wall, leukocyte activation, intrafollicular distension, appearance of proteolytic enzymes, namely plasminogen activator (PA) and matrix metalloproteinase (MMP). These enzymes are

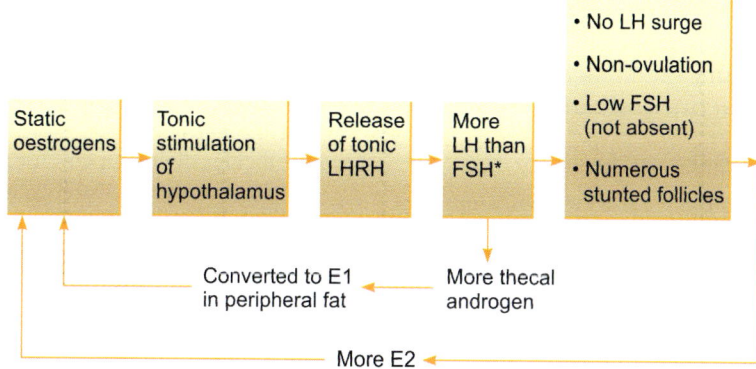

Fig. 12.8: Main events in non-ovulation

induced by follicular fluid prostaglandins which in turn is generated by rising level of LH.

- Absence of these enzymes and prostaglandins lead to clinical situation of anovulation and luteinised unruptured follicle (LUF) syndrome.
- There is a secondary rise of FSH prior to ovulation—brought about by rising progesterone level. Secondary rise of FSH induces granulosa cell to produce the proteolytic enzymes like plasminogen activator and matrix metalloproteinase. These enzymes cause digestion/disintegration of wall of follicles for follicular rupture.

Main Events in Non-ovulation

As stated earlier, in an ovulatory cycle the level of oestradiol should be fluctuating—this means that oestrogen must decline once in late luteal phase when FSH starts rising. And also oestradiol must rise once in the mid-menstrual cycle for ovulation to occur. On the other hand, if the level of oestrogen remains static throughout the menstrual cycle, non-ovulation is the consequence.

Static elevated level of oestrogen is the main cause of non-ovulation, e.g. in PCOS women. Static elevated oestrogen results from contribution of oestradiol from numerous small and semi-matured follicles in the ovary and in addition from estrone generated from conversion of excess androgen in the peripheral fat which is commonly observed in PCOS women. This elevated static level of oestrogen exerts a continuous tonic effect on hypothalamus. Hypothalamus in response releases tonic elevated LHRH. As LHRH is more luteinising hormone releasing than FSH releasing, an elevated static level of LH continues to persist. There is no LH surge typical of ovulatory cycle, and because of absence of LH surge there is non-ovulation. Pituitary also releases FSH, but less than LH (LHRH is more LH than FSH releasing). A low level of static FSH continuously stimulates the follicles in the ovary. The follicles try to become mature, but cannot become fully mature because of the inadequate amount of FSH.

Excess LH from pituitary leads to more thecal androgen production. This androgen is converted in peripheral fat to estrone. Excess estrone combined with excess oestradiol produced by numerous immature stunted follicles in the ovary result in an elevated level of static elevated oestrogen throughout the cycle. This leads to a vicious cycle in non-ovulatory women who frequently present with oligomenorrhoea or secondary amenorrhoea.

The sequence of events have been illustrated in Fig. 12.8.

Conclusion

Therefore, it may be concluded that the ovary, specifically the fluctuating level of E2, is the band master of endocrine orchestra for a normal ovulatory menstrual cycle.

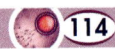

With intact hypothalamic-pituitary-ovarian axis, ovulation is under the control of delicately balanced regulatory "feedback" mechanism of endocrine, paracrine and autocrine factors.

REFERENCES

1. Baker T. A quantitative and cytological study of germ cells in human ovaries. Proc R Soc Lond [Biol] 1963; 158: 417–433.

2. Block E. Quantitative morphological investigations of the follicular system in women: variations at different ages. Acta Anat 1952; 14: 108–123.

3. Gougeon A. Regulation of ovarian follicular development in primates: facts and hypotheses. Endocr Rev 1996; 17: 121–155.

4. Gougeon A. Ovarian follicular growth in humans: Ovarian ageing and population of growing follicles. Maturitas 1998; 30: 137–142.

5. Hansen KR, Knowlton NS, Thyer AC, Charleston JS, Soules MR, Klein NA. A new model of reproductive aging: the decline in ovarian non-growing follicle number from birth to menopause. Hum Reprod 2008; 23: 699–708.

6. Gougeon A. Influence of cyclic variations in gonadtrophin and steroid hormones on follicular growth in the human ovary. In: De Brux J, Gautray J (eds). Clinical Pathology of the Endocrine Ovary. Lancaster, UK: MTP Press, 1984.

7. McNatty KP, Hillier SG, Boogaard AMVD, Trimbos-Kemper TC, Reichert LK, Hall EVV. Follicular development during the luteal phase of the human menstrual cycle. J Clin Endocrinol Metab 1983; 56: 1022–1031.

8. Baerwald A, Adams G, Pierson R. A new model for ovarian follicular development during the human menstrual cycle. Fertil Steril 2003b; 80: 116–122.

9. Craig J, Orisaka M, Wang H, Orisaka S, Thompson W, Zhu C, Kotsuji F, Tsang BK. Gonadotropin and intra-ovarian signals regulating follicle development and atresia: The delicate balance between life and death. Front Biosci 2007; 12: 3628–3639.

10. Weenen C, Laven J, Von Bergh A, Cranfield M, Groome N, Visser J, Kramer P, Fauser B, Themmen A (2004). "Anti-Müllerian hormone expression pattern in the human ovary: potential implications for initial and cyclic follicle recruitment" (abstract). Mol Hum Reprod 10 (2): 77–83. doi:10.1093/molehr/gah015. PMID 14742691).

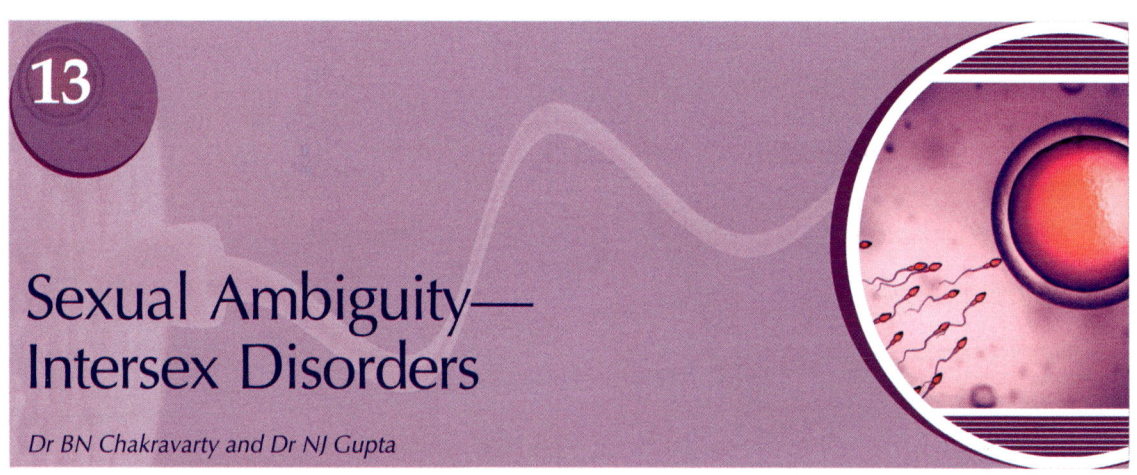

13

Sexual Ambiguity— Intersex Disorders

Dr BN Chakravarty and Dr NJ Gupta

INTRODUCTION

The clinical situation in which there is existence of both male and female genital organs in the same individual is defined as sexual ambiguity. Ambiguity may involve only external genital organs or both internal and external genital organs.

Sexual Ambiguity and Intersex

Sexual ambiguity of external genital organs is an usual but not invariable marker of all intersex problems. Three major intersex problems are:

- Female intersex
- Male intersex
- True intersex.

In Allen's classification (1985), 'Mixed' gonadal dysgenesis with sexual ambiguity has also been included under the heading of intersex disorders.

For evaluation and treatment of sexual ambiguity, it is important to recapitulate briefly the normal embryology leading to development of male and female genital organs.

Sequence of Events in Embryologic Development of Genital Organs

Sexual differentiation either to male or to female type occurs in an embryo around 7–8 weeks of intrauterine life. There are two phases of sex organ differentiation.

First Phase

First phase consists of formation of gonads. This depends on chromosomal make up of the embryo. When the chromosomal make up is 'XX', ovary forms; if it is 'XY', testis develops. Chromosomal arrangement is completed at the time of fertilisation.

The molecular basis of gonadal development is complex. The gene sequence known as "testis determining factor (TDF)" on the Y chromosome appears to be responsible for testis development. In its absence ovary forms (Wiener and Gonzales, 1996). In addition to TDF, other sex-determining genes have been identified, e.g. SRY, DSS, DOX-9, DOX-3 etc. When either TDF or other sex determining gene(s) is absent or mutated testis cannot function properly even if Y chromosome is present. This leads to a clinical situation of intersex.

Immediately following development of gonads, external and internal genital organs start developing (Flowchart 13.1). This brings about the second phase of sexual development. The external genital organs continue to develop up to 20 weeks, whereas the development of internal genital organs is completed within 10 weeks of intrauterine life.

Second Phase

With the formation of gonads, external and internal genital organs start developing

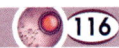

Flowchart 13.1

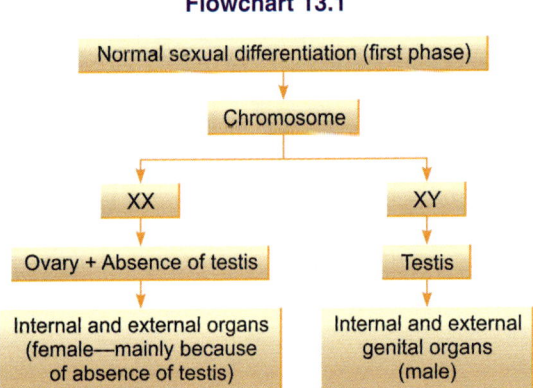

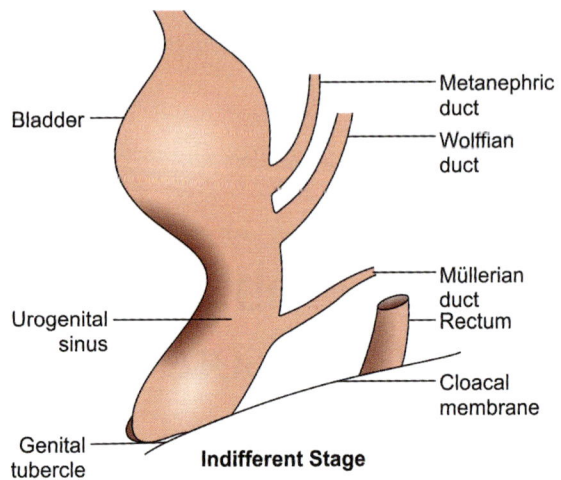

Fig. 13.1: Embryologic source of development of external genital organs and the site of its communication with internal genital organs (*Adapted from* "Intersexual Disorders". Dewhurst and Gordon, 1969)

from two different sources. These two sources are:

    a. Urogenital sinus derivatives (external genital organs)

    b. Mesodermal derivatives (internal genital organs)

A communication is established between external and internal genital organs, through urogenital sinus.

External genital organs in association with urinary bladder and urethra (commonly known as urogenital organs), develop from primitive cloaca, which becomes subdivided to form:

    a. Ventral urogenital sinus

    b. Dorsal cloaca.

Ventral urogenital sinus is again anatomically subdivided into two parts: (i) Cephalic (ii) Caudal. Cephalic end is the embryologic source of origin of bladder and ureteric diverticulum (metanephric duct) in both male and female (Fig. 13.1).

The caudal part of the urogenital sinus in the male develops into prostate, prostatic and membranous urethra into which the structure derived from wolffian duct (the vas deferens) will drain. The site of drainage into the urethra is known as prostatic utricle (embryologic homologue of uterus).

In male, testis produces two types of hormones, testosterone and müllerian inhibitory substance (MIS). In the foetal testis, MIS leads to regression of müllerian ducts, which otherwise form fallopian tubes, uterus and vagina.

In the female, the caudal part of urogenital sinus forms the entire urethra and the vestibule into which the lower part of müllerian duct opens forming the lower vagina. The site of contact between the lower part of müllerian duct and dorsal wall of the caudal part of urogenital sinus will form the sinovaginal bulb. Following canalisation, this area (sinovaginal bulb) develops into lower vagina, hymen and vestibule (Flowchart 13.2).

Therefore, the caudal part of urogenital sinus contributes mostly to the development of a communicating channel between the internal and external genital organs both in males as well as in females. But the more important components of external genital organs have an origin from structures which lie in close proximity to urogenital sinus (Flowchart 13.3). These are:

    a. Genital tubercle: This is the embryologic source of origin of penis in the male and clitoris in the female.

    b. Genital fold: In the male, it forms the penile urethra and in the female, it contributes to the formation of labia minora.

    c. Genital swelling: In the male, it leads to formation of scrotum; whereas in female, it contributes to the development of labia majora.

Flowchart 13.2

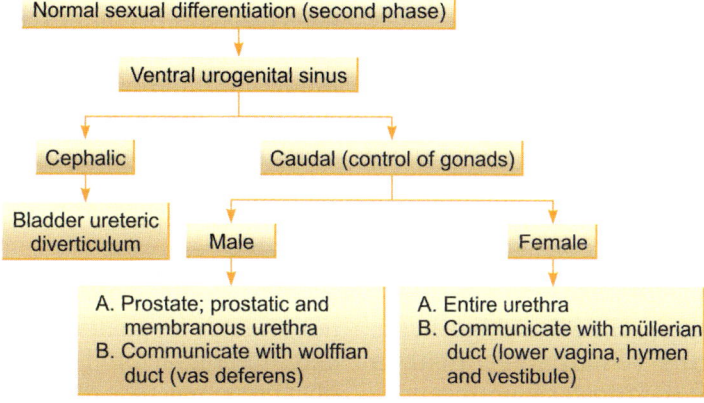

Flowchart 13.3

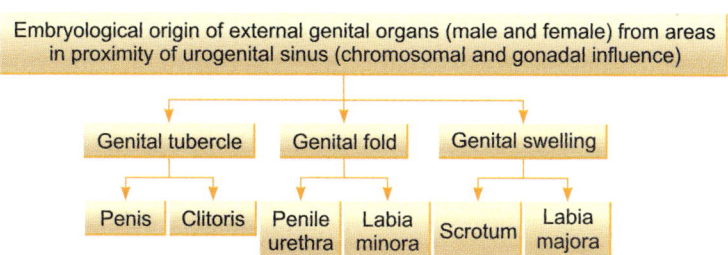

Development of external genitalia towards male or female direction primarily depends on presence or absence of androgens and androgen receptors, and not on chromosomes. Excess of androgen leads to the development of external genitalia more towards male side (e.g. virilising influence of CAH) even when the chromosome pattern is 46XX. On the other hand, with presence of adequate amount of androgens but absence of androgen receptors, the development of external genitalia will be more towards female side (testicular feminising syndrome) in individuals with 46XY chromosomes.

Development of Internal Genital Organs

Simultaneously, with the development of external genital organs, internal genital organs start developing. Normally the development of internal genital organs is completed by 10 weeks, whereas the external genital organs continue to develop till 20 weeks of intrauterine life.

The source of origin of internal genital organ is primary mesoderm covered by coelomic epithelium situated in the lumbar region cephalad to cloaca. Three ridges appear from medial to lateral side, they are:

a. Gonadal ridge or genital ridge
b. Mesonephric ridge
c. Paramesonephric ridge or müllerian ridge.

Internal genital organs originating from these embryologic areas

a. Gonadal ridge or Genital ridge: This is the area of development of primitive gonads. In male, testis develops whereas in female, this is the area of development of ovaries. Germ cells migrate to this area from hind gut to form either male or female gametes (spermatocytes or oocytes) within the gonads.

b. Mesonephric ridge: In the male, this ridge forms the testicular duct which gives rise to epididymis, seminal vesicles and vas deferens. This duct connects testis with prostatic part of

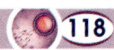

urethra. On its way, it receives collections from seminal vesicles and prostate, which contribute to the bulk of semen volume.

In female, this structure becomes atrophic and remains as a vestigial structure in between the leaves of broad ligament as epoophoron, paroophoron, and duct of Gartner. The terminal end of the duct of Gartner ends at the introitus on either side of the lateral vaginal wall. Sometimes, this duct is converted into a vaginal cyst known as "duct of Gartner cyst".

c. Paramesonephric or müllerian ridge: In the male, this structure remains vestigeal as prostatic utricle in the prostatic urethra into which ejaculatory duct formed by union of seminal vesicle and vas deferens drain. In female, this structure forms the fallopian tubes, uterus and upper two-thirds of vagina.

Hence to summarise, development of external and internal sex organs depend on following factors:
  a. Chromosomal
  b. Gonadal
  c. Genetic
  d. Endocrinological.

Sexual Ambiguity

Abnormality in one or more of the factors mentioned above lead to sexual ambiguity. Clinical situations in which these factors may become relevant for development of sexual ambiguity are briefly discussed below.

Chromosomal anomalies: Chromosomal anomalies do not always lead to sexual ambiguity. For example, in Turner's syndrome (45XO) or in Klinefelter's syndrome (47XXY), there is no sexual ambiguity.

In classic variety of testicular feminizing syndrome (male intersex), there is no ambiguity of external genitalia. But in incomplete variety of testicular feminising syndrome, (another variety of male intersex) and in true intersex, there may be ambiguity of external genitalia.

Gonadal factors: Testis produces two types of hormones, viz. testosterone and anti-müllerian hormone (AMH). Presence of testosterone with absence of AMH leads to presence of uterus and fallopian tube with male phenotype and male external genitalia. Such uterus with fallopian tubes are sometimes accidentally detected in hernial sac in male intersex individuals.

Similarly, deficient Leydig cell function leads to subnormal testosterone production with may lead to a clinical situation of micropenis with cryptorchidism (a variety of male intersex).

Genetic factor: Presence of 'Y' chromosome is not enough for maleness. Presence of testis-determining factor (TDF) is essential. A 46XX phenotype boy (sex-reversed boy) can develop into a phenotypic male individual without sexual ambiguity. In this variety, translocation of male determining genetic material (TDF) would lead to male phenotype even in the absence of 'Y' chromosome (Blyth and Churchill, 1996; Donahoe, 1987; Federman and Donahoe, 1995). Similarly, even in the presence of 'Y' chromosome, mutation or deletion of sex determining genes lead to the development of 46XY female (classic testicular feminising syndrome, male intersex). Though these individuals have no ambiguity of external genitalia, they have ambiguity between chromosomal, gonadal sex on one side and phenotypic sex on the other.

In addition, genetically determined enzymatic deficiency which is a receptor defect leads to sexual ambiguity. Examples of sexual ambiguity due to enzymatic deficiency are 5α-reductase deficiency in male intersex and several enzymatic blocks in congenital adrenal hyperplasia (CAH), the commonest one being 21-hydroxylase deficiency. Example of target organ androgen receptor block is testicular feminizing syndrome.

Endocrine factor: Abnormal androgen production from hyperactive adrenal cortex virilises a female foetus with ambiguity of external genitalia.

Similar ambiguity is also observed due to a virilising tumour in a female foetus or following administration of progestogens or androgens to the mother in her early months of pregnancy.

CLINICAL FINDINGS AND DIAGNOSIS OF DIFFERENT TYPES OF INTERSEX

Female Intersex

Apart from tumour and iatrogenic causes, the commonest cause of female intersex is congenital adrenal hyperplasia (CAH). This is also the commonest cause of sexual ambiguity observed in clinical practice. The basic endocrinologic problem is a defect in the biosynthesis of cortisol.

If the cortisol production is less or absent, the negative feedback control on the pituitary decreases resulting in increased pituitary output of ACTH. The adrenal gland reacts to ACTH stimulation by increased production of androgens and oestrogens from zona reticularis. Androgen in intrauterine life of a female foetus virilises external genitalia. Depending on the time of onset, amount of androgen secreted and duration of exposure, there will be varying grades of labio-scrotal fusion, clitoral enlargement and anatomical occlusion of urethra and vagina (Figs 13.2 to 13.7).

The vagina and urethra share a common urogenital sinus formed by fusion of labial folds. Complete vaginal suppression due to virilising effect of congenital adrenal hyperplasia has rarely been reported. This is an important point of advantage during surgical correction. In the commonest variety, i.e. in 21-hydroxylase deficiency, there is accumulation of dihydroepiandrosterone (DHEA) which is a weak androgen. Consequently these affected girls are less masculinised. Therefore, in majority, a separate vaginal and urethral opening can be easily identified.

Degrees of virilisation of external genitalia originating from urogenital sinus in congenital adrenal hyperplasia

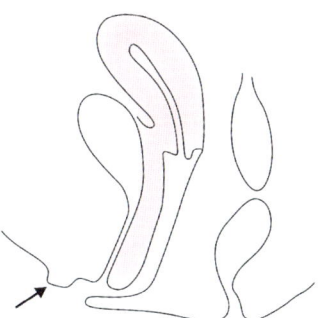

Fig. 13.2: Slight enlargement of phallus; urethral and vaginal orifices are easily identified

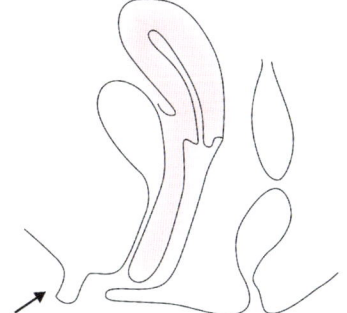

Fig. 13.3: Moderate enlargement of phallus; urethral and vaginal orifices are difficult to locate

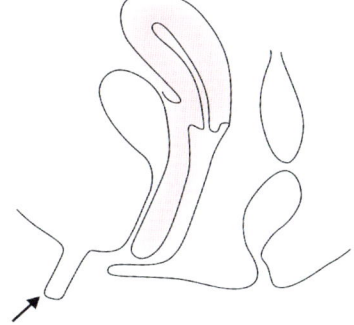

Fig. 13.4: Gross enlargement of phallus, total concealment of urethral and vaginal opening, occasional absence of communication between lower end of müllerian duct and upper end of urogenital sinus (extremely rare situation)

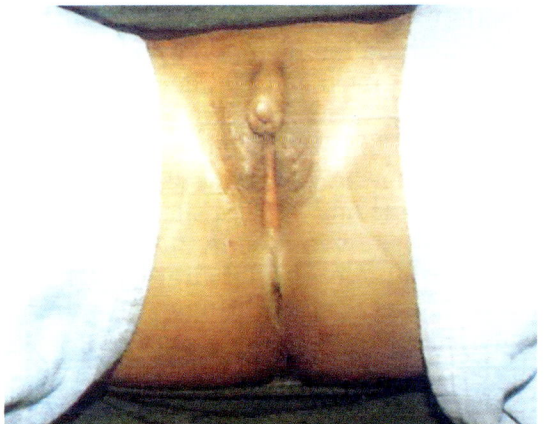

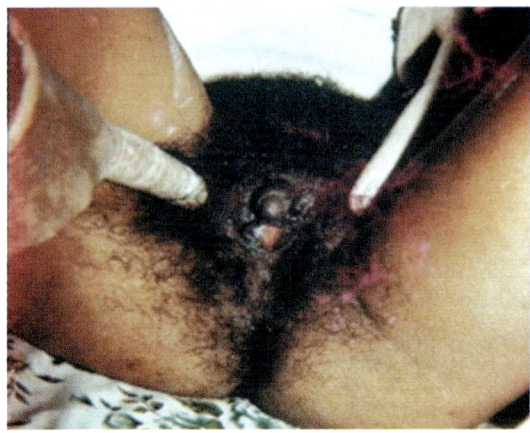

Fig. 13.5: Sexual ambiguity: Congenital adrenal hyperplasia in child aged 7 years (common opening of urethra and vagina through urogenital sinus with fusion of labioscrotal folds, phallus is enlarged)

Fig. 13.6: Sexual ambiguity: Congenital adrenal hyperplasia in an adolescent; note the degree of virilisation. Common opening of vagina and urethra through urogenital sinus with fusion of labioscrotal fold; phallus is enlarged

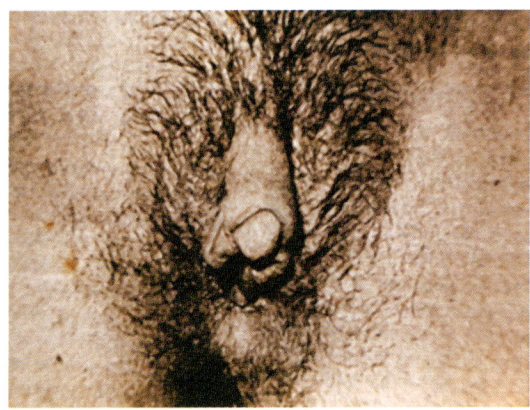

Fig. 13.7: Congenital adrenal hyperplasia (late onset), gross enlargement of phallus, minimum labio-scrotal fusion; urethral and vaginal opening are visible (not in the figure); obviously time of onset of syndrome in this case was delayed. Clitoral hypertrophy depends on amount of androgen exposure and not on time of onset of the syndrome

Internal genital organs are not affected in CAH. This is because development of internal genital organs is completed by 10–12 weeks, whereas significant amount of androgen secretion from adrenal cortex starts after 10–12 weeks. Moreover, there is no anomalous secretion of anti-müllerian hormone in females, affected with congenital adrenal hyperplasia.

In addition to ambiguity of external genitalia, excess androgens and oestrogens have undesirable metabolic side effects. During infancy and childhood, bone growth is markedly stunted and epiphyseal fusion occurs before attaining adult height. Static oestrogen excess puts a negative feedback effect on the gonadotropin function resulting in absence of breast development and amenorrhoea. Increased androgen levels may be responsible for increased hair on face and body.

More than half of the patients with CAH will have a deficiency of the enzyme 21-hydroxylase which leads to elevated serum levels of 17-hydroxyprogesterone (17-OHP) and increased urinary pregnanetriol (Allen, 1985).

Diagnosis of CAH is confirmed by estimation of serum 17-OHP. Normal level of serum 17-OHP in the morning should be less than 200 ng/dl. Level of serum 17-OHP more than 800 ng/dl is diagnostic of CAH.

Level between 200 ng/dl and 800 ng/dl requires ACTH stimulation test for confirmation of diagnosis of CAH. In infants immediately after birth, 17-OHP level is elevated (1000–3000 ng/ml). This declines to a value of 100–200 ng/dl after 24 hours. In affected infants the value of 17-OHP ranges between 3,000 and 40,000 ng/dl. Many infants are at a risk of salt wasting, and therefore, to the risk of dehydration and hypotension. Deficiency of 11-hydroxylase (another variety of CAH), on the other hand, may be associated with salt retention and hypertension (Robertson and Walker, 1975). 3-OL dehydrogenase deficiency is the rarest form of defect in CAH and these infants do not usually survive becasue of severe salt wastage.

Prenatal Diagnosis of CAH

Amniocentesis and Chorion Villous biopsy may be helpful for prenatal diagnosis (Reindoller et al., 1988). The objective is to initiate treatment with dexamethasone before the female foetus is affected by genital ambiguity (Mulaikal et al., 1987; Meyer et al., 1996).

But as the prenatal diagnosis is not 100% accurate and there are potential hazards for such empirical therapy with dexamethasone, this type of prenatal treatment has remained controversial and questionable (Pang et al., 1992; Mercado et al., 1995).

Male Intersex

In this group, the chromosomal pattern is 46XY and the gonads are invariably testes. 80% of affected individuals have an altered phenotype caused by genetically determined abnormal target organ response to testosterone (testicular feminising syndrome or "feminised males"), but mostly with normal response to anti-müllerian hormone (absence of müllerian system). Remaining 20% have deficient testosterone and anti-müllerian hormone production in their testes (Rubenstein and Mandell, 1993). Therefore, in majority of male intersex individuals (80%), the normal hypothalamic pituitary feedback loop is impaired resulting in elevated gonadotropin and excess production of testosterone and androgens. But in this variety of male intersex, androgens cannot work because of deficient cellular response in the target organs. In the other variety, production of either testosterone, or anti-müllerian hormone or both are less, resulting in a clinical state of under-masculinised males with or without existence of müllerian system.

Etiological Background of Male Intersex

The are two steps in the etiological background of male intersex; one is linked with the other. These steps are:

Direct etiology: Deficiency of two hormones produced by testes namely:
  i. Testosterone
  ii. Anti-müllerian hormone (AMH).

Background etiology: In the background of these defects, there is either deletion or mutation of the sex determining gene(s).

Clinical Classification based on Etiology

There are two broad groups, viz.
A. Under-masculinised males
B. Feminised males or 46XY females.

Each group has two subgroups.

A. Under-masculinised males, usually reared as men

The two subgroups are:
  a. The first subgroup consists of individuals who have deficiency of anti-müllerian hormone and mild deficit of testosterone. External genitalia, therefore, are more masculine in appearance, but occasionally with unilateral or bilateral undescended testes. They have persistence of müllerian system in the form of uterus and tube occasionally found in inguinal hernial sac (hernia uteri inguinalis). In this group, ambiguity of external genitalia is rare and sex of rearing is male, which is not in doubt. Fertility is possible in these individuals with at least one testis in the scrotal sac.

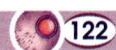

b. Individuals in other subgroup in this category have moderate to severe grades of testosterone deficiency with or without deficit of anti-müllerian hormone. Majority of individuals in this group are grossly under-masculinised and in more than 50%, external and internal genital organs are ambiguous. In this subgroup, deficiency of testosterone with or without anti-müllerian hormone may be due to several reasons. Some of the clinical evidence is given below.

Deficiency of testosterone in these individuals may be due to:

i. Abnormal pituitary (counterfeit) gonadotropin secretion (Park et al., 1975; Siler-Khodar et al., 1974): These patients do not survive beyond neonatal period, though they may have ambiguity of external genitalia. Therefore, they are not clinically significant.

ii. Subnormal testicular testosterone biosynthesis due to enzymatic deficiency (Dagenhart, 1972; Bongivanni, 1961; Cravioto et al., 1986): These patients are under-masculinised without any evidence of müllerian system. Some may have micropenis with cryptorchidism. Breast development is variable.

iii. Defective biological expression (failure of testosterone being converted to dihydrotestosterone (DHT)) at the target organ level due to deficiency of enzyme 5α-reductase (Peterson, Imperato-Mcginley et al., 1988): DHT is more potent and more biologically active than testosterone. Wolffian duct derivatives namely, epididymis, vas deferens and seminal vesicles are normally developed because these organs develop under the influence of testosterone. Urogenital sinus derivatives like prostate and membranous urethra are not well-developed because they are under the influence of DHT. Urethra opens into urogenital sinus giving appearance of hypospadias. Penile development is moderate because this is controlled by both testosterone and DHT. There is no facial hair indicating that facial hair is also under control of DHT. Majority have sexual ambiguity of external genitalia.

iv. Inadequacy of Leydig cell function (Jones, 1992): External genitalia are feminised; ambiguity of external genitalia will depend on the degree of Leydig cell inadequacy. Müllerian system is inhibited, because anti-müllerian hormone (AMH) is normal.

v. Familial gonadal destruction leading to deficiency of both testosterone and anti-Müllerian hormone has been reported in the literature (Park and Jones, 1970; Rios et al., 1974): These individuals had testes in embryonic life, but subsequently were destroyed by genetic influence. When seen in adult life, there is hardly any evidence of identifiable testis. They are 46XY individuals. Phenotype, appearance of external and internal genitalia depends on the time in embryonic life when testicular function was suppressed. Therefore, in these individuals, there may be müllerian remnants, ambiguity of external genitalia and the phenotype will be under-masculinised.

B. Feminised males or 46XY females

Individuals in this group have defect in target organ cellular response to testosterone, but normal response to anti-müllerian hormone. Common variety in this group is "testicular feminising syndrome".

Morris (1953) collected several cases from literature and added two of his own and coined the term "Testicular Feminising syndrome". Keenan et al. (1974) showed that the basic defect was an inability of the cytosol receptors to bind testosterone. Therefore, the target organs are unable to recognise testosterone and translate it into a biological reality. This is the reason why this syndrome is also known as "Androgen insensitivity syndrome". But the current view is that there are a number of different mutations in sex determining genes that may result in androgen insensitivity (Brown, 1986).

There are two subgroups of this syndrome

i. Majority in the first subgroup have external genitalia; typical feminine in appearance; breasts are well-developed. Pubic and axillary hairs are absent and gonads are externally palpable. Total absence of müllerian system is the characteristic finding but in a few cases we have found existence of müllerian tissue. In addition, we have also observed evidence of ovarian stromal cells and testicular seminiferous tubules or dysgenetic gonads (unpublished). In these cases, during laparoscopy, gonads are found within abdominal cavity. This category has been specially designated as "46XY sex reversed females".

ii. The other subgroup has typical ambiguous external genitalia with total absence of müllerian system. They have phallic enlargement with variable grades of urogenital sinus opening suppression. Pubic hairs though sparse are present. Breasts are usually absent, and if present are very ill-developed (incomplete variety of testicular feminising syndrome).

Based on these information, phenotype and external genitalia in male intersex can be broadly grouped as given in Flowchart 13.4.

In this chapter, we are more concerned with individuals who are born with typical or more towards female external genitalia. This group has been further subclassified as given in Flowchart 13.5.

Flowchart 13.4

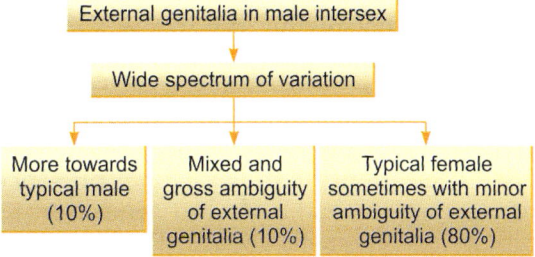

Table 13.1: Differences between complete (classic) and incomplete variety of testicular feminising syndrome

	Complete (classic)	*Incomplete (partial)*
Karyotype	46XY	46XY
Phenotype	Female	Female
Gonads	Testes (ectopic)	Testes (ectopic)
Müllerian system	Inhibited	Inhibited
Secondary sex characters	Well-developed	May not be well-developed
External genitalia	Typical female	Ambiguous
Vagina	Short blind	Usually blind (remnant of UGS)
Pubic and axillary hair	Absent	May be present

In the incomplete variety, secondary sex characters are not well-developed. Pubic and axillary hair may be present, which are totally absent in the complete variety. Moreover, in incomplete variety, external genitalia is more often ambiguous sometimes with suppression of vaginal opening. But an urogenital sinus opening always exists in this incomplete variety and vaginal reconstruction is possible.

Flowchart 13.5

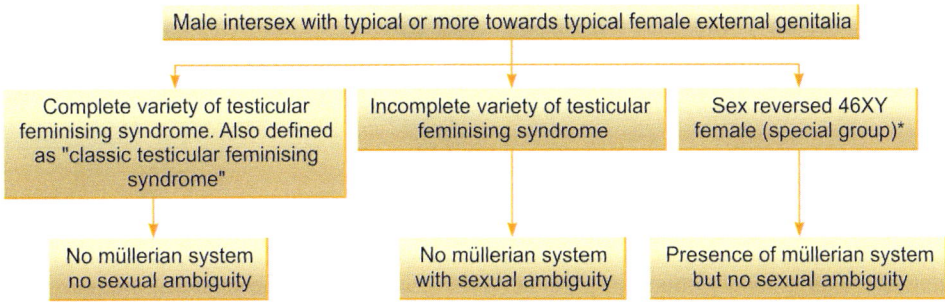

* This special group has been identified more in members of the same family and designated by us (in collaboration with Center for Cellular and Molecular Biology, Hyderabad) in the category of "46XY sex reversed female".

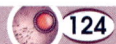

Tables 13.1 and 13.2 illustrate the differences amongst complete, incomplete varieties of testicular feminising syndrome and sex-reversed 46XY females.

In sex reversed 46XY females (Fig. 13.9), rudimentary to normal-sized uterus and tubes have been found with occasional presence of ovarian stromal cells and seminiferous tubules or dysgenetic gonads. They were not cases of true intersex because mosaicism either in peripheral blood or in gonads was not detected.

Background etiology

The basic defect leading to various clinical abnormalities in male intersex is due to either deletion or mutation of sex determining gene(s).

Table 13.2: Differences between classic testicular feminising syndrome and 'sex reversed' 46XY females

	Typical TFS	Sex reversed XY females
Karyotype	46XY	46XY
Phenotype	Feminine	Feminine
Secondary sex characters	Well-developed	Well-developed
External genitalia	Feminine	Feminine
Vagina	Short blind	Normal
Gonads	Testes (ectopic)	Ovaries, sometimes ovaries and testes (normal situation for ovaries)
Müllerian tissues	Absent	Present (uterus and tubes—usually rudimentary, sometimes normal in size)

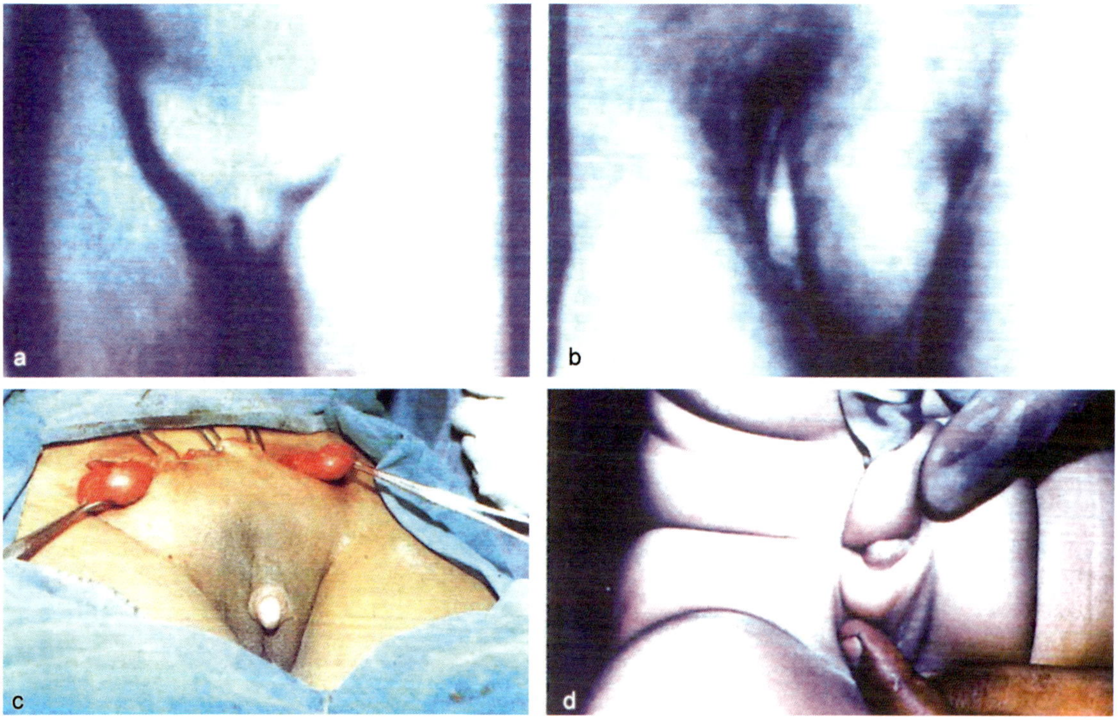

Figs 13.8a to d: (a) Complete variety of testicular feminising syndrome, typical feminine external genitalia, no pubic hair, bilateral inguinal gonads; (b) and (c) Incomplete variety of testicular feminising syndrome in two adolescent girls. Mildly enlarged phallus, labial gonad in (b) and bilateral inguinal gonads with markedly enlarged phallus in (c); (d) Another case of incomplete testicular feminising syndrome in child-bilateral labial gonads with phallic enlargement, larger than clitoris, but smaller than penis; karyotype 46XY

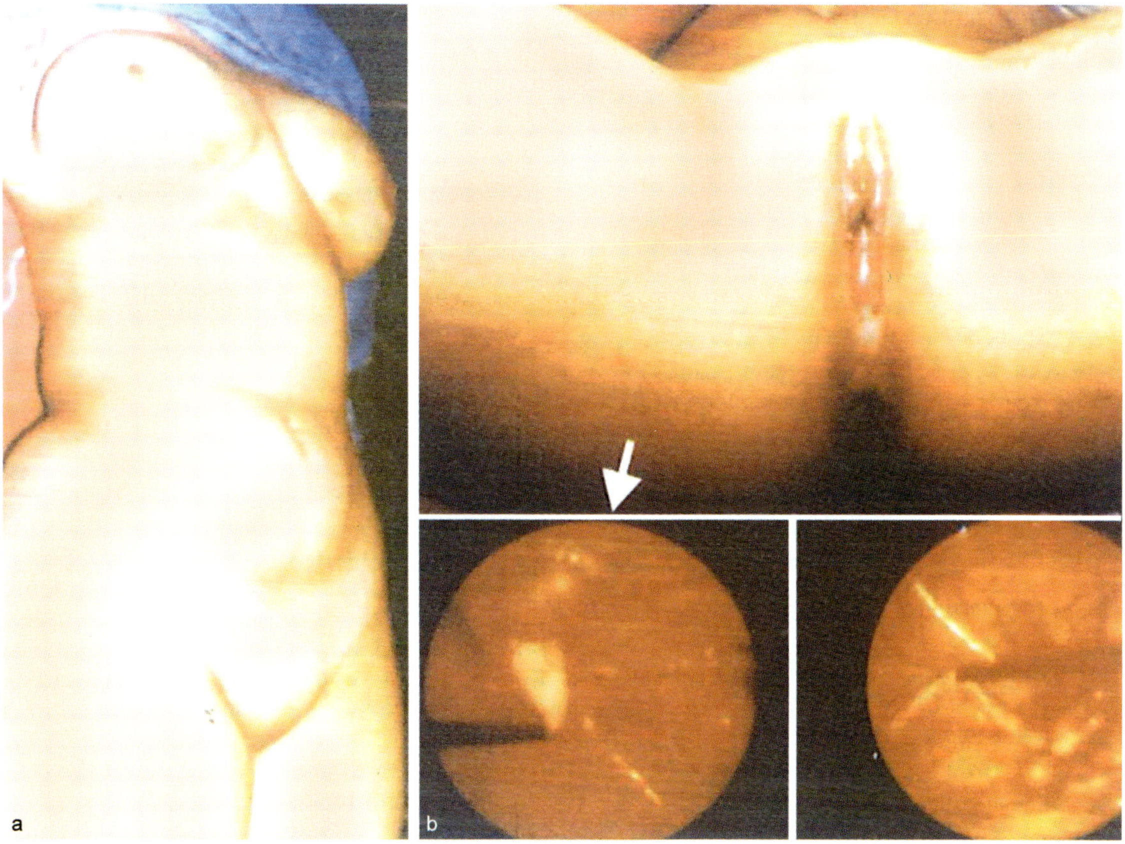

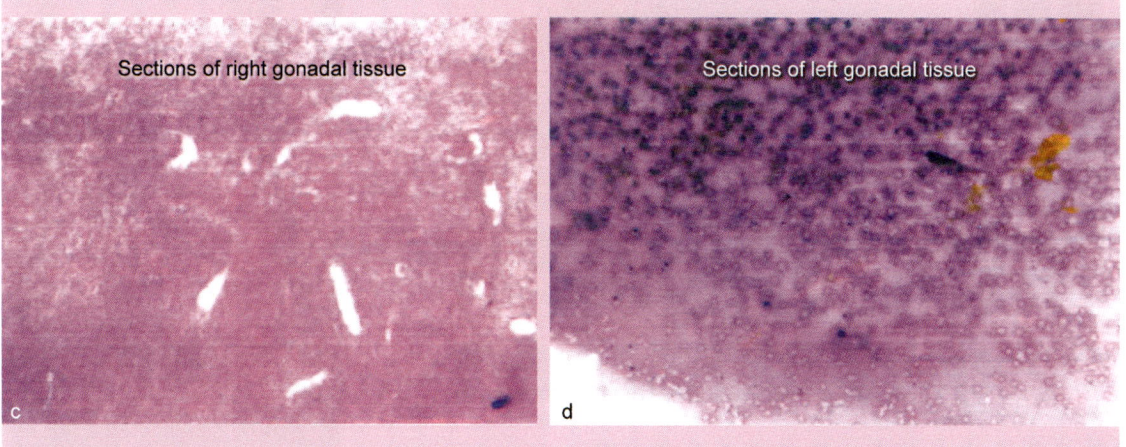

Figs 13.9a and b: (a) Phenotype of sex reversed 46XY females shows typical feminine external genitalia, absence of pubic hair with well developed breasts. (b) Inset shows laparoscopic view of internal genital organs. Biopsy revealed ovarian stroma on one side and seminiferous tubules containing Sertoli cells on the other side. Hypoplastic uterus is seen in the inset on the left side (marked by arrow)

Figs 13.9c and d: Histopathology report: (c) Sections of right gonadal tissue show histologic features compatible with ovarian stroma, (d) left sided gonadal tissue revealed occasional seminiferous tubule containing Sertoli cells only

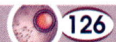

Sex-determining Genes

The following are the known sex-determining genes:

SRY, SOX3, SOX9, DSS, ZFY, TDF

Literature survey (Rubenstein and Mandel, 1993) reveals that in 46XY females, müllerian system is totally inhibited and the sex-determining gene is either deleted or mutated.

But our observation based on evaluation of 52 cases of 46XY females (testicular feminising syndrome, Table 13.3), suggested that:

i. Except in 3, in all other cases of 46XY females, these genes were intact
ii. In 13 cases, there was evidence of müllerian system and/or presence of ovaries (sometimes streak/dysgenetic gonads)
iii. They had no sexual ambiguity.

Table 13.3: Our observation (Jan 1999–Dec 2003)

Cases of XY ♀ studied at Institute of Reproductive Medicine, Calcutta and CCMB, Hyderabad, India

Total no.	52
Testicular feminisation	42
Sex reversed XY females	9
*XXY (female Klinefelter)	1

*(Published in Lancet, 1998)

In this group, there was one case of 47XXY female Klinefelter (Fig. 13.10) which has been reported for the first time in the world literature (Thangaraj et al., 1998).

46XY Sex Reversed Females

In the present study, we had 13 cases of so called "Testicular Feminising Syndrome" who had existence of müllerian system with evidence of dysgenetic gonads or presence of seminiferous tubules and ovarian stromal cells in their gonads. This specific group of feminising male intersex does not fall in the category of "typical or classic testicular feminising syndrome". We (in collaboration with Center for Cellular and Molecular Biology, Hyderabad) have, therefore, subgrouped them in a special category which has been designated as "46XY sex reversed female". Successful pregnancies have been reported in this group following ovum donation and IVF (Kan et al., 1997).

Figure 13.11 illustrates the family tree pattern of 3 families of the subgroup.

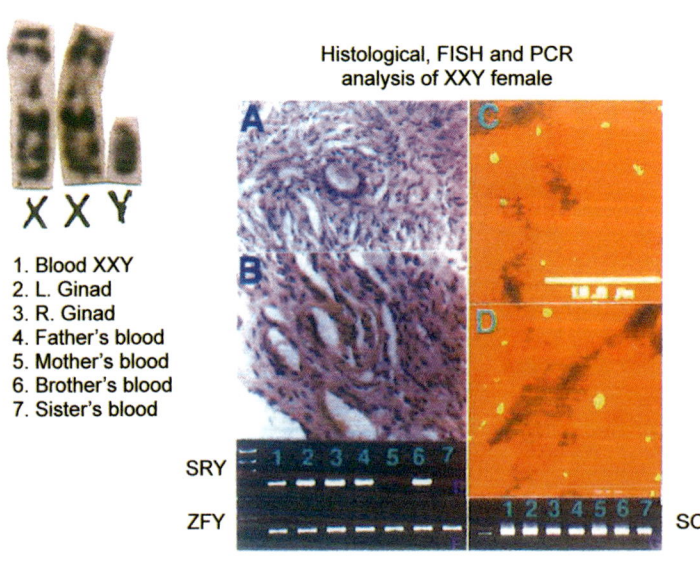

Histological, FISH and PCR analysis of XXY female

X X Y

1. Blood XXY
2. L. Ginad
3. R. Ginad
4. Father's blood
5. Mother's blood
6. Brother's blood
7. Sister's blood

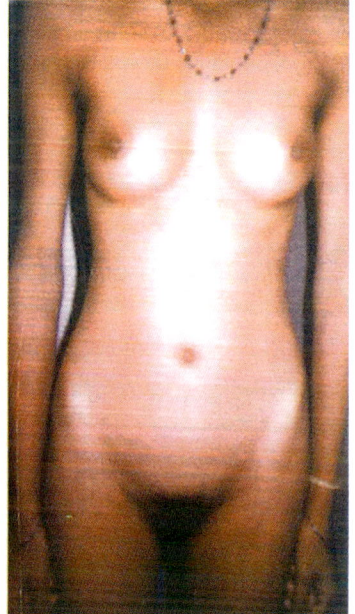

Fig. 13.10: A case of sex reversal (47XXY female Klinefelter) showing female secondary sex characters (Lancet, Vol. 352; 1998)

Figure 13.11 illustrates the proposed theory of inheritance of 46XY sex reversed female.

Figure 13.12 reveals that mother is the carrier of the affected gene. If the offspring is a female child, she becomes a carrier. If the offspring has 46XY component, then the child is affected as "sex reversed XY female".

Findings of current study on genetic background of 46XY female is as follows:

A marker loci has been observed by PCR technique in all cases, which is located on X chromosome. Size of this loci is still not determined and this could involve many genes. Depending on the mutation/deletion in these genes, there may be variety of

Three families of sex reversed XY females

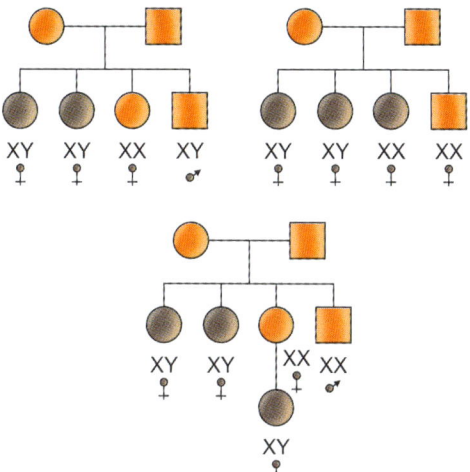

Fig. 13.11: Three families of sex reversed XY females

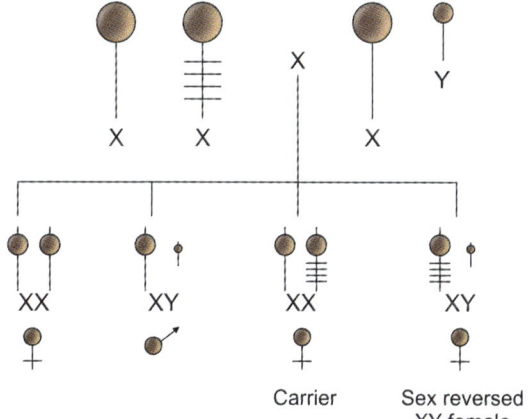

Carrier   Sex reversed
             XY female

Fig. 13.12: Proposed theory of inheritance of XY ♀

phenotypic differentiation in 46XY females like typical testicular feminising syndrome, incomplete variety of testicular feminisation with ambiguous genitalia and total sex reversed XY females with presence of müllerian system.

True Intersex

These patients form the rarest group accounting for less than 10% of all intersex disorders. Though majority of individuals reported as true intersex have been reared up as boys and men, the commonest chromosomal pattern is 46XX. The common chromosomal finding in true intersex is of great interest, as it is very rare proof that a testis can develop without an apparent Y chromosome. 10% have male genotype (46XY) and remaining are either mosaic (46XX/46XY) or chimeras with elements from two zygotes (Sivan and Reece, 1995). These individuals may have either an ovary on one side and testes on the other or an ovary opposite to an ovotestis on the contralateral side. Bilateral ovotestis may exist in 20% of true intersex, while 10% of patients may have ovary and testis or ovotestes on the same side and no gonad on the other side. Though in majority, sex of rearing is male, breast development and menstruation occur in substantial number of true intersex individuals. Those patients who are reared up as male will have external genitalia more towards male side and those reared up as female will have ambiguous external genitalia. In all individuals with true intersex, the internal genital organs are of mixed variety. Uterus and tubes are found on the side on which ovary is present. Uterus may sometimes be malformed with evidence of haematometra. Vas deferens and Seminiferous tubules are found on the side on which testis is present. This may not be always true specially in the presence of ovotestis. In these cases, remnants of müllerian and wolffian duct structures may exist on the same side.

Mixed Gonadal Dysgenesis

These patients have a phenotypic appearance of classic Turner's syndrome but with

ambiguous external genitalia. They have chromosomal mosaicism (45XO/46XY). Internal findings consist of streak gonad associated with ipsilateral fallopian tube and uterus with a contralateral dysgenetic testis.

Evaluation

Evaluation of ambiguous genitalia and sex assignment begins in the delivery room.

It will be a mistake to assign the sex casually immediately after birth. Because the hint of gender by the physician immediately after birth and then it been subsequently changed, may be harmful and disastrous for the family. Therefore, in the immediate neonatal period, gender-specific terms are to be avoided till the sex of rearing has been properly evaluated following collection of as many information as possible.

Evaluation, for assignment of appropriate sex of rearing, depends on following parameters:

   a. Physical examination

   b. Imaging: By ultrasonography, genitogram and MRI

   c. Chromosome analysis

   d. Biochemical assessment

Physical Examination

The presence or absence of externally palpable gonad helps in establishing a working diagnosis. Only a palpable gonad externally excludes female intersex and strongly suggests that the patient is either a male intersex or a true intersex.

Flowchart 13.6 illustrates the provisional diagnosis in individuals with ambiguous external genitalia based on palpation of at least one gonad externally.

Apart from gonads, other features of external genitalia have a similar appearance whether the condition is due to masculinisation of a female foetus or undermasculinisation of male or due to true intersex. The phallus may be too large for female and perhaps too small for a male. In case of doubt, therapeutic trial with injection of depot testosterone may be helpful. If size of phallus increases after depot

Flowchart 13.6

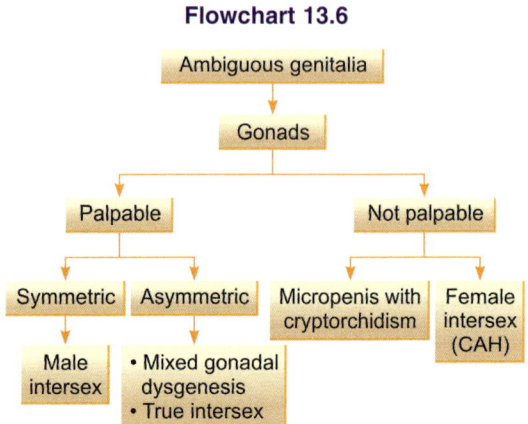

testosterone sex of rearing is male otherwise sex assignment is female with subsequent plan for female genitoplasty. The scrotum either looks like normal or fused labia. The urethra usually opens onto the perineum but may be prolonged along the ventral surface of the phallus (Fig. 13.13).

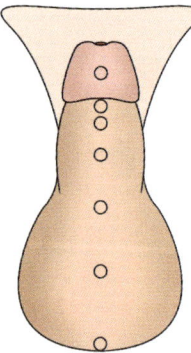

Fig. 13.13: Various potential locations for the urethral meatus in boys with hypospadias (*Adapted from Abnormalities of the External Genitalia; Zaontz and Packer, 1997*)

However, the exact diagnosis of the cause of sexual ambiguity based on physical examination alone may not be possible.

Hence additional information by imaging, Karyotype and biochemical assessments are essential.

Imaging

I. *Ultrasonography*

Ultrasonographic imaging helps in identifying internal genital organs like uterus and ovaries

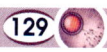

(Kutteh et al., 1995) and also enlarged adrenal glands in congenital adrenal hyperplasia (Wiener and Gonzales, 1996).

II. *Genitogram*

Sometimes there may be a single opening of urogenital sinus into which both vagina and urethra open. Genitogram can identify urethra and bladder and the level of entry of vagina and presence of other müllerian structures like cervix, uterus and fallopian tubes. This may help in planning female genitoplasty specially in congenital adrenal hyperplasia.

III. *Magnetic resonance imaging (MRI)*

Though a more expensive technology, MRI will be more useful for morphologic evaluation of internal organs (Secaf et al., 1994).

Chromosomal Analysis

Karyotype may help in confirmation of diagnosis of intersex, but does not necessarily help in identifying the sex of rearing. Nor does it help in deciding the type of surgical reconstruction required. Chromosomal findings, however, help in decision making regarding dysgenetic gonads and their risk of malignancies.

Appropriate Biochemical Assessment

This is essential specially in newborn with suspicion of congenital adrenal hyperplasia (CAH). Estimation of 17-hydroxyprogesterone (17-OHP) for confirmation of diagnosis and measurement of serum electrolytes are essential for immediate medical management, if necessary. The salt losing variety of AGS (adrenogenital syndrome) will have hyperkalaemia and hyponatraemia.

In some cases of male intersex, when decision has been taken in favour of feminising genitoplasty, measurement of serum testosterone before and after stimulation with human chorionic gonadotropin (hCG) may be helpful in establishing presence or absence of functional testicular tissue (Griffin and Wilson, 1992). If present, this organ is to be removed.

Practical Criteria for Assignment of Sex of Rearing

Hence, the decision of sex of rearing at the neonatal age depends on availability of as many of the above-mentioned information as possible. Of these, the following two criteria are of practical importance. The first criteria is whether gonads are externally palpable or not. As a general rule, when gonads are not palpable externally, the assigned sex of rearing should be female irrespective of other findings.

The second criteria is size of phallus. If it is more than 2.5 cm (except in CAH), sex of rearing should be male. In case of doubt as has already been suggested, therapeutic trial with depot testosterone is helpful.

Objectives of Surgical Correction

The following are the objectives of surgical correction:
   a. Acceptable gender assignment
   b. Better chance of coital function
   c. And if possible, improvement of reproductive potential.

Types of Surgery Performed

   a. Excision of unwanted genital organs and gonads
   b. Construction of external genitalia in the desired line of sex of rearing.

Timing of Surgery

This depends on the age of the individual at the time of first visit. If the child is seen in the neonatal period and the decision regarding sex of rearing has been confirmed, external genitalia should be constructed in the desired line of sex of rearing within 24 months of birth. This approach is likely to avoid psychological conflict and embarrassment for the child as well as for the family.

Following are the exceptions:
   a. Introitoplasty/vaginoplasty specially in CAH or incomplete variety of testicular feminising syndrome should be performed when child grows to the age of adolescence, for better exposure and handling.

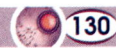

b. Gonadectomy—when the sex has been assigned as female like testicular feminising syndrome, testis should be removed in adolescence after secondary sex characters have developed.

c. Similarly, in true intersex, when sex has been assigned as male, mastectomy should be performed during adolescence. Because, in majority of true intersex reared up as male (46XX) breasts are well-developed.

Surgical Approach

This chapter primarily deals with surgical approach towards feminising genitoplasty. In fact majority of individuals with sexual ambiguity in intersex problems require feminising genitoplasty. Also feminising genitoplasty is a relatively simpler procedure than masculinising genitoplasty.

For better understanding of surgical approach it is worth while to describe briefly surgical anatomy in sexual ambiguity problems.

Surgical Anatomy

The nature of defect in the urogenital sinus derivatives are remarkably constant regardless of the etiology of the anomaly.

This will be clear when embryology of the genitalia is recalled. It is essential to remember that without a virilising factor, either from normal embryonic testis or from an abnormal virilising source as in congenital adrenal hyperplasia, the urogenital sinus develops in the female line. In the presence of a virilising source, there will be fusion of scrotolabial folds in such a manner that the vaginal opening is suppressed completely or concealed from the outside.

Vaginal communication is almost always in relation to caudal urogenital sinus derivatives (Fig. 13.14). This means that vagina communicates with that part of urogenital sinus which in male forms membranous part of urethra and in female this forms the vestibule. Vagina (müllerian duct) never communicates with that part of urogenital sinus which in male forms the prostatic urethra and in female forms the entire urethra (Bargy et

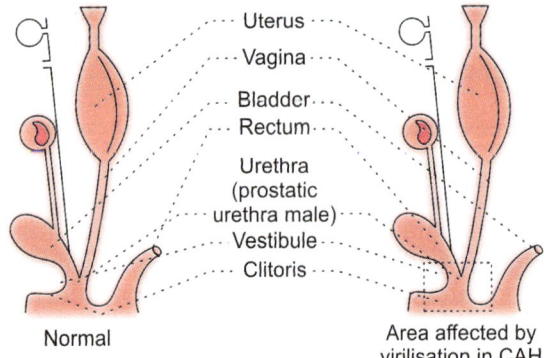

Fig. 13.14: Area affected by virilisation in CAH

al., 1989). This is of considerable surgical importance because anomalously persistent urogenital sinus may be boldly incised without apprehension of disturbing the urinary sphincteric continence.

With this knowledge of surgical anatomy, surgical correction of sexual ambiguity in different intersex problems are now briefly outlined.

Surgical Correction of Female Intersex: Commonest is Congenital Adrenal Hyperplasia (CAH)

Surgical correction consists of:

a. Phalloplasty

b. Introitoplasty or vaginoplasty.

In addition to surgical repair, all individuals with CAH require dexamethasone or hydro-cortisone throughout their life.

Phalloplasty

This can be performed in two ways:

i. Amputation

ii. Amputation of corpus and preservation of glans.

Amputation

Amputation of the phallus and reconstruction of the redundant part of the corpus to provide the shape for clitoris. Care should be taken not to injure the urethra, which lies just below the base of enlarged phallus (Figs 13.15a to c).

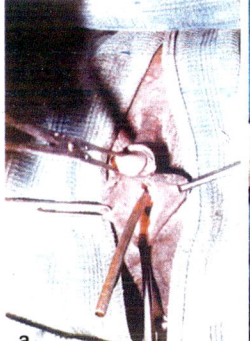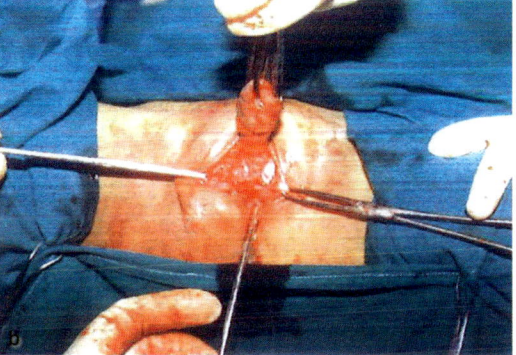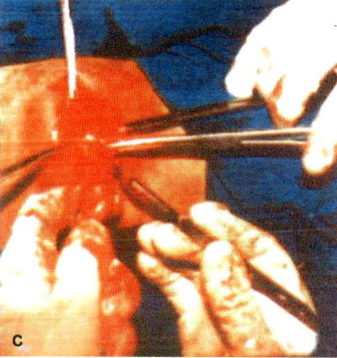

Figs 13.15a to c: (a) Enlarged phallus, urethra and vaginal opening are clearly visible. Metal catheter inside the bladder, (b) Elliptical incision; dissection of corpus, (c) Clamping and excision of phallus

Amputation of Corpus with Preservation of Glans (for Cosmetic Reasons)

The primary incision is same. A broad clitoral flap is preserved to maintain the blood supply of the glans. Shaft of the phallus is removed. The space from which corpus was removed is closed. This is followed by fixing the flap containing the preserved glans on the base of the shaft which has been left behind following removal of corpus (Fig. 13.16).

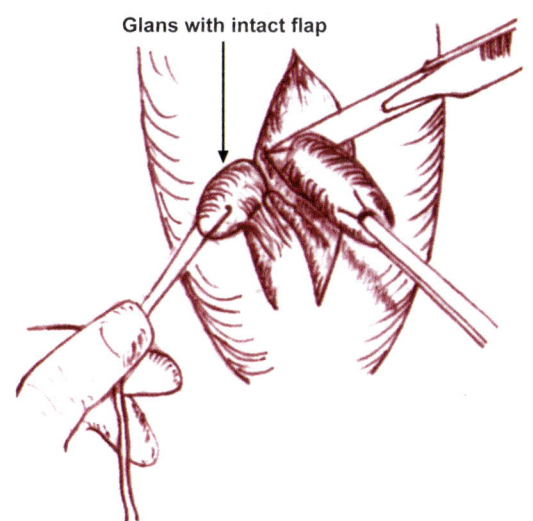

Glans with intact flap

Fig. 13.16: Amputation of corpus with preservation of glans (*Adapted and Modified from* "Female Reproductive Surgery"; (ed). Rock, Murphy and Jones, 1992)

Vaginoplasty

Vaginoplasty depends on the degree of virilisation. Because, in majority of individuals affected by CAH there will be a single opening of urogenital sinus, into which both urethra and vagina open. Depending on degree of virilisation, the sites of urethral and vaginal opening may be either easy or difficult to identify at the time of reconstructive surgery.

Type I

In this group, through a narrow common urogenital sinus opening, vaginal and urethral orifices are easily identified. The steps of operation are similar to those of Fenton's introitoplasty (Fig. 13.17a). In some cases there may be labial fusion which may conceal urethral and vaginal openings. The fused area is usually very thin and can be vertically incised under guidance of a probe or an artery forceps. The probe or artery forceps can be negotiated through anterior opening of fused labia (marked by arrow below the enlarged phallus, Fig. 13.17b). The hidden urethral and vaginal orifices are then clearly visible. A few interrupted stitches may be necessary to cover the raw edges of the incised portion. Additional introitoplasty may not be necessary.

Type II

In this group, vaginal and urethral orifices are difficult to locate due to more aggressive scrotolabial fusion. An operative endoscope may be used to identify separately the urethral and vaginal openings (Fig. 13.18).

Even without using an endoscope, the urogenital sinus can be enlarged by midline perineal incision after putting a double-gloved finger in the rectum. The urethral and

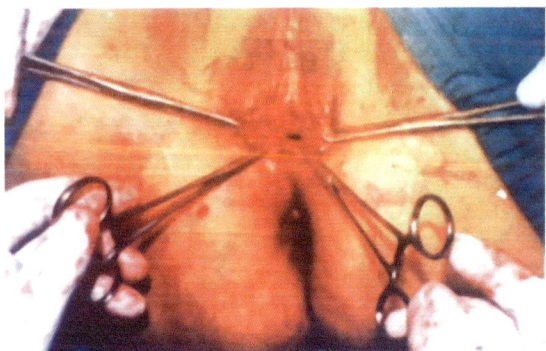

Fig. 13.17a: Vaginoplasty in CAH in an adolescent girl (vaginal and urethral orifices are easily identified); phalloplasty was performed at the age of 2 years in this girl

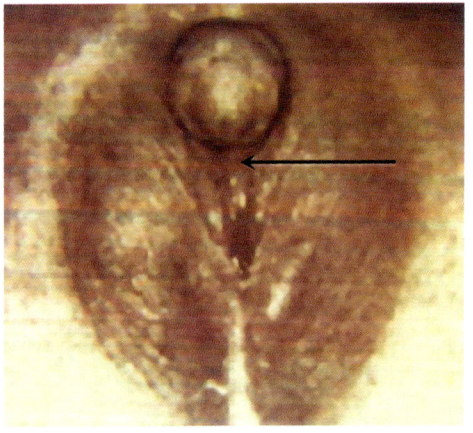

Fig. 13.17b: Fused labio scrotal fold conceals vaginal and urethral orifices but there is small opening below the enlarged phallus through which urine escapes

vaginal openings may then be seen separately. The vaginal mucous membrane is dissected to a variable distance upwards. Again keeping the double-gloved finger in the rectum, perineal muscles are incised in the midline followed by apposition of vaginal mucous membrane with skin.

Type III

Vagina remains imperforate, i.e. failure of communication between lower end of müllerian duct and caudal end of urogenital sinus. This is an extremely rare situation.

Abdomino-perineal approach has been recommended (Jones, 1992). The abdominal route of approach is either through laparotomy or through laparoscopy. We prefer open laparotomy. A sound or guide is to be negotiated through the uterus or through the cervix (following bladder dissection). The tip of the sound or guide after passing through cervix and upper vagina pushes the perineal skin and is palpated through perineum.

With the guide still in place the skin and underlying urogenital sinus, through the perineum, can be palpated and incised (marked by arrow in the diagram). Edges of vaginal epithelium, which can be identified, can be brought down and sutured to the perineal skin (Fig. 13.19).

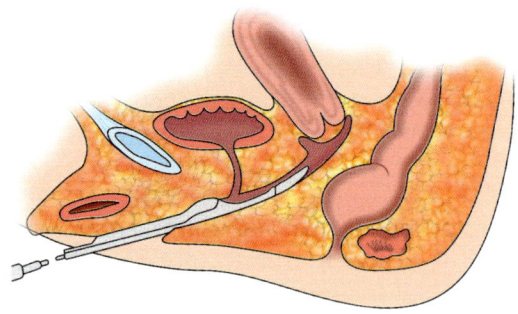

Fig. 13.18: Vaginal and urethral orifices are difficult to identify. This can be identified with endoscope or through midline perineal incision after placing a double-gloved finger in rectum (*Adapted and Modified from* "Female Reproductive Surgery". Ed. Rock, Murphy and Jones, 1992)

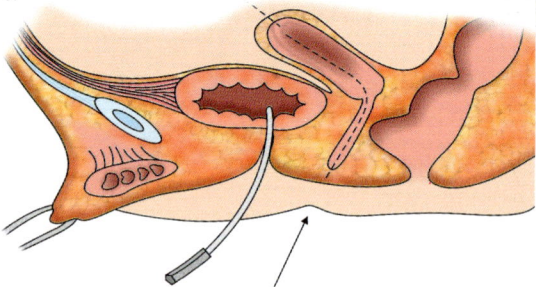

Fig. 13.19: Vagina is imperforate (very rare situation). A guide is negotiated through fundus after laparotomy or laparoscopy. The guide pushes urogenital sinus and perineal skin (marked by arrow). This is the point of incision of perineal skin. Through this incision, vaginal mucous membrane can be brought down and sutured to perineal skin. (*Adapted and Modified from* "Female Reproductive Surgery"; (Ed.) Rock, Murphy and Jones, 1992)

Obviously such operation can only be performed in the adolescent age when uterus and cervix have become reasonably big in size.

Surgical Approach in Male Intersex

It has already been described that, in nearly 80% of male intersex, phenotype is feminine (46XY females—testicular feminising syndrome). Sex of rearing is also in the female line and external genitalia is typically feminine. Therefore, majority do not require surgical correction of external genitalia. A small group (incomplete variety of testicular feminising syndrome) may have ambiguity of external genitalia with phallic enlargement. They require surgical correction of enlarged phallus as has been described in the section of congenital adrenal hyperplasia. Vaginoplasty in these individuals may not be that easy as in congenital adrenal hyperplasia. They do not have müllerian system; but certainly they have an urogenital sinus below the orifice of external urethral meatus. This can be widened surgically up to a depth of 2.5 to 4 cm and subsequently, the length can be increased by regular use of a plastic mould. However, in all these cases, gonads are testes and gonadectomy should be performed after the age of puberty (Fig. 13.20). Oestrogen substitution is essential for a few years.

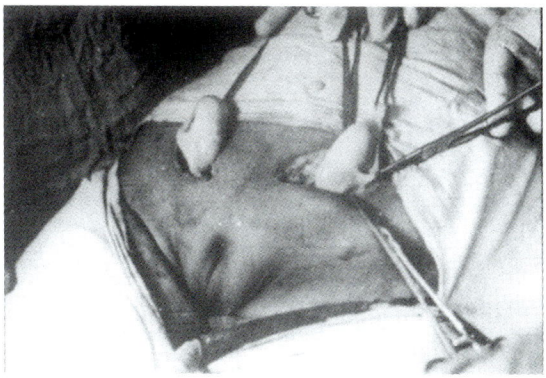

Fig. 13.20: Complete variety of testicular feminising syndrome—feminine external genitalia—no pubic hair, ectopic gonads are testes: Gonadectomy is being performed

The second group consisting of 10% individuals are reared up as males and external genitalia are more towards male (under-masculinised males). This group consists of those who may have Leydig cell insufficiency or deficiency of anti-müllerian hormone. They may have remnants of müllerian tissue either in abdomen or in inguinal region. These organs are to be removed.

The third group of male intersex (10%) may exhibit evidence of sexual ambiguity. Surgical correction depends on length of phallus primarily and secondarily on sex of rearing. Phallus size more than 2.5 cm indicates a male genitoplasty while size less than 2.5 cm is the indication for female genitoplasty. If the size is doubtful, depot testosterone may be used as therapeutic trial. If the response is adequate, male genitoplasty is considered. If inadequate, female genitoplasty should be the surgical approach.

The entire plan of surgical approach for sexual ambiguity in male intersex can be outlined in Flowchart 13.7.

True Intersex

Surgical approach in true intersex is more or less similar to those of male intersex. This includes removal of contradictory organs and reconstructing the external genitalia in keeping with the sex of rearing. Majority of these individuals are reared up as males with average to normal penile development (may be with minor grade of hypospadias) with unilateral testis located anywhere between the deep inguinal ring and scrotum (Fig. 13.21).

However, in this group there may be a problem in some cases during surgery and that is to establish the characteristic of the gonad. This refers to ovotestis where recognition by gross morphologic characteristic may be inaccurate. At the time of exploration, a biopsy as well as bisection of the gonad should be made and inspected so as not to miss the contradictory gonad.

Mixed Gonadal Dysgenesis

These individuals have a Y chromosome with streak gonad on one side and dysgenetic testis on the other side.

Flowchart 13.7: Surgical approach to male pseudohermaphroditism.

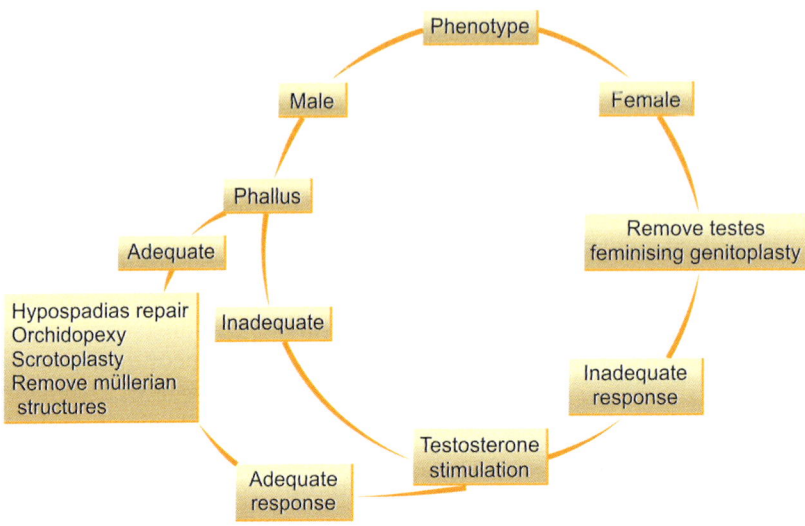

(*Adapted from* Abnormalities of the External Genitalia, Zaontz and Packer, 1997)

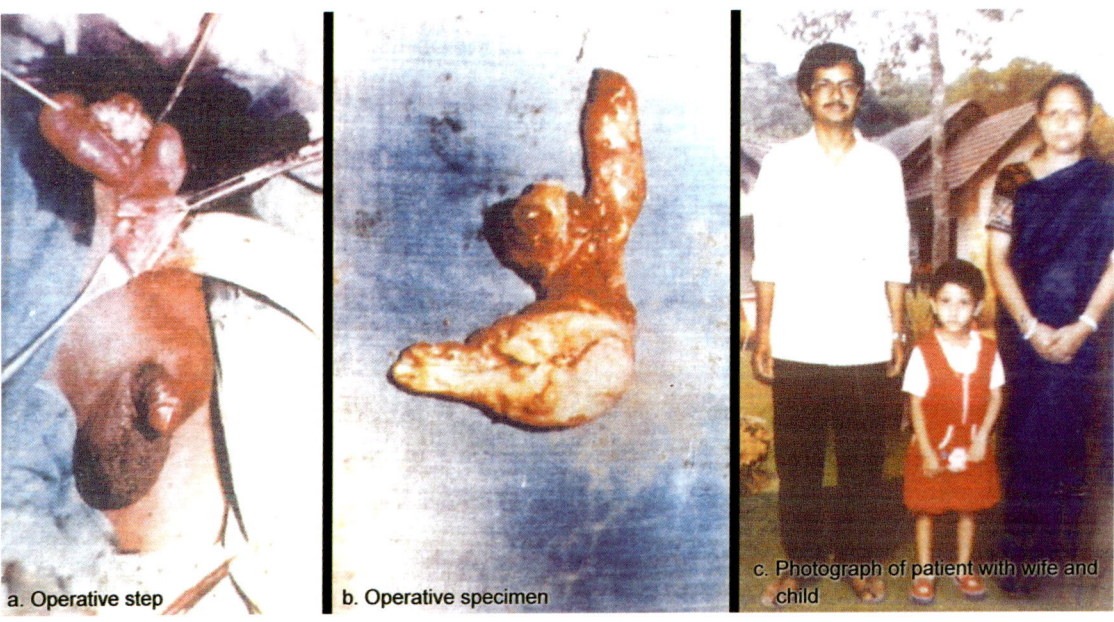

a. Operative step

b. Operative specimen

c. Photograph of patient with wife and child

Figs 13.21a to c: True intersex: Surgical removal of unwanted genital organs; uterus, unilateral tube (hydrosalpinx) and ovary. The individual was reared up as male with male external genitalia, unilateral testis, the other scrotal sac was empty. He presented at the age of 22 with periodic haematuria. He had history of mastectomy at the age of 14, and reconstructive surgery of genital organs at the age of 23. Subsequently married and got a child by AID

Conventional treatment is gonadectomy to avoid risk of malignancy with sex organ reconstructed in the female line. Very rarely some of them have been reconstructed as boys with testes left in place, but they need very careful monitoring (Sivan et al., 1995).

Summary

Sexual ambiguity, though rare, is a challenging clinical problem. Identification of exact etiology and correct management often becomes problematic and embarrassing. Commonest cause of sexual ambiguity encountered in clinical practice is due to congenital adrenal hyperplasia (female intersex) followed by testicular feminising syndrome (male intersex). True intersex and mixed gonadal dysgenesis are rare observations. The objectives of surgical correction are primarily to assign the appropriate sex of rearing and secondarily to offer the scope of coital, and if possible, the reproductive function. In addition, unwanted organs and undesirable (which may be harmful) gonads are to be removed.

FURTHER READING

1. Allen TD. Disorders of sexual differentiation: In Kelalis KP, King LR, Belman BA (eds); Clinical pediatric urology, ed. 2 Philadelphia, WB Saunders, P 904, 1985.

2. Bargy F, Lande F, Barbet JP and Houtte A. The anatomy of intersexuality. Surg Radiol Anant 11: 103–107, 1985.

3. Blyth B and Churchill BM. Intersex. In Gillenwater JY, Grayhack JT, Howrads SS, et al. (eds). Adult and pediatric Urology, ed-3. St Louis, CV mosby, P-2591, 1996.

4. Bongiovanni AM. Unusual steroid pattern in Congental adrenal hyperplasia: Deficiency of 3-hydroxydehydrogenase. J Clin Endocrinol Metab 21: 860–862, 1961.

5. Brown TR, Migeon CJ. Androgen receptors and abnormal male sexual differentiation. Adv Exp Med Biol; 196: 227–255, 1986.

6. Cravioto MD, Ulloa-Aguirre A, Bermudez JA, et al. A new inherited variant of the 3-hydroxysteroid dehydrogenase-isomerase deficiency syndrome evidence for existence of two isoenzymes. J Clin endoe Metab 63: 360–367, 1986.

7. Degenhart HJ, Visser HKA, Boon H, et al. Evidence for dificient 20-cholesterol-hydroxylase activity in adrenal tissue of patients with lipoid adrenal hyperplasia. Acta Endocrinol 71: 512–518, 1972.

8. Donahoe PK. The diagnosis and treatment of infants with intersex abnormalities, Pediatric Clin North Am 34: 1333, 1987.

9. Federman Dd, Donahoe PK. Ambiguous genitalia: Etiology, diagnosis and therapy ADV Endocrinol Metab 6: 91, 1995.

10. Griffin JE, Wilson JD. Disorder of sexual differentiation. In Walsh PC, Retik AB, Stamey TA, et al (eds). Campbell's Urology, ed 6. Philadelphia, WB Saunders, P-1509, 1992.

11. Imperato-Mcginley J, Gautier T, Peterson RE, et al. The prevalence of 5-reductase deficiency in children with ambiguous genitalia in the Dominican Republic. J Urol; 136: 867–873, 1986.

12. John AR, Murphy AA, Jones Jr. HW, Female Reproductive Surgery, Williams and Wikins, p 311, 1992.

13. Kan AK, Abdalla HI, Oskarsson T. Two successful pregnancies in a 46XY patient; Hum Reprod (1997) Jul; 12(7): 143–5.

14. Keenan BS, Meyer WJ III, Hadian AJ, et al.: Syndrome of androgen insensitivity in man: Absence of 5 alpha-dihydrotestosterone binding protein in skin fibroblasts; The Journal of Clinical Endocrinology and Metabolism; Volume 38, Issue 6 (1974).

15. Kutteh WH, Santos-Ramos R, Eramel LD: Accuracy of ultrasonic detection of the uterus in normal newborn infants: implication for infants with ambiguous genitalia. Ultrasound obstet Gynecol: 5: 109, 1995.

16. Mercado AB, Wilson RC, Cheng KC, Wei J-Q. New MI. Prenatal treatment and diagnosis of congenital adrenal hyperplasia owing to steroid 21-hydroxylase deficiency. J. Clin Endocrinol Metab 80: 2014, 1995.

17. Meyer-Bahlburg HF, Green RS, New MI, Bell JJ, Morishima A. Shimshi M, Bueno Y, Vargas I, Baker SW. Gender Change from female to male in classical congenital adrenal hyperplasia, Horn Behav 30: 319–1996.

18. Morris JM. Syndrome of testicular feminisation in male pseudohermaphrodites. Am J. Obstet Gynecol 1953; 65: 1192–1211.

19. Mulaikal RM, Migeon CJ, Rock JA. Fertility rates in female patients with congenital adrenal hyperplasia due to 21 hydroxylase deficiency, New Engl J Med 316: 178, 1987.

20. Pang S, Clark AT, Freeman LC, Dolan LM, Immken L, Mueller OT, Stiff D, Shueman DI, Maternal Side effects of prenatal dexamethasone therapy for foetal congenital adrenal hyperplasia. J Clin Endocrinol Metab 75: 249, 1992.

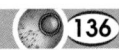
21. Park IJ, Aimakhu VE, Jones HW Jr. An etiologic and pathogenetic classification of male hermaphroditism. Am J obstet gynecol; 123: 505–518, 1975.

22. Park IJ, Jones HW Jr. Familial male hermaphrodite with ambiguous external genitalia. Am J obstet Gynecol; 108: 1197–1205, 1970.

23. Reindoller RH, Lewis JB, White PC, Fernhoff PM, McDonough PG, Whitney III JB: Prenatal diagnosis of 21-hydroxylase deficiency by the omplementary deoxyribonucleic acid probe for cytochrome P-450C 210 H, Am Jobstet Gynecol 158: 545, 1988.

24. Rios EP, Herrera J, bermudez JA. Endocrine and metabolic studies in an XY Patient with gonadal agenesis. J Clin Endocrinol Metabl 39: 540–547, 1974.

25. Rubenstein SC, Mandell J: Ambiguous genitalia in newborns. Contemporary pediatrics 10: 83, 1993.

26. Siler-khodr TM, Morgenstern LL, Greenwood FC. Hormone synthesis and release from human fetal adenohypophysis in vitro. J Endocrine Metab 39: 891–905, 1974.

27. Sivan E, Koch S, Reece EA. Sonographic Prenatal diagnosis of ambiguous genitalia: Fetal Diagnosis and Therapy 10: 311, 1995.

28. Secaf E, Hricak H, Gooding CA: Role of MRI in the evaluation of ambiguous genitalia. Pediatr Radiol 24: 231, 1994.

29. Thangaraj K., Gupta N. J., Chakravarty B.N. and Singh L.: A 47XXY female; the lancet: 352, 3, 1121, 1998.

30. Wiener JS, Gonzales ET. Intersex, curr opin Urol 6: 320, 1996.

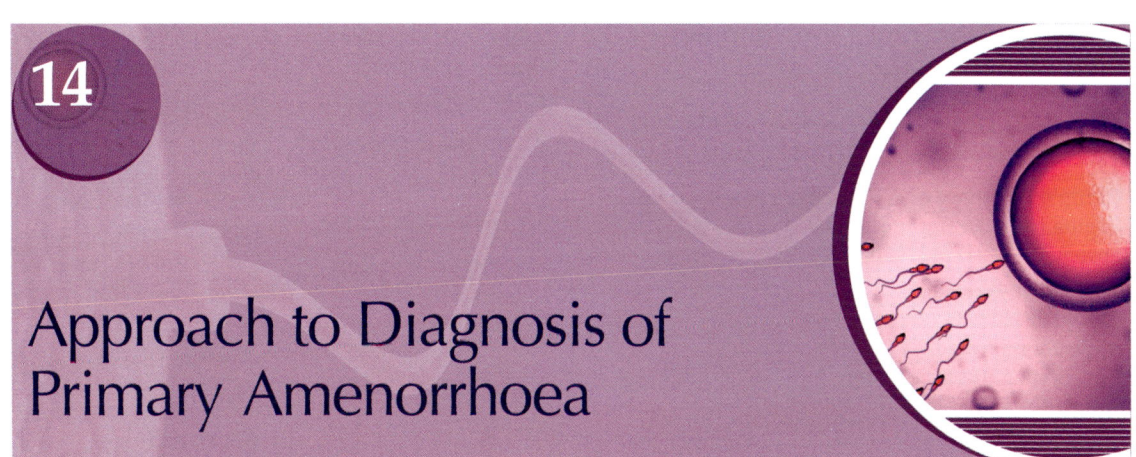

14

Approach to Diagnosis of Primary Amenorrhoea

INTRODUCTION

Girls have experienced menarche at increasingly younger ages during the past century and age limitations defining primary amenorrhoea have been lowered. Primary amenorrhoea is now defined as absence of menses at the age of 13 years when there is no visible secondary sexual characteristic development or age of 15 years in the presence of normal secondary sexual characteristics.[1]

During evaluation of a girl with primary amenorrhoea, physicians should conduct a comprehensive patient history and a thorough physical examination.[2–4]

In an apparently normal looking girl (with secondary sexual characteristics) presenting with primary amenorrhoea the initial clinical investigation suggested is the test for withdrawal bleeding either with medroxy-progesterone acetate or with combination of oestrogen-progesterone pills. Additional investigation consists of abdominal ultrasound scan for presence and size of uterus and ovaries.

Basic Factors Involved in Onset and Continuation of Normal Menstruation

A complex hormonal interaction must take place for normal menstruation to occur. The primary stimulus for triggering pubertal manifestations including menarche comes from coordinated functioning of an intact hypothalamic-pituitary-ovarian (HPO) axis.

In addition to HPO axis, there are other factors as well contributing to onset and continuation of menstrual cycles from puberty to menopause. Menstruation is one of the clinical landmarks of onset of puberty. Initiation of menstruation at puberty is known as 'menarche'. Defect in one or more than one of these factors is responsible for either primary or secondary amenorrhoea. The factors are:

a. Anatomical patency of genital tract
b. Normal female chromosomal pattern (46XX)
c. Coordinated hypothalamic-pituitary-ovarian axis
d. Active support by two other endocrine glands namely, adrenal cortex and thyroid
e. Responsive endometrium, e.g. absence of endometrium or uterine synechiae may be responsible for primary or secondary amenorrhoea.

These factors are discussed in further detail.

Anatomical Patency of Genital Tract

The specific defects of genital tract which may cause amenorrhoea is an obstruction located in the lower genital tract usually in the vagina and cervix. Outflow obstruction of menstrual blood is associated with cryptomenorrhoea. Rarely true amenorrhoea has also been observed with lower müllerian duct obstruction. The types of defect and the probable diagnosis of either true amenorrhoea

or cryptomenorrhoea are summarised in Table 14.1.

Table 14.1: Types of defect and probable diagnosis

Types of defect	Probable diagnosis
Complete absence of vagina (functioning uterus absent)	True amenorrhoea
Transverse septum, partial absence of vagina, imperforate hymen (functioning uterus present)	Cryptomenorrhoea
Annular constriction upper 1/3rd of vagina with cervical stenosis	True amenorrhoea
Imperforate hymen	Cryptomenorrhoea

Further details of each type of defect have been described in subsequent sections of this chapter (*see* Table 14.4).

Chromosomal and Hypothalamic-Pituitary-Ovarian Axis Defect

There are two types of chromosomal defect which can cause primary amenorrhoea—(a) Turner's syndrome and its variants (mosaicism) and (b) testicular feminising syndrome (46XY females—androgen insensitivity syndrome).

Similarly, hypothalamic-pituitary-ovarian axis defect may exist either in the: (a) central nervous system (CNS), (b) ovaries or (c) dysregulation in the feedback mechanism amongst hypothalamic-pituitary-ovarian axis. Table 14.2 briefly describes the types of these defects.

Adrenocortical thyroid Defects and Unresponsive Endometrium

The specific defects related to adrenocortical anomalies are: (a) Congenital adrenal hyperplasia (CAH) and (b) Cushing's syndrome, whereas that involving thyroid gland responsible for primary amenorrhoea is cretinism or primary congenital hypothyroidism. Subclinical hypothyroidism is not responsible for primary amenorrhoea.

Endometrial defects leading to absence of menstruation are: (a) Congenital receptor

Table 14.2: Chromosomal and hypothalamic-pituitary-ovarian axis defect

Pathological lesions	Diagnosis
Abnormal chromosomal pattern	Turner's syndrome with variants Testicular feminising syndrome (46XY female)
Hypothalamic-pituitary-ovarian axis defect	Defect in CNS—may be of two types: (a) Functional (b) Organic, Genetic (Kallmann's), Hypogonadotropism, PCOS, androgen Producing tumours in ovary

defect and (b) Uterine synechiae—the commonest cause in our country is tubercular synechiae. Table 14.3 illustrates the cause-effect relationship of these anomalies.

Table 14.3: Adrenocortical thyroid defects and unresponsive endometrium

Pathological lesions	Diagnosis
Dysfunction of thyroid and adrenal cortex	Adrenogenital syndrome Cushing's disease Cretinism
Unresponsive or absent endometrium	Congenital receptor defect Uterine synechiae—tubercular

Lower Müllerian Duct Anomalies Leading to Primary Amenorrhoea

In the category of genital tract defect, lower müllerian duct (cervical and vaginal) anomalies are the commonest causes of primary amenorrhoea. This section requires an elaborate description and a separate classification.

The classification which is being presented here is based on therapeutic prognosis. Lower müllerian duct malfunctioning is commonly associated with simultaneous anomalies of internal genital organs as well. For example, complete absence of vagina is usually associated with agenesis or dysgenesis of the entire müllerian system. This suggests that these girls have true amenorrhoea. On the other hand, partial vaginal agenesis or

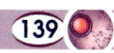

septum in the vagina is associated with the presence of a normally functioning uterus. Obviously these girls have cryptomenorrhoea. This differentiation has a considerable impact on outcome of therapeutic approach. The objectives of therapeutic approach in these girls are basically to restore: (a) Menstrual function, (b) reproductive function and (c) sexual function.

In the first variety (complete absence of vagina and a non-functioning uterus only müllerian knobs) surgical correction may only restore sexual function, but not the menstrual and reproductive functions, whereas in the second and third varieties (vaginal malformation with a functioning uterus) with proper patient selection and skilled expertise all the three functions can be reasonably reestablished.

The specific types of müllerian anomalies described above, clinical diagnosis and coexisting malformations of internal genital organs are given in detail in Table 14.4.

Therapeutic Approach of Vaginal Anomalies with Primary Amenorrhoea

From therapeutic outcome point of view we have made a new classification of vaginal malformations. Vaginal malformation has been classified in two broad groups: (a) Obstructive and (b) non-obstructive. In this chapter, we only present the obstructive varieties of vaginal malformations leading either to true amenorrhoea or crytomenorrhoea.

The classifications have already been described in the previous section of this chapter. The following paragraphs highlight the specific surgical approach in the different types of vaginal malformations.

i. **Group A:** Complete absence of vagina and uterus (Mayer-Rokitansky-Küster-Hauser syndrome—MRKH syndrome). In this group, only vaginoplasty is possible. Different approaches have been discussed in the literature. Our preference is vaginal approach. Only sexual function can be restored. Recently surrogacy is being advocated after marriage. The anatomical abnormalities of external and internal genital organs are presented in Figs 14.1a and b.

The details of surgical correction have been presented in some other chapter of this book.

ii. **Group B:** Complete absence of vagina, but with a functioning uterus. This is a small subgroup of Group A. Because with complete absence of vagina, only 5% women have a functioning uterus resulting in haematometra. In this group also, preservation of menstrual and reproductive function in addition to sexual function may be possible. The problem is that, in addition to complete

Table 14.4: Types of müllerian anomalies

Types of malformation	Clinical diagnosis	Coexisting abnormalities
Complete absence of vagina	True amenorrhoea	Functioning uterus absent; two solid müllerian knobs connected by fibromuscular band; fallopian tubes normal, gonads are ovaries. Otherwise normal female (46XX) very rarely (5%), they have a functioning uterus—leading to haematometra
Transverse septum of vagina	Haematocolpos and haematometra	Functioning uterus may be normal or malformed (bicornuate); cervix, tubes and ovaries normal
Partial agenesis of upper part of vagina	Haematometra only	Functioning uterus may be normal or malformed, cervix is ill developed, cord like and non-canalized
Annular constriction of upper part of vagina	Isthmial stenosis	

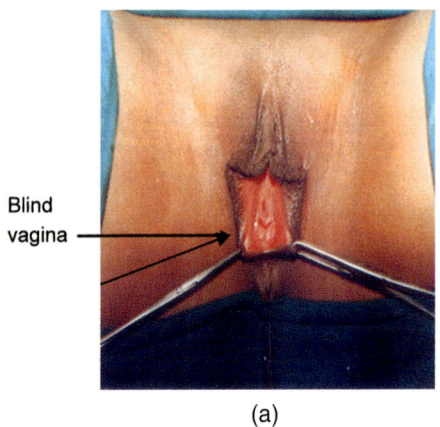

Blind vagina

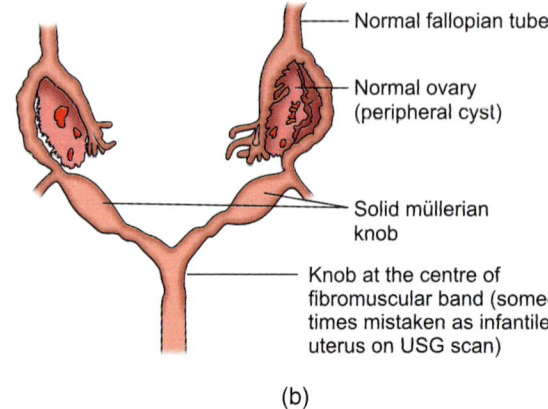

Normal fallopian tube

Normal ovary (peripheral cyst)

Solid müllerian knob

Knob at the centre of fibromuscular band (sometimes mistaken as infantile uterus on USG scan)

(a)

(b)

Figs 14.1a and b: *Group A*: Blind vagina with absence of functioning uterus—two müllerian knobs on either side connected by fibromuscular band—tubes and ovaries normal

vaginal atresia, the cervix is also stenosed. Cervical reconstruction and prevention of restenosis becomes difficult following reconstructive surgery.

The approach of cervicovaginoplasty consists of simultaneous abdominal and vaginal route. Currently, we have been performing a modified version of this surgery with laparoscopy-guided vaginal approach. Details have been described in some other chapter (Fig. 14.2).

iii. **Group C:** Agenesis of upper third of vagina and cervix with a normal functioning uterus (haematometra). This group resembles the previous one, with

the difference that vagina is partially occluded. The operative steps, outcome and the difficulties are similar to those which have been mentioned in Group B. (Fig. 14.3).

iv. **Group D:** Agenesis of only the lower third of the vagina (colpohaematometra) (Fig. 14.4). This is relatively a commoner type of malformation than the previous types. Only septal resection by either vaginal approach or abdominovaginal approach (when the septum is thick) may correct the specific defect and bring about the normal functions. The procedure is relatively easier than in the other variety. (Fig. 14.4).

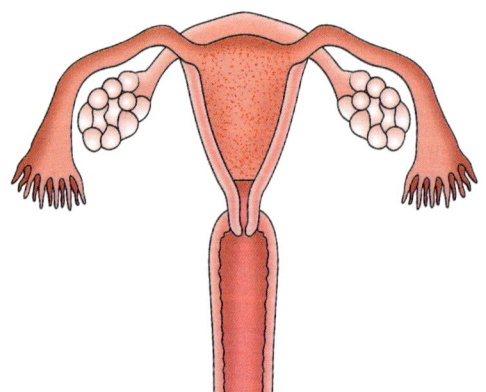

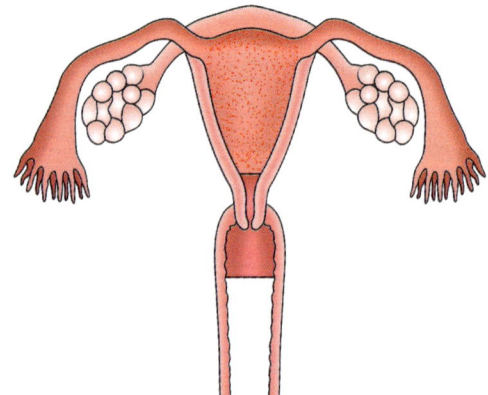

Fig. 14.2: *Group B*: Complete absence of vagina, but with a functioning uterus (haematometra). Cervicovaginoplasty; abdominovaginal approach

Fig. 14.3: *Group C*: Agenesis of upper 1/3rd of vagina and cervix (haematometra). Cervicovaginoplasty; abdominovaginal approach

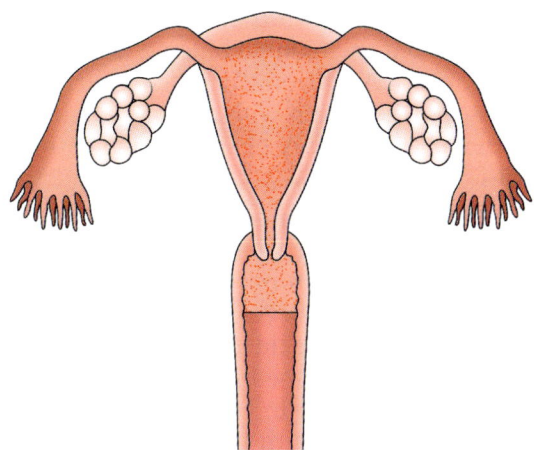

Fig. 14.4: *Group D*: Agenesis of only lower part of vagina (colpohaematometra). Septal resection—vaginoplasty; vaginal or abdominovaginal approach

v. **Group E:** Transverse septum of vagina—the defect is similar to the previous one, but the approach of surgical treatment may be difficult. This is because the obstructing membrane is situated at a higher level and approachability and visualisations during surgical correction may be difficult. However, currently with laparoscopic guidance this problem may be simplified to some extent. It is reemphasised that the correct timing and skill of surgery are both essential for the final outcome of the therapeutic approach. (Fig. 14.5).

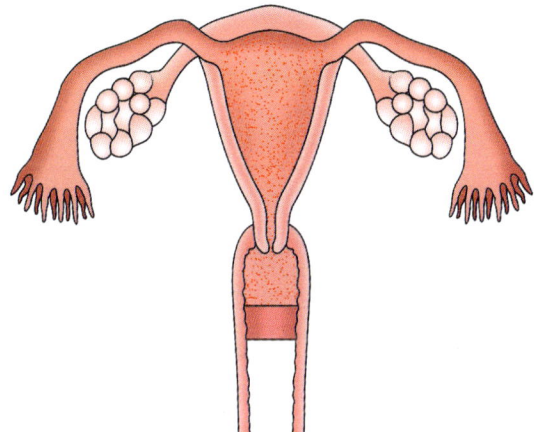

Fig. 14.5: *Group E*: Transverse septum of vagina (colpohaematometra). Septal resection—vaginoplasty; vaginal or abdominovaginal approach

vi. **Group F:** Isolated cervical atresia (Fig.14.6) with haematometra—this is the rarest type of malformation encountered amongst all types of cervicovaginal atresia. Correction is always performed by abdominovaginal approach. Though vaginal approach may be tempting, but invariably there is a risk of creation of a false passage. Hence it is always advisable to have an abdominovaginal approach or a vaginal approach under laparoscopic guidance. The most common problem following this type of surgery is restenosis leading to formation of haematometra and haematosalpinx resulting in pelvic peritonitis. Therefore, in recurrent restenosis it is always advisable to perform hysterectomy.

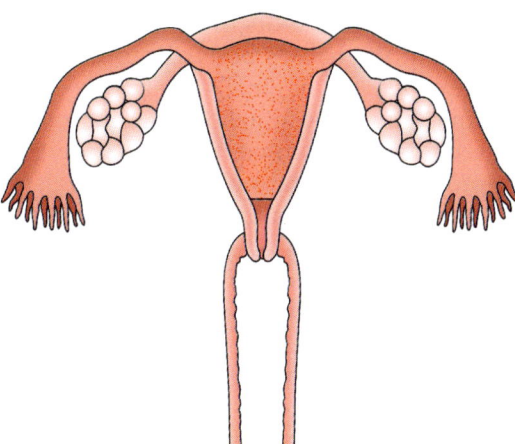

Fig. 14.6: *Group F*: Isolated cervical atresia

Differential Diagnosis of Absence of Vaginal Opening

Many anxious mothers observe the absence of vaginal opening in their young daughters and bring it to the notice of physicians usually between the age of 2 and 7 years.

The causes of such abnormality in the child may be: (a) Labial adhesion—due to low grade chronic vulvitis, (b) labial fusion—may be due to congenital adrenal hyperplasia (CAH) or incomplete variety of testicular

feminising syndrome, (c) imperforate hymen and (d) complete absence of vagina.

Labial adhesion (Fig. 14.6) is commonly due to low grade vulval infection. The consequent vulvitis leads to labial skin adhesion leaving behind a small opening which is seen at the upper fused end of labia majora. This is the common opening for urethra and vagina (urogenital sinus) through which the urine escapes. Low grade infection in these small girls occurs with sudden withdrawal of maternal oestrogen. Oestrogen in the newborn girl babies is derived from the mother and continues to persist till she is between 6 months and 2 years. Oestrogen induces production of glycogen from the vaginal epithelium. The glycogen is converted to lactic acid by Döderlein's bacillus, a normal inhabitant of vagina. The lactic acid thus produced makes the vaginal secretion acidic which prevents the occurrence of any infection. After the age of 2 years, maternal oestrogen existing in the baby's body disappears and consequently the vaginal secretion becomes alkaline. Alkaline vaginal discharge provides a favourable environment for the growth of streptococcal and staphylococcal organisms. If the external genitalia of these small girls are not kept clean, such infections may occur leading to low grade vulvitis and labial adhesion. This occludes the vaginal orifice. The treatment is separation of labia majora either by mild digital pull or by a probe. Mother should be instructed to keep the parts clean specially after voiding (urination or defaecation).

Labial fusion may also be due to androgenic hyperactivity as in congenital adrenal hyperplasia. The area of fusion is at the level of labia minora. The diagnosis can be confirmed by coexisteance of phallic enlargement. Another condition leading to labial fusion at the level of labia minora is incomplete variety of testicular feminising syndrome. Adolescent girls, with this syndrome, present with true amenorrhoea (absence of müllerian system).

In imperforate hymen the level of obstructing membrane is at the level of introitus. When found in adolescent girls, a clear evidence of crytomenorrhoea (haematocolpos with distended bluish-coloured bulging membrane) is observed. Additionally, she experiences intense periodic pain with occasional urinary problems and urinary obstruction in extreme cases.

In complete absence of vagina (MRKH syndrome), the external evidences are similar to those observed in imperforate hymen. In adolescent girls, however, there is no evidence of cryptomenorrhoea. In prepubertal girls, the obstructing membrane in congenital absence of vagina is pinkish in colour with marks of rugosity whereas with imperforate hymen, the obstructing membrane is pearly white with no rugosity. Moreover, the obstructing membrane in imperforate hymen is convex outwards whereas in absence of vagina the membrane is convex inwards. Table 14.5 illustrates differences between imperforate hymen and complete absence of vagina (MRKH syndrome). The final diagnosis in the prepubertal girl is confirmed either by high resolution USG scan or by MRI.

Figures 14.7 to 14.10 illustrate the clinical landmarks of external genitalia observed in a girl presenting with absence of vaginal opening.

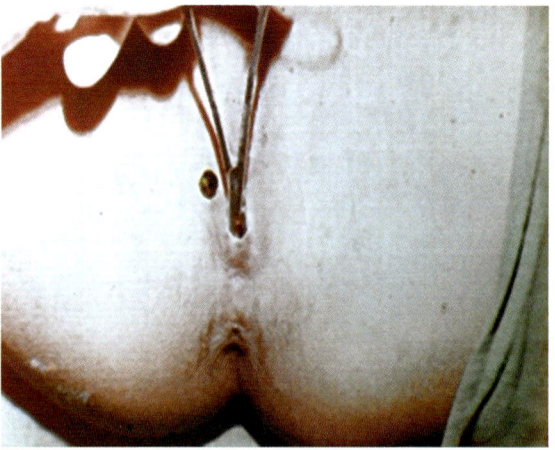

Fig. 14.7: Labial adhesion

ABNORMAL CHROMOSOMAL PATTERN

These girls have female phenotype but show chromosomal abnormalities on karyotyping.

Table 14.5: Differences between imperforate hymen and complete absence of vagina

	Imperforate hymen	*Complete absence of vagina*
Colour of the obstructing membrane	Pearly white, smooth	Pinkish with rugosity of obstructing membrane
Concavity or convexity of the obstructing membrane	Convex inwards	Concave inwards
Syringing and needle puncture test	Saline introduced through obstructing membrane can be reaspirated. Microscopic examination reveals squamous epithelium.	Saline injected cannot be aspirated
Rectal examination	Uterus palpable	Uterus not palpable

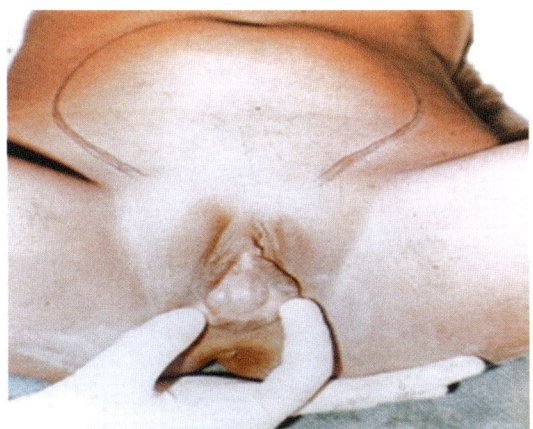

Fig. 14.8: Imperforate hymen

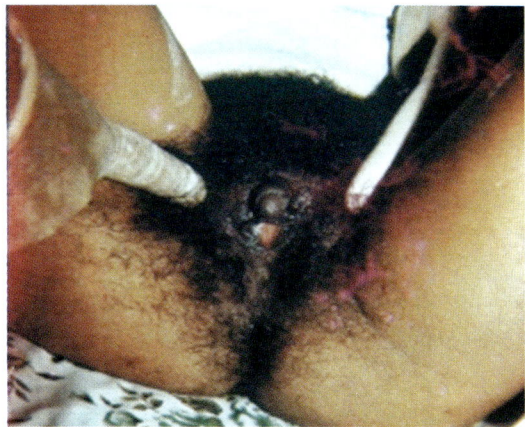

Fig. 14.9: Congenital adrenal hyperplasia (girl aged 14 years)

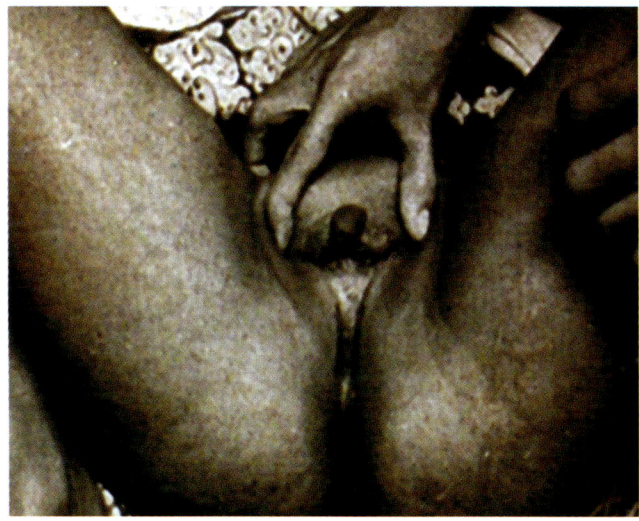

Fig. 14.10: Incomplete variety of testicular feminising syndrome in girl aged 12 years

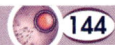

The presenting symptom is primary amenorrhoea. There are two subtypes: (a) Turner's syndrome[5-11] and (b) testicular feminising syndrome.

Turner's Syndrome

The classical features as described by Turner in 1938 are: (i) Sexual infantilism, (ii) neck webbing, (iii) retardation of growth and (iv) bilateral cubitus valgus.

Since then many other somatic and chromosomal abnormalities have been observed in patients simulating Turner's syndrome, and various terminologies have been coined to describe the syndrome. Wilkins (1944) described Turner's syndrome as individuals who had no ovaries. They had only 'streak' gonads. Therefore, syndrome was renamed as 'ovarian agenesis'.

Subsequent publications (1950s) suggested that these girls lacked nuclear chromatin "Barr Body"—therefore, chromosomally these individuals were termed by new terminologies:

   a. Gonadal agenesis
   b. Gonadal dysgenesis
   c. Gonadal aplasia

Simultaneously, other abnormal physical 'stigmas' were identified. These abnormal stigmas included: (a) Shield chest, (b) high arch palate, (c) low set ears, (d) lymphoedema, (e) deafness, (f) pigmented moles and (g) coarctation of aorta (Figs 14.11 to 14.13).

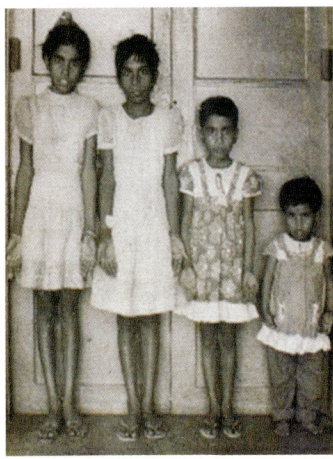

Fig. 14.11: Four sisters with features of Turner's syndrome; Youngest one has hypothyroid also

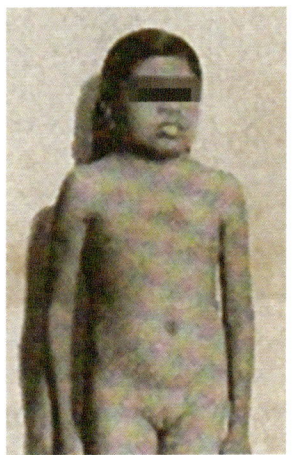

Fig. 14.12: Phenotypic abnormalities of Turner's syndrome (absence of secondary sex character, shielding of chest)

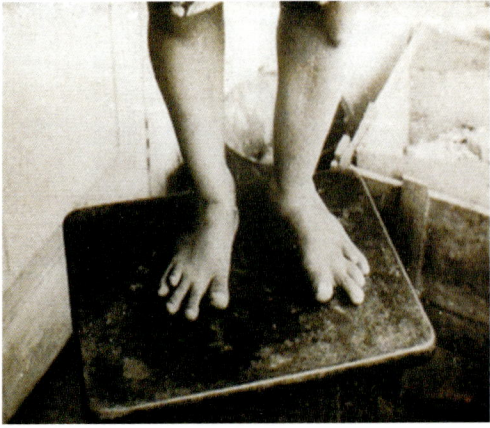

Fig. 14.13: Short 4th metatarsal bone in girl with Turner's syndrome

Male/Female Turner's Syndrome

This is a special variety of Turner's syndrome. They are phenotypically and chromosomally male individuals but with Turner's stigma. The chromosomal pattern is 45XO/46XY. The gonads may be in the inguinal canal or in the labioscrotal fold. Once diagnosed—gonadectomy is offered as there is a risk of development of gonadoblastoma. Whenever Y chromosome is detected in phenotypic girl with primary amenorrhoea, gonadectomy is always indicated.

Criteria for Diagnosis of Turner's Syndrome—Reasons for Confusions

There are three basic criteria for the diagnosis of Turner's syndrome. These criteria may not be typically present in all individuals presenting with primary amenorrhoea with either numerical or structural anomaly of sex chromosomes. In addition, in all of these women the gonads (ovaries) may not be typically 'streak'. Confusion in the precise diagnosis of Turner's syndrome may arise when some of the features are present and others are absent in women presenting with primary amenorrhoea either with abnormal sex chromosomal pattern with normal gonads or abnormal gonads with apparently normal sex chromosomal pattern. Table 14.6 demonstrates the reasons for this confusion.

Table 14.6: Confusing criteria for precise diagnosis of Turner's syndrome

Physical stigma	None/some/all
Gonads	Streak/follicular/male or female
Karyotype	Normal/mosaic/45XO

Embryologic and chromosomal background for genesis of Turners' Syndrome

Classical Turner's syndrome is a consequence of accident during fertilisation. There is a missing X chromosome (45XO) during fertilisation. Embryologically, in these individuals, ovarian development proceeds normally up to 20 weeks of intrauterine gestation because of absence of Y chromosome. Thereafter, oocyte maturation stops because this requires presence of two X chromosomes. Oocytes undergo accelerated atresia.[12] At this stage, ovary consists of mostly stroma—unable to produce oestrogen. Uterus, tubes and ovaries develop because of absence of Y chromosome. Short stature is a result of absent X chromosome, as height determining genes on the X chromosome are also omitted.

In mosaic Turner (45XO/46X; 46XX/46^^), the proportion of each cell line determines the intensity of manifestation of the condition. For example, individuals with higher percentage of 45XO or 46^^ cells have more features of Turner's syndrome.

Presence of a small percentage of normal 46XX chromosome indicates some degrees of normal ovarian differentiation. This results in development of normal secondary sex characters. A few cases with early normal menstrual cycles and occurrence of spontaneous pregnancy have been recorded in the literature.

Therefore, all Turner women are not amenorrhoeic. This depends on the amount of genetic material loss on X chromosome. Loss of short or long arm may be complete or partial. Amount of genetic material loss in these arms determines the impact of Turner's features on the patient. Incidence of primary amenorrhoea is about 35% with long arm deletion and about 15% with short arm deletion.

Other rare varieties of primary ovarian failure (simulating Turner's syndrome) may be due to:

a. Rare undetectable deletion of gene in X chromosome leading to mosaicism

b. Receptor defect in the ovarian follicles (genetically determined) may exist in a syndrome known as 'Savage' syndrome—causing primary amenorrhoea with normal sized ovaries and normal follicular stock. This syndrome is also known as ovarian insensitivity syndrome.

c. Occasionally metabolic defect may also occur due to genetically determined deficiency of an enzyme responsible for galactose metabolism—which leads to galactossaemia and primary amenorrhoea. Some of these syndromes with case presentation are described below.

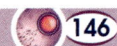

Tall Turner—A variety of Mosaic Turner

These girls are relatively tall (eldest one is more than 65 inches in height). In addition to primary amenorrhoea they have other features of hypo-oestrogenism—absence of secondary sex characters, hypoplastic genital organs and streak gonads.

The genesis of tall Turner is due to minute undetectable sex chromosome deletion (loss of height controlling gene). There is failure of epiphyseal closure because of absence of oestrogen. Tallness is also due to unopposed effect of growth hormone. This syndrome is due to autosomal recessive transmission.

The following photograph is from a family of five sisters who had the specific syndrome (tall Turner, 'Mosaic Turner'). The youngest sister is 14-year-old and has evidence of hypothyroidism as well (Fig. 14.14).

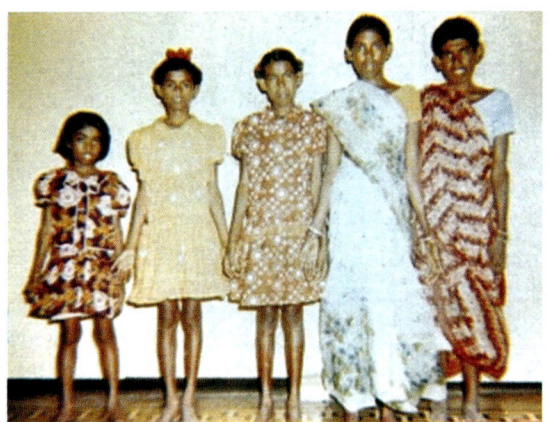

Fig. 14.14: Five sisters tall in stature and the youngest sister has evidence of hypothyroidism; Turner's syndrome may run in families

Ovarian Insensitivity Syndrome (Savage Syndrome)

The criteria for diagnosis are: (a) Primary amenorrhoea, (b) the build and height are normal, (c) normal secondary sex characters, (d) gonadotropin levels are elevated and (e) on ultrasound scan variable number of primordial follicles are present.

The probable etiology is follicular wall membrane receptor defect (genetically determined) to circulating gonadotropin.

Galactossaemia[13–16]

This is a rare cause of hypergonadotropic primary amenorrhoea. This is due to inborn error of galactose metabolism because of deficiency of galactose-1-phosphate uridyl transferase. Deficiency of this enzyme causes damage of germ cells at the time of migration from hind gut to genital ridge.

Testicular Feminising Syndrome (46XY Female)[16–22]

This is a subgroup of male intersex. Male intersex may be broadly classified into two groups: (a) under masculinised males and (b) feminized males. Testicular feminising syndrome is a variety of feminised male intersex.

The clinical features of testicular feminising syndrome are:
- Phenotype—feminine
- Breasts—well-developed
- Pubic and axillary hairs—absent
- External genitalia—feminine
- Vagina—short blind—sometimes normal
- Uterus and tubes—absent
- Bilateral testes—always present, may be in the inguinal canal, labia majora or near deep inguinal ring.

Development of Vagina in Testicular Feminising Syndrome

In normal embryology, a part of vagina develops from urogenital sinus, and rest develops from fused müllerian duct. In normal female this part is not closed as in males, because of absence of androgenic influence (testes is absent). In testicular feminising syndrome, in spite of presence of testes and normal androgen production, this part of urogenital sinus is not closed because of insensitivity to androgen. However, in incomplete variety of testicular feminising syndrome there is a variable degree of closure of this part of urogenital sinus because of partial sensitivity to androgen.

Histological, Biochemical and Chromosomal Features in Testicular Feminising Syndrome (TFS) (Figs 14.15 to 14.17)

a. Histological feature of gonads; there is normal testicular tissue, immature germ

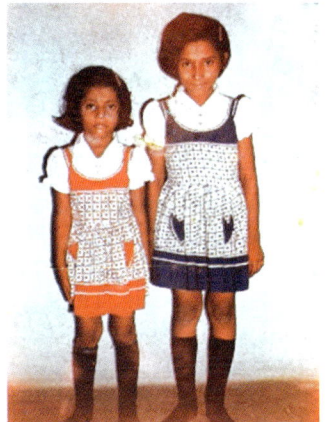

Fig. 14.15: Two sisters in the same family; elder one affected, younger normal

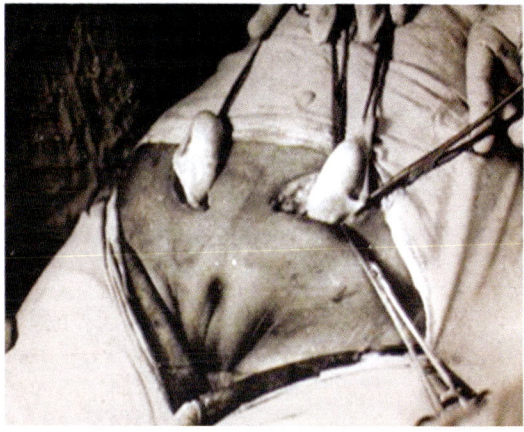

Fig. 14.16: Testes in the inguinal region (operative photograph), normal feminine external genitalia, absence of pubic hairs

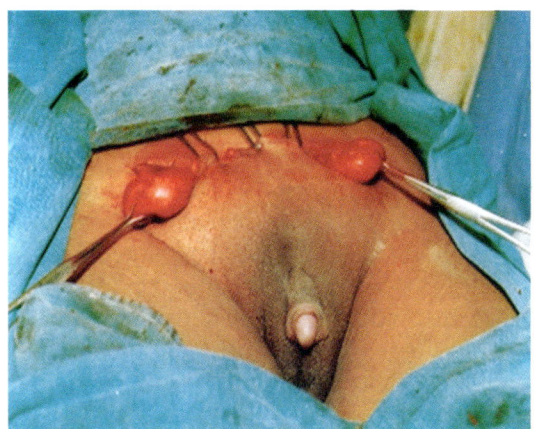

Fig. 14.17: Incomplete variety of testicular feminising syndrome (phallic enlargement, pubic hair present), testes in inguinal region

cells and Sertoli cells, but Leydig cells are prominent.

b. Androgens and LH are normal and are of postpubertal range. They may be marginally elevated because target organs are insensitive.

c. Anti-müllerian hormone (AMH) is normal. This causes suppression of müllerian system. Therefore, in this syndrome, uterus, tubes and upper part of vagina are invariably absent.

d. Karyotype is 46XY.

Explanation of Feminine Phenotype at Puberty

Feminine phenotype in testicular feminising syndrome is due to oestrogen which is synthesised and released from normal adrenal and testicular tissue acting on end organs which are resistant to androgens.

In some individuals with TFS, androgen resistance may be partial or in other words, few organs may be sensitive to androgen. These individuals may have some degree of pubic and axillary hairs and variable grades of phallic enlargement with closure of urogenital sinus and consequently of vaginal orifice.

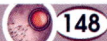

Breasts are ill-developed in incomplete variety of TFS. They have been included in the category of incomplete variety of testicular feminising syndrome. The differences between complete and incomplete varieties of TFS have been illustrated in Table 14.7.

Table 14.7: Differences between complete and incomplete varieties of TFS

	Complete	Incomplete
Phenotype	Feminine	Feminine
Karyotype	46XY	46XY
Gonads	Testes	Testes
Müllerian system	Absent	Absent
Breasts	Well-developed	Ill-developed
Pubic hamir	Absent	Scanty, present
External genitalia	Feminine	Ambiguous

Etiology of Testicular Feminising Syndrome

This is due to deficiency of cytosol receptor in the target organ. These defects are genetically determined. The defect primarily involves male-determining gene (mainly SRY segment) located on short arm of Y chromosome.

In some individuals with TFS, deletion or mutation of sex-determining gene at SRY segment of Y chromosome has not been detected. In these individuals, there may be a gene on X chromosome or autosome which may control the function of sex-determining gene in SRY segment. Perhaps these controlling genes which are yet to be identified are deleted or mutated.

Depending on the number of genes involved (mutated), individuals with testicular feminising syndrome may have presence of variable grades of müllerian tissue. These individuals have been designated as 'Sex reversed XY' females (for details, see chapter on Intersex).

Management of Testicular Feminising Syndrome

In short, the management of testicular feminising syndrome is gonadectomy. Because these gonads ectopically situated are susceptible to risk of malignancy. Gonadectomy should be performed after puberty. This allows development of secondary sex characters following which replacement therapy with oestrogen is required for a shorter period.

The management, in general, of all varieties of male intersex is diagrammatically represented in the following diagram (Fig. 14.18). For details, chapter on intersex or Sexual Ambiguity is to be consulted.

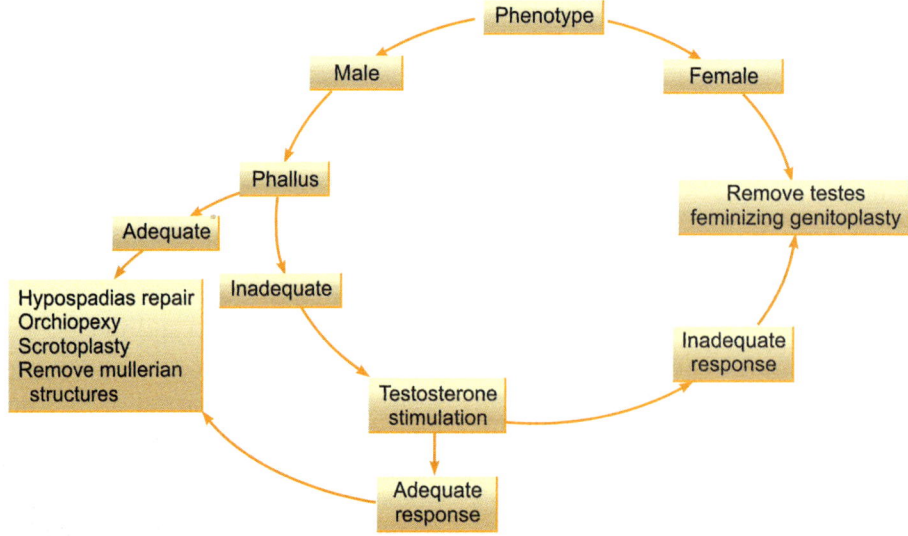

Fig. 14.18: Surgical approach to male intersex

DYSFUNCTION OF HYPOTHALAMIC-PITUITARY-OVARIAN AXIS

Dysfunctions are sequentially discussed as follows:

Amenorrhoea due to Hypothalamic Dysfunction

The dysfunction may be of two types—(a) Functional or (b) organic.

Hypothalamic functional defect may again be divided into two subgroups: (i) Anorexia nervosa,[23] and (ii) sustained emotional stress.

Similarly, organic hypothalamic defect may be subclassified into two types: (i) 'ill-defined' genetic etiology and (ii) 'well-defined' genetic etiology.

The etiologies are summarised in Fig. 14.19.

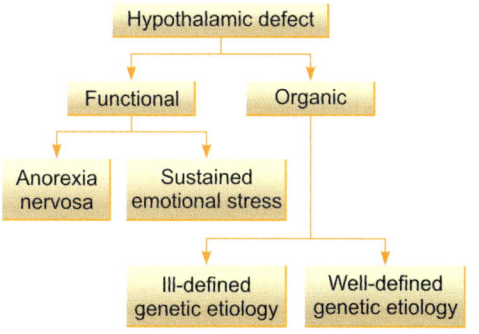

Fig. 14.19: Etiologies of hypothalamic defect

Functional hypothalamic defect: A brief description of each specific defect is given below.

Anorexia Nervosa

These girls have a low body mass; meaning thereby that they have low levels of leptin. Leptin is a fat cell hormone. Because of deficient adipose tissue in girls with anorexia nervosa, the level of leptin is low. Hypothalamus has leptin receptors. Because of low level of leptin, there is fault in pulsatile release of gonadotropin leading to amenorrhoea and anovulation.

Hypothalamic leptin receptors are modified by neuropeptide 'Y' gene. This gene is modulated through dietary intake and exercise which in turn modifies hypothalamic release of GnRH. This phenomenon is also observed in athletes, because of excessive exercise and restricted dietary intake. They finally develop a condition known as 'anorexia nervosa'. This results in functional hypogonadotropic hypogonadism leading to amenorrhoea.

Sustained Emotional Stress

This may also be a cause of hypothalamic amenorrhoea. The mechanism involved is through release of neurotransmitters from cerebral cortex in consequence of stress.

There are two types of neurotransmitters: (a) Catecholamines and (b) indolamines. Catecholamines comprise acetylcholine, epinephrine and norepinephrine. Indolamines comprise serotonin, melatonin and dopamine. These neurotransmitters are generated from amines (dietary intake) and psyche. Amines come from food and psyche is driven by environment in which the girl is surrounded.

Catecholamines and indolamines have opposite releasing action on hypothalamus. Catecholamines lead to secretion of gonadotropins whereas indolamines inhibit secretion of gonadotropin. This inhibition of secretion of gonadotropin is brought about by inhibition of prolactin inhibitory factor (dopamine—PIF) and release of ACTH.

It is well-known that both PIF and ACTH inhibit synthesis and release of GnRH from hypothalamus. This is the basic cause of amenorrhoea in young girls who become victims of anorexia nervosa or sustained emotional stress.

Inhibition of PIF (dopamine) leads to hyperprolactinaemia leading to clinical manifestation of galactorrhoea. At the same time hyperprolactinaemia also leads to suppression of hypothalamic synthesis and release of GnRH leading to primary amenorrhoea.

On the other side, excess indolamine leads to release of ACTH resulting in over-production of adrenocortical androgen through stimulation of adrenal cortex. Hyperandrogenism thus created, causes ovarian enlargement resulting in clinical

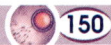

manifestation of polycystic ovarian syndrome (PCOS)—amenorrhoea and anovulation. The following photographs illustrate extreme examples of sequence of events resulting from sustained emotional stress. Four photographs arranged in chronological order depict clinical manifestation of sustained emotional stress (Fig. 14.20).

Organic Hypothalamic Defect (Poorly-defined Etiology)

These defects are usually due to 'poorly-defined' genetic etiology. Occasionally in these individuals presenting with primary amenorrhea, a space occupying lesion (SOL) is detected in cerebral region. This may be due

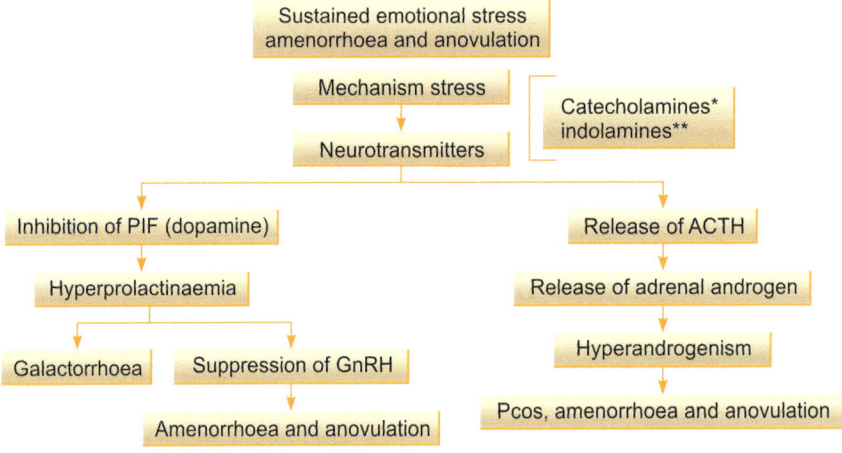

*Acetylcholine, epinephrine, nor-epinephrine
**Serotonin, melatonin, dopamin

Diagrammatic representation of clinical effect of sustained emotional stress

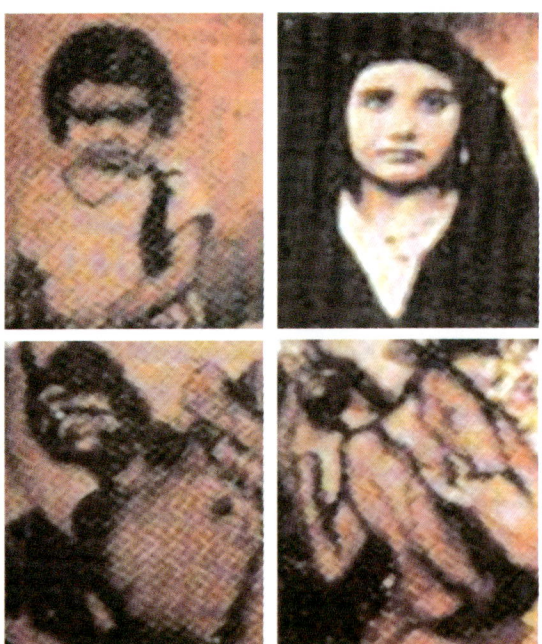

Fig. 14.20: Clinical effect of sustained emotional stress—PCOS, anorexia nervosa (infertility and subsequent divorce). Chronological photographs of the same girl: 4 years, during marriage, subsequent to divorce

to defective embryogenesis based on genetic defect. Some of the examples are:

a. Laurence-Moon-Biedl syndrome[27]—they have mental retardation, polydactyly, coarctation of the aorta, retinitis pigmentosa.

b. Prader-Willi syndrome[28]—clinical features are more or less similar to the previous one. They are abnormally obese.

c. Pineal gland tumour[29, 30]—these individuals have gonadotropin inhibitory hormone or an enzyme that produces melatonin which suppresses gona-dotropin—resulting in amenorrhoea (Fig. 14.21).

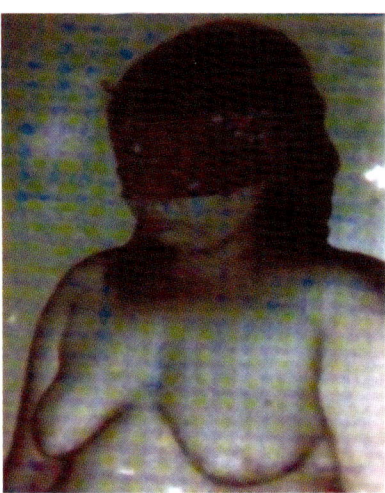

Fig. 14.21: Primary amenorrhoea due to hypothalamic tumour (poorly-defined etiology)

Organic Hypothalamic Defect (Well-defined Etiology)

There are groups of women who present with primary amenorrhoea and the etiology can be detected as inherited genetic defect. This refers to a syndrome—anosmia amenorrhoea syndrome (Kallmann's syndrome). In these girls, hypothalamus is unable to generate GnRH hormone leading to a hypogonadotropic state. The background etiology is a gene deletion at the Xp, 22.3 site (single KAL gene defect). This defect results in inability of the cells that produce GnRH to migrate during embryogenesis to the hypothalamic area from the olfactory region. Embryologically olfactory area and hypothalamic area producing GnRH

have the same origin. Hence the syndrome is sometimes known as olfactogenital syndrome.

Primary Amenorrhoea due to Pituitary Defect

These defects may also be due to organic or functional abnormality:

The organic pituitary defects

a. **Hydrocephalus:** The defect is more in hypothalamus than in pituitary. This means that synthesis and release of GnRH is deficient.

b. **Trauma:** Like in hydrocephalus, amenorrhoea may be more hypothalamic than pituitary in origin.

c. **Empty-sella syndrome:** This may be due to congenital incompleteness of sellar diaphragm, for which pituitary is flattened. This leads to a hypogonadotropic state. Galactorrhoea and elevated prolactin may be present because of coexisting prolactin secreting adenoma.[24-26]

The condition is benign: Does not progress to pituitary failure. Empty-sella syndrome may develop following surgery, radiotherapy or infarction of a pituitary tumour.

Because of possibility of coexisting adenoma, annual surveillance is essential. This may be done by periodic prolactin assay and imaging. The condition is totally benign. Treatment is possible by hormones; pregnancy may be achieved by ovulation induction.

d. **Pituitary tumours:** Three types of tumours are significant with primary amenorrhoea. These are: (i) **Craniopharyngioma**, (ii) **acromegaly** and (iii) **pituitary adenoma**. Individuals with these types of intra-cranial lesions present with neurologic and ophthalmic problems, and therefore, may not present to a gynaecologist. However, occasionally they may be encountered in the gynaecological outpatients department.

i. *Craniopharyngioma:*[31, 32] It is a Rathke's pouch tumour. The tumour originates from the embryonic squamous cell

which persists after upward migration of stomodial epithelium to anterior pituitary.

This is a non-pituitary suprasellar mass. The tumour is found commonly in children and adolescents, but may occur at any age. The presenting symptoms are visual and neurological symptoms—variable features of hypopituitarism leading to amenorrhoea and anovulation.

Diagnosis is confirmed by CT scan and MRI. Treatment consists of surgical approach through craniotomy and removal of the tumour. Morbidity and mortality are very high. Tumours are relatively radioresistant.

ii. *Acromegaly*: This is a pituitary adenoma. The tumour produces excess growth hormone. If the tumour occurs before puberty, there may be linear acceleration of growth leading to gigantism.

Apart from neurological lesion, the tumour may produce gonadal dysfunction leading to amenorrhoea and anovulation. Hyperprolactinaemia may be associated in 40% of cases. Galactorrhoea even without hyperprolactinaemia may be present due to lactogenic effect of GH.

Treatment consists of surgical excision followed by radiotherapy. Medical treatment has to be continued for a long time even after surgical excision. Medical treatment consists of bromocriptine and somatostatin analogues.

iii. *Pituitary adenoma, prolactinoma*:[24–26] This is the commonest type of pituitary adenoma. The condition is associated with galactorrhoea, amenorrhoea and elevated level of serum prolactin (> 50 ng/ml). The condition is diagnosed by CT scan or MRI of pituitary. The treatment consists of bromocriptine and/or surgical excision. Sometimes radiotherapy may be helpful.

Malignant Tumours of Pituitary are Almost Never Encountered

Other non-neoplastic organic pituitary defect:

i. *Non-neoplastic intrasellar masses*: Occasionally such types of intrasellar lesions may be associated with primary amenorrhoea. Though rare, the examples are—tuberculoma, fat deposits, syphilitic gumma which may cause pituitary compression leading to hypogonadotropic amenorrhoea and anovulation.

ii. *Pituitary necrosis*: This is also a rare cause of primary amenorrhoea in young girls. This commonly occurs as a result of ischaemia or infarction as a late sequelae of obstetric haemorrhage. The condition is known as "Sheehan's syndrome".

Primary amenorrhoea as a result of pituitary necrosis in adolescent girl may be a consequence of tuberculosis.

Functional Pituitary Defect

it is also known as unexplained hypogonadotropism leading to primary amenorrhoea.

This variety of hypogonadotropism without any apparent cause, like tumor or necrosis, is commonly found in clinical practice. The probable etiological factors may be: (a) defect in the pituitary receptor for GnRH or (b) defective or deficient production of GnRH by the hypothalamus.

In the first group, the synthesis and release of hypothalamic GnRH is normal, but as the receptor in the pituitary is defective, the pituitary production of FSH and LH are subnormal. The clinical features consist of short stature, absent secondary sex characteristics, absent pubic and axillary hair and other features suggestive of hypo-oestrogenism. They are usually nonresponsive to progesterone challenge test. Baseline serum FSH and LH are below 3 mIU/ml. Hypothyroidism and hyperprolactinaemia are often coexistent. The clinical features are similar to those of Turner's syndrome. Differentiation can be done by estimation of baseline FSH and LH.

Prognosis with regard to restoration of menstrual and reproductive function is relatively unsatisfactory than those in the second group.

The girls in the second group are less critical than those in the first group. They have normal height and normal secondary sex characters. Hypo-oestrogenic state is not as severe as in the first group. Baseline FSH and LH are between 3 and 5 mIU/ml. TSH and prolactin values are within normal limits. Presenting features are amenorrhoea, anovulation and infertility. They respond more favourably to conventional treatments.

Diagnosis is mainly by exclusion of positive signs of organic defect which is confirmed by CT scan or MRI of brain and karyotype. Basal FSH and LH are the primary markers for diagnosis of hypogonadotropic hypogonadism. The two groups of unexplained hypo-gonadotropism as defined in the previous paragraphs can be differentiated by 'GnRH challenge test'. The GnRH challenge test involves: (a) estimation of basal FSH which is usually less than 3 mIU/ml, (b) injection of a bolus dose of GnRH (Luprolide acetate, 0.5 to 1 mg IV), (c) estimation of blood serum samples for FSH at 15 min, 30 min, 45 min and 60 min and (d) if subsequent values show incremental levels at least by 2–4 mIU compared to the basal level, then it may be presumed that the hypogonadotropic condition in the individual is due to GnRH deficiency and she may be treated with GnRH analogue for ovulation and menstruation. Alternatively, if there is no elevation of the level of gonadotropin (FSH) in subsequent estimations (receptor defect), then the cause is probably organic. In these cases pulsatile GnRH pump administration may not be effective. Gona-dotropin injections for ovulation induction may be attempted for IVF or IUI. Half-life of GnRH is so short that the hormone cannot be directly estimated from serum by RIA or EIA.

Probable Etiology of Hypogonadotropic Hypogonadism

There are two possible etiological factors which may explain this variety of hypo-gonadotropism in young adolescent girls. This may be due to suppression of release of pulsatile GnRH secretion which consequently remains below the critical range. Etiology is probably an underlying genetic defect.

Alternatively, GnRH secretion may be normal, but there may be receptor defect in the pituitary, and therefore, pituitary cannot respond even in the presence of adequate amount of GnRH secretion. In clinical practice, exact etiology remains uncertain because GnRH cannot be estimated by RIA or EIA as half-life of GnRH is very short.

Management of Functional Hypogonadotropism

Previously treatment of this condition was attempted with pulsatile, programmable GnRH pump which was attached to the body by a belt (called 'Policeman's Belt'). This allowed release of defined amount of GnRH at prefixed intervals in a pulsatile fashion. But as the procedure was cumbersome it was found impractical for clinical use, and therefore, has been discarded.

On the contrary, gonadotropin stimulation of ovary has been found to be more suitable in these women followed by IUI and IVF. The only disadvantage is that huge amount of gonadotropin (both FSH and LH) is required and sometimes ovaries (if they have become very small) do not always respond properly. In these cases IVF with donor's egg is indicated, provided size of uterus and endometrial receptivity are satisfactory.

Amenorrhoea–Galactorrhoea Syndrome

This is synonymous with previously described syndromes in the literature as—Forbes' syndrome, Chiari-Frommel syndrome, del Castillo's syndrome, etc.

The background etiology of these specific syndromes may be either: (a) functional defect (hypothalamic pituitary unit) or (b) space occupying lesion (SOL) like pituitary adenoma.

Mechanism of Amenorrhoea and Glactorrhoea

Synthesis and release of prolactin is mainly controlled by hypothalamic dopamine, known as prolactin inhibitory factor (PIF) which causes prolactin inhibition. Prolactin release is also controlled partly by thyroid-releasing hormone (TRH). Therefore, when TRH is elevated, there is elevation of both TSH (thyroid-stimulating hormone) as well as of prolactin. This explains the clinical features associated with amenorrhoea–galactorrhoea syndrome in which there is not only elevation of prolactin leading to galatorrhoea, involving primarily PIF (dopamine) or PRF (TRH) the condition is also associated with sub-clinical hypothyroidism. In addition, elevated level of prolactin has a negative impact on GnRH leading to low level of FSH resulting in amenorrhoea. Elevated level of prolactin also has a positive effect on adrenal cortex resulting in overproduction of adrenal androgen. Adrenal androgen has an impact on ovarian steroidogenesis leading to PCO like mani-festation, ultimately ending in clinical situation of amenorrhoea and anovulation. The third impact of elevated prolactin is on the receptors of the ovarian follicles. Hyperprolactinaemia makes ovaries less sensitive to pituitary gonadotropin which may also be responsible for amenorrhoea and anovulation. The entire mechanism of excess prolactin leading to amenorrhoea and anovulation has been represented in Fig. 14.22.

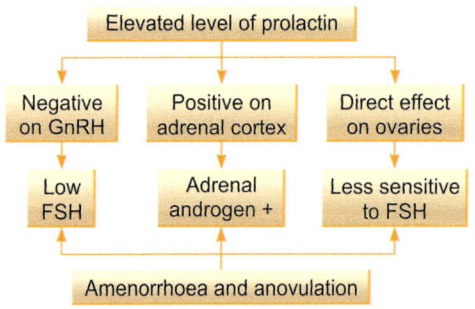

Fig. 14.22: Mechanism of amenorrhoea anovulation

Ovarian Causes of Primary Amenorrhoea

The individual causes have been described before and are summarised as follows:

a. Ovarian dysgenesis—the mechanism of amenorrhoea has been discussed under the heading of Turner's syndrome.

b. PCOS—this is a common cause of secondary amenorrhoea. Rarely, a girl with PCOS may present with primary amenorrhoea.

c. Androgen producing tumours of the ovary like arrhenoblastoma (Sertoli-Leydig cell or hilus cell tumour)—apart from amenorrhoea they produce marked features of hirsutism and virilisation. 1/3rd of these tumours are malignant.

d. Germ cell tumours like dysgerminoma may also cause primary amenorrhoea. These tumours may be malignant as well.

e. Embryonic carcinoma may lead to primary amenorrhoea, but these tumours are virulently malignant.

DEFECTS IN ADRENAL CORTEX

Two types of adrenocortical defects are associated with primary amenorrhoea: (a) Congenital adrenal hyperplasia (CAH) and (b) Cushing's syndrome.[33–36]

Congenital Adrenal Hyperplasia (CAH)

Basic defect in CAH is genetically determined enzymatic defect in adrenal cortex—leading to defective cortisol synthesis. Because of less amount of cortisol released by adrenal cortex, there is no negative feedback of anterior pituitary resulting in increased release of ACTH. This primarily attempts to release more cortisol from the adrenal cortex. As a result there is adrenal enlargement.

While trying to do so, increased ACTH stimulation of adrenal cortex leads to over-production of other adrenocortical hormones like androgens and oestrogens which cause virilisation of the female fetus. Excess static oestrogen has an impact on adolescent girl, resulting in stunted growth and amenorrhoea because of early epiphyseal fusion and static negative impact on hypothalamus. Aldosterone which is produced by zona glomerulosa of the adrenal cortex is not much under pituitary control—yet due to disturbance of sodium metabolism, there is reduction of serum sodium because of salt loss in urine.

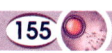

The clinical features are amenorrhoea, ambiguous genitalia, sometimes salt loss, wasting and hypotension.

(*It is worthwhile to recapitulate that adrenal cortex has got three zones—outer zone is known as zona glomerulosa which produces mineralocorticoids, involved in control of salt and water metabolism; intermediate zone known as zona fasciculata produces glucocorticoids which controls carbohydrate metabolism and maintains homeostasis; inner zone known as zona reticularis produces sex steroids—androgen and oestrogens. Fasciculata and reticularis are under ACTH control and are largely involved in CAH, whereas zona glomerulosa is relatively an autonomous zone*).

The entire mechanism of genesis of CAH is represented in Fig. 14.23.

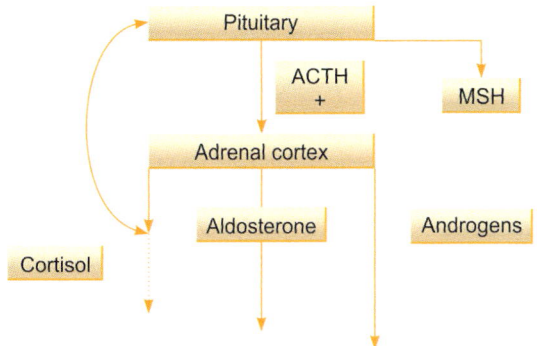

Fig. 14.23: Genesis of CAH

Types of Enzymatic Defects in CAH

It has already been mentioned that overproduction of cortisol and sex steroids in CAH is due to enzymatic defects in adrenal cortex. Broadly there are three types of defects.

They are all genetically determined defects. The defects are:

   a. 21-hydroxylase deficiency—this is the commonest variety found in clinical practice.
   b. 11β-hydroxylase deficiency.
   c. 3β-hydroxysteroid dehydrogenase deficiency.

Subtypes of 21-hydroxylase deficiency: Of all CAH cases, 21-hydroxylase deficiency is found in 95% of women. This specific defect has got three clinical subtypes:

   i. Salt wasting—this is rarely seen presenting with primary amenorrhoea because they do not survive up to the adolescent age.

   ii. Simple virilising—this variety is commonly observed as female intersex at birth.

   iii. Non-classical CAH—this variety was previously known as late onset, attenuated or acquired CAH—the clinical features of which become apparent at adolescence and in reproductive years with manifestations of hirsuitism, menstrual irregularity and infertility.

Other two varieties of CAH (apart from 21-hydroxylase deficiency) are less significant and a short description of these two rare varieties is given below:

11β-hydroxylase deficiency: This variety constitutes 5% of all CAH cases. In this variety zona glomerulosa is affected resulting in increased release of aldosterone. In addition to virilisation, hypertension and volume overload are the other consequences.

Defect in 3β-hydroxysteroid dehydrogenase: Infants with this type of enzyme deficiency are born with decreased synthesis of glucocorticoids, mineralocorticoids, androgens and oestrogens. They rarely survive in neonatal period.

Clinical Significance of Sexual Ambiguity in CAH

During 6–7 weeks of intrauterine life, in the absence of a virilising source like testis or CAH, the urogenital sinus of a female fetus develops in female pattern. But when virilising source (like hyperactive adrenal) is present, there may be fusion of labioscrotal folds in such a manner that vaginal opening is suppressed completely or concealed from outside. The genital tubercles which form clitoris in female enlarge to form an enlarged phallus as in male. These features found in a virilised female fetus in case of CAH are represented in Fig. 14.24.

Embryologically vagina communicates with lower part of urogenital sinus. Vagina

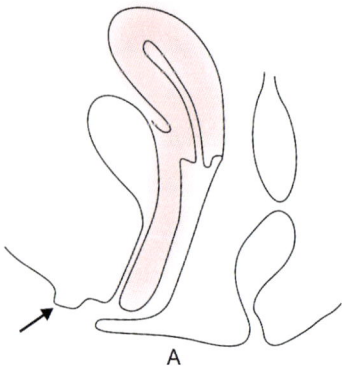 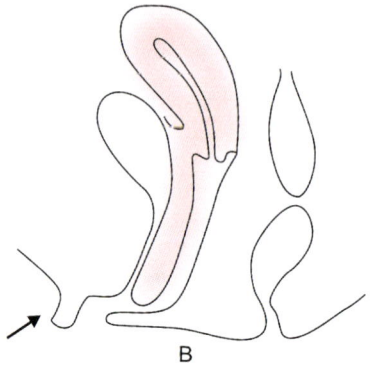 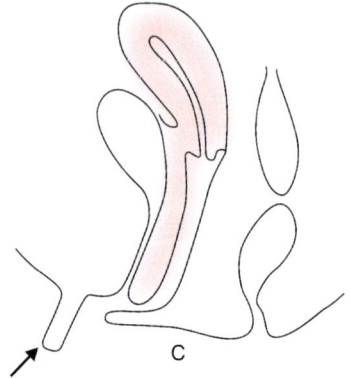

A

B

C

- Minimal clitoral enlargement
- Minimum degree of labial fusion

- Moderate clitoral enlargement
- Intermediate grade of labial fusion with partial concealment of vaginal orifice

- Gross clitoral enlargement
- Maximum concealment of vaginal orifice with a small opening at the upper end of fused labia for escape of urine
- Blind contact at the junction of lower end of fused müllerian duct and at the point of opening into urogenital sinus leading to vaginal obstruction—very rare

Fig. 14.24: Different degrees of virilisation of external genital organs of a female fetus in CAH

communicates with that part of urogenital sinus which in male forms membranous part of urethra and in female, the vestibule.

Vagina never communicates with that part of urogenital sinus which in male forms the prostatic urethra and in female the entire urethra (Fig. 14.25).

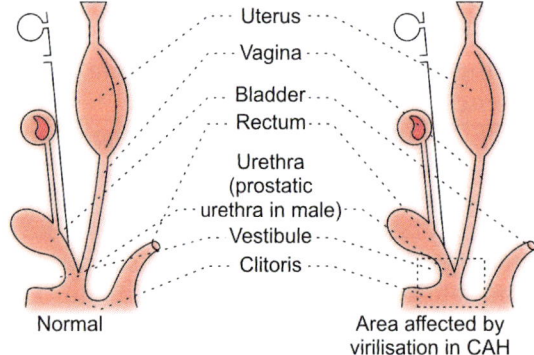

Uterus

Vagina

Bladder

Rectum

Urethra (prostatic urethra in male)

Vestibule

Clitoris

Normal

Area affected by virilisation in CAH

Fig. 14.25: Area affected by virilisation in CAH

This is of surgical significance because anomalous persistence of urogenital sinus may be boldly incised without apprehension of urinary incontinence.

In CAH—why are only external genital organs affected and not the internal genital organs?

This is because

Internal genital organ development is completed by 10 to 12 weeks but androgen secretion from adrenal cortex starts after 10–12 weeks. The common clinical variety is 21-hydroxylase deficiency. And the common form of androgen produced is DHEA-SO$_4$ which is not a very potent androgen. Salt losing variety is also not commonly encountered in clinical practice. Because they do not usually survive up to adolescent age.

Ambiguity of external genitalia is restricted only at the lower part of urogenital sinus. In late onset of CAH there may not be labioscrotal fusion. Only phallic enlargement and coarse pubic hair may be seen. This is because the impact of excess androgen secreted by adrenal cortex due to genetically determined enzymatic deficiency is manifested at the age of puberty.

There is no anomalous secretion of anti-müllerian hormone, and therefore, there is no abnormality of internal genital organs even in late onset of CAH (Fig. 14.26).

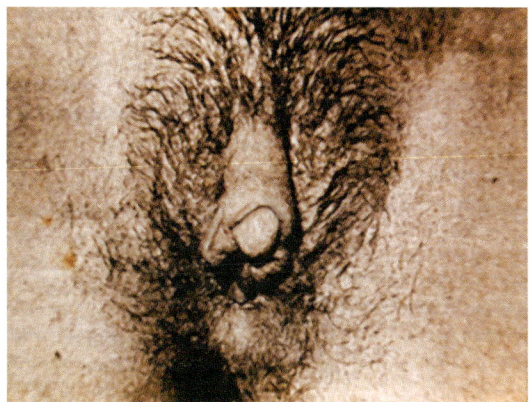

Fig. 14.26: Congenital adrenal hyperplasia (late onset), gross enlargement of phallus, minimum labio-scrotal fusion

Why are there amenorrhoea, stunted growth and absence of breast development in CAH?

This is because of:

a. Excess androgen and static oestrogen production from zona reticularis

b. This causes early epiphysial fusion—short stature

c. Static elevated oestrogen—exerts negative feedback effect on pituitary—leading to absence of breast development

d. Excess androgen leads to development of body and facial hairs.

Diagnosis of CAH

The main confirmatory diagnostic parameter is estimation of 17-OHP (hydroxyprogesterone in the morning blood sample). If the level is more than 800 ng/dl, diagnosis of CAH is confirmed. Value less than 200 ng is the normal baseline level of 17-OHP. Values between 200 and 800 ng/dl of 17-OHP is a doubtful range which may indicate an overlapping value with PCOS. Confirmation requires ACTH stimulation test (*see* under diagnosis of PCOS)

To distinguish between 21-hydroxylase deficiency and other varieties of enzymatic disorders, in addition to 17-OHP, the following estimations should be made at 0 and 60 minutes after ACTH stimulation.

a. Pregnenelone

b. 17-hydroxylase pregnenelone

c. DHEA

d. 11-deoxycortisol

e. Cortisol

f. Testostorene

In 11β-hydroxylase deficiency, the diagnosis is confirmed when there is elevation of 11-deoxycortisol in addition to 17-OHP.

However, in 3β-hydroxysteroid dehydrogenase deficiency 17-OHP is not elevated. DHEA and DHEAS are to be elevated.

Treatment

Medical treatment consists of administration of hydrocortisone (cortisol 10 mg/day) or 9-fluorohydrocortisone—100 mg/day. This therapy is to be continued throughout the life. The objective is to maintain the level of 17-OHP between 400 and 500 ng/dl and to avoid over- and undertreatment.

The surgical correction of anomalous external genitalia consists of clitoroplasty (*see* Chapter on Intersex) in neonatal period and vaginoplasty or introitoplasty, if necessary, during adolescent period.

Subsequent Reproduction

Pregnancies have been reported provided corticosteroid therapy is continued religiously. During pregnancy and labour, the steroid therapy should be continued. There is a risk of transmission of the disease from the mother to the offspring. There is also a possibility of steroid crossover through placenta which may lead to suppression of fetal adrenal in utero leading to fetal shock after delivery. So there is a debate regarding treatment of unborn baby in women who conceive following treatment of CAH.

Diagnosis of 21-hydroxylase Deficiency in Newborn

Normally, 17-OHP is elevated in cord blood (1000–3000 ng/dl). The level rapidly decreases within 24 hours of delivery. Therefore, accurate and reliable measurement can be assured 24–48 hours after delivery.

In affected infants the level of 17-OHP ranges between 3000 and 4000 ng/dl. Incidence of neonatal CAH is one in 16,000 babies.

Prenatal Diagnosis of 21-hydroxylase Deficiency

In suspected pregnancies, the diagnosis can be confirmed by: (a) elevated 17-OHP in amniotic fluid and (b) molecular genetic diagnosis by PCR-CVS (Chorionic-villus sampling).

The Plan of Diagnosis

During pregnancy in these women, chorionic villus sampling is performed which is subjected to two types of testing—(a) karyotype and (b) DNA analysis. If the karyotype suggests male fetus and DNA analysis shows normal result—there is no need of treatment. Similarly, amniocentesis can be performed around 14–15 weeks of pregnancy submitting the cells in the amniotic fluid for karyotype and DNA analysis. The subsequent treatment depends on the result of the analysis. The entire diagnostic procedure in suspected cases is represented in Fig. 14.27.

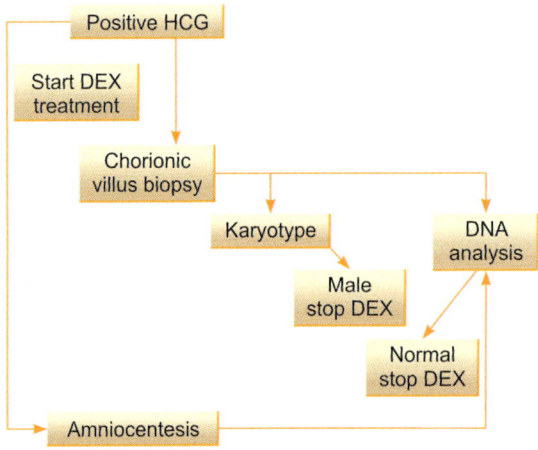

Fig. 14.27: Plan of diagnosis 21-hydroxylase deficiency

Treatment with Dexamethasone for the Mother with Affected Female Child

The treatment starts from 4–5 weeks of pregnancy. The daily dose of dexamethasone should not be more than 1.5 mg. Complete prevention of the disease has been achieved with no teratogenic effect in the newborn while the patient was on cortisol therapy throughout the pregnancy. However, the dose is to be reduced during later part of pregnancy.

In spite of the advantages claimed, prenatal treatment with dexamethasone has not been very popular, because primarily there may be many maternal side effects and secondly diagnosis is not always 100% accurate. Maternal side effects consist of hypertension, hyperglycaemia, gastrointestinal symptoms and permanent abdominal striae. Regarding accuracy of diagnosis and advantages—one out of 8 fetuses actually require the treatment. Therefore, 7 fetuses are being unnecessarily exposed to prenatal glucocorticoid therapy. In addition, as has already been stated, prenatal diagnosis of CAH is not 100% correct.

Cushing's Syndrome

The basic etiology of Cushing's syndrome is oversecretion of cortisol. The causes of oversecretion of cortisol are:

a. ACTH overproduction by pituitary—commonest
b. Autonomous cortisol secretion by ovarian tumours
c. Ectopic ACTH production by tumours other than in pituitary or in adrenal cortex—as in bronchogenic carcinoma.
d. Also secretion of corticotrophin releasing hormone (CRH) by a tumour
e. Autonomous cortisol secretion by the adrenal.

Diagnosis

Clinical Manifestations of Cushing's Syndrome

Manifestations are—(a) primary amenorrhoea, (b) obesity—typical sites of distribution of fat are—facial, nuchal, truncated girdle area, 'buffalo' obesity, 'moon facies', (c) skin striae—because of protein wastage—pink or purple striae, (d) hypertension, (e) diabetes and (f) clitoromegaly may or may not be present.

In addition to clinical features, the diagnosis is confirmed by

   i. *Single dose overnight dexamethasone (DXM) suppression test*: In this test DXM (1 mg) is given orally at 11 PM and sample of blood for estimation of cortisol is collected at 8 am next morning. If the value of cortisol in the sample is less than 5 µg/dl, the diagnosis of Cushing's syndrome can be ruled out. Also if the value is between 5 and 10 µg/dl diagnosis of Cushing's syndrome is doubtful—but unlikely. But, if the value is more than 10 µg/dl, the diagnosis of Cushing's syndrome or adrenal hyperfunction is confirmed.

In case of doubt, i.e. value between 5 and 10 µg/dl—the next investigation is given as follows.

ii. *Low dose DXM—(for two days) suppression (test) which*: Provides final confirmation. The procedure consists of—(a) 24 hours basal urinary cortisol excretion is measured—normal level is 10–90 µg/dl, and (b) DXM 0.5 mg is given every six hours for two days. 24 hours urinary cortisol is again measured. If the level of free cortisol is more than 250 µg/dl, the diagnosis of Cushing's syndrome is confirmed.

iii. *Other types of investigations consist of*: (a) Imaging adrenal with ultrasonograpy, CT scan and MRI for hypertrophy, tumours, etc.; (b) to confirm pituitary origin for excess ACTH—bilateral venous sampling from the inferior petrosal sinus for the measurement of ACTH before and after CRH stimulation (1 µg/kg) is an effective method for accurate diagnosis of pituitary origin of ACTH; (c) 15 min plasma cortisol level greater than 1.4 µg/dl, and if it is positive—she requires further evaluation for pituitary origin of ACTH and (d) in suspected cases chest and abdominal imaging is recommended.

Finding out the basic cause is important because treatment of etiology of different origin is different (Fig. 14.28).

Thyroid Disorders[37]

Though thyroid is basically associated with regulation of menstrual and reproductive functions, primary amenorrhoea is not a feature with thyroid disorders. Oligomenorrhoea may be associated with subclinical hypo-

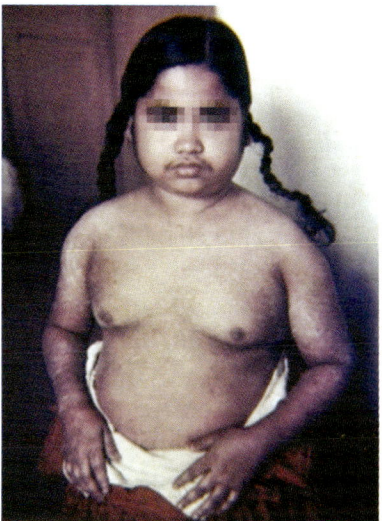

Fig. 14.28: Typical clinical features of Cushing's syndrome girl aged 16 years

thyroidism. Very rarely primary amenorrhoea may be associated with primary hypothyroidism. Primary hypothyroidism indicates loss or atrophy of thyroid tissue resulting in decreased production of thyroid hormone—though TRH production is normal.

Primary hypothyroidism may also be a result of postablative hypothyroidism and sporadic athyreotic cretinism. Primary hypothyroidism may be associated with hyperprolactinaemia. Majority of them have thyroid autoantibodies (Hashimoto's disease) (Fig. 14.29).

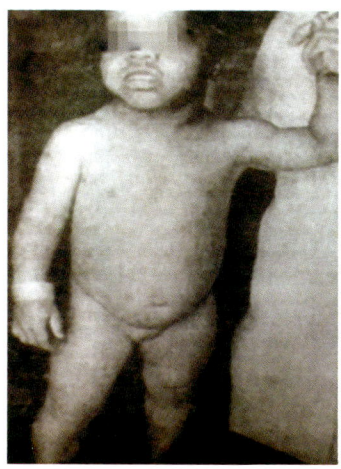

Fig. 14.29: Girl aged 16 years with athyreotic cretinism

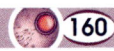

Treatment consists of L-thyroxine and not with bromocriptine (BRC) except when prolactin level is more than 50 ng/ml.

Primary amenorrhoea is not a feature of hyperthyroidism (Graves' or Plummer's disease)

Endometrial Defect

Endometrial defect leading to primary amenorrhoea may be due to two basic abnormalities:

a. Uterine synechiae—commonest complication of endometrial tuberculosis
b. Patchy or absent endometrium is a rare cause—may be a consequence of genetic defect.

Treatment is very unsatisfactory in uterine synechiae. Hysteroscopic synechiolysis may be attempted, but the results are unrewarding. In these cases surrogacy is advocated.

Apparently Unexplained Primary Amenorrhoea

A step wise approach for provisional diagnosis of the etiology is summarised in the subsequent paragraphs.

In an adolescent girl aged between 13 and 17 years presenting with primary amenorrhoea, a physical examination should be performed with two additional investigations provided the physical examination does not reveal any abnormality. These additional investigations consist of ultrasound scan of pelvic organs for presence and size of uterus and ovaries, and if no abnormality is detected, the second investigation which is recommended is progesterone challenge test. Progesterone challenge test consists of administration of medroxyprogesterone acetate (MPA), 5 mg twice a day for 10 days. The positive result of the test indicates not only the presence of the uterus but also the presence of functioning ovaries and endometrium. Following administration of MPA, there may be two consequences:

a. Withdrawal bleeding within 10 days
b. No withdrawal bleeding even after 15 days

Interpretation for—(a) withdrawal bleeding means she has got a functioning uterus and ovaries. Even if anatomically and functionally these organs are intact, defect in regulation of coordinated functioning of hypothalamic-pituitary-ovarian uterine axis is suspected, because there is a delay in onset of menarche. Sometimes the defect is transient and reversible. But occasionally this may have far-reaching consequences and may not be easily correctable. To clarify these doubts, estimation of FSH and LH on Day 1 or Day 2 of withdrawal bleeding should be performed.

Interpretation of the result with regard to relative values of FSH and LH are:

i. FSH > LH—delayed menarche
ii. LH > FSH—PCOS
iii. LH and FSH in modest elevation (15–30 IU/l)—incipient ovarian failure

However, prognosis of the second group (b), where withdrawal bleeding does not occur is desperately poor. In these cases, further investigation consists of administration of oestrogen along with progesterone (OC pill); 1 tab daily for 20 days and withdrawal bleeding is awaited for next 10 days.

The interpretation of outcome is as follows:

a. Withdrawal bleeding present—FSH (D1/D2) is to be estimated. If the level of FSH is very high (more than 15 miu/ml), it suggests primary ovarian failure. A diagnosis of hypogonadotropic hypogonadism is made when the FSH level is very low (less than 3 miu/ml).

In such cases, if the uterus and ovaries are very small, there is hardly any scope of restoration of menstrual and reproductive functions even IVF with gamete donation may not be successful. On the other hand, if there is:

b. No withdrawal bleeding—diagnosis is in favour of uterine synechiae, non-responsive endometrium or patchy endometrium

In these cases, there is a scope for surgical correction, especially in mild or moderate uterine synechiae. But in clinical practice they are very unrewarding. If the ovarian function is normal—surrogacy may be advised.

The stepwise approach for diagnosis of apparently unexplained primary amenorrhoea is represented in Figs 14.30 and 14.31.

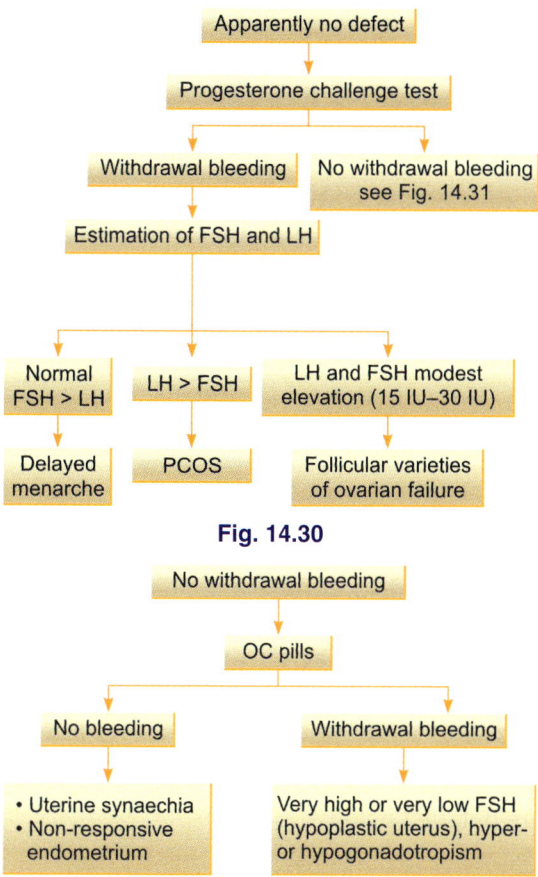

Fig. 14.30

Fig. 14.31

Figs 14.30 and 14.31: Diagrammatic representation of approach for diagnosis of unexplained primary amenorrhoea

In summary, some of the significant clinical landmarks for identification of etiology— while evaluating a case of primary amenorrhoea are outlined below:

a. *History*

i. History of delayed menarche in the family, e.g. mother, sister or cousin

ii. Periodic pain with urinary problems and sometimes with urinary outflow obstruction—the possible etiology is suggestive of imperforate hymen or lower müllerian duct anomaly leading to cryptomenorrhoea.

iii. History of tuberculosis either in the patient or in the family or history suggestive of tuberculosis like neck gland swelling in childhood, ascitis in childhood, emergency laparotomy in childhood for acute abdomen, etc.

iv. History of mumps in childhood

v. History of absence of 'smell sensation'— Kallmann's syndrome or olfactogenital syndrome

vi. History of headache, vomiting or disturbance of vision—suggests CNS abnormality responsible for primary amenorrhoea.

vii. History of galactorrhoea—suggestive of pituitary adenoma.

b. *General Examination*

i. **Short stature:** Indicates one of the following possibilities—(a) Turner's syndrome, (b) hypogonadotropic hypogonadism, (c) cretinism, and (d) congenital adrenal hyperplasia (not abnormally short as in other three groups). Differentiation of the individual etiological factors has already been discussed under individual categories of abnormalities.

ii **Abnormally tall:** *Gigantism* suggests possibility of acromegaly. Sometimes abnormally tall features with absence of secondary sex characters is observed in special type of Turner's syndrome known as 'Tall Turner's' syndrome.

iii **Obesity:** Abnormal obesity with amenorrhoea is observed in some varieties of hypothalamic amenorrhoea with 'ill-defined, etiology which may be associated with a space occupying lesion (SOL). Examples are—Prader-Willi syndrome, Forbes' syndrome, Laurence-Moon-Biedl syndrome, etc. Modest obesity is found in Cushing's syndrome, PCOS and hypothyroidism. The special features of obesity in Cushing's syndrome are— moon facies and 'buffalo obesity' and that in PCOS is central (android obesity). Obesity in hypothyroidism is modest associated with rough skin.

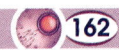

iv. **Thin and lanky:** This feature is commonly associated with—(a) Turner's syndrome, (b) premature ovarian failure, (c) tuberculosis and (d) anorexia nervosa.

v. **Hirsuitism:** Commonly associated with congenital adrenal hyperplasia (coarse hairs), Cushing's syndrome, PCOS, virilising tumours of ovary like arrhenoblastoma.

vi. **Other skeletal abnormalities:** Like kyphosis, scoliosis, shielding of chest, short metacarpal and short metatarsal bones, coarctation of the aorta are commonly found associated with 'Turner's syndrome'.

c. Examination of Secondary Sex Characteristics

i. **Pubic and axillary hair absent, breast absent:** Turner's syndrome, hypogonadotropic hypogonadism and cretinism

ii. **Pubic and axillary hair absent, breast present:** Testicular feminising syndrome (classic or complete variety)

iii. **Pubic and axillary hair present, breast absent:** (a) Incomplete variety of testicular feminising syndrome and (b) late onset CAH. In CAH, the hairs are more coarse and dense. In both conditions phallic enlargement may be present but more prominent in CAH than incomplete variety of testicular feminising syndrome.

iv. **Normal feminine phenotype with normal stature and build, and normal secondary sex characters including normal looking feminine external genitalia:** Probable diagnosis is Mayer-Rokitansky-Küster-Hauser (MRKH) syndrome.

d. Examination of External Genitalia

i. **Clitoral (phallic) enlargement:** (a) CAH, (b) Cushing's syndrome, (c) incomplete variety of testicular feminising syndrome, and (d) virilising tumour of ovary. The differentiating points have already been discussed.

ii. **Absence of vaginal opening:** (a) Imperforate hymen, (b) labial fusion, (c) congenital adrenal hyperplasia (CAH) and (d) MRKH syndrome. Points for differential diagnosis have already been discussed in detail.

iii. **Presence of a lump in the labial/inguinal region sometimes resembling inguinal hernia with absence of pubic hairs:** Diagnosis in testicular feminising syndrome. The lump palpated is gonad.

e. Abdominal Examination

i. **Palpation of an abdominopelvic lump:** (a) Haematometra and haematocolpos, (b) ovarian tumour—dysgerminoma, virilizing tumour of the ovary, embryonic cell carcinoma and (c) encysted ascitis—the commonest diagnosis is encysted tubercular ascitis, sometimes resembling an ovarian cyst; but without a definite margin. Rarely, a kidney may be palpated in the pelvic region—commonly found in association with MRKH.

If no abnormality is detected on clinical examinations outlined above, supplemented with USG evaluation of pelvic organs—progesterone challenge and OC withdrawal tests are to be performed.

Summary of the defects detected in a girl with primary amenorrhoea which are correctable are detailed below:

Objectives of correction are:

a. To restore menstrual function

b. To restore reproductive potential

c. To optimise sexual function and gender correction

These objectives may be fulfilled either completely or partially. Complete fulfillment can be achieved in:

i. **Genital tract abnormalities:** Imperforate hymen, lower müllerian duct obstruction, but not in MRKH syndrome. In MRKH syndrome, only restoration of sexual function is possible. Pregnancy has been achieved through surrogacy.

ii. **Chromosomal anomalies:** In general, restoration of menstrual function is possible only by replacement in some of the cases of Turner's syndrome. Pregnancy has also been achieved in few cases either spontaneously or through IVF and egg donation. In testicular feminising syndrome (TFS), rehabilitation only by gonadectomy and clitoroplasty in incomplete variety is possible. Sexual function restoration may be necessary in some cases of incomplete variety of TFS.

iii. **Hypothalamic-pituitary-ovarian axis defect:** A few functional hypothalamic-pituitary-ovarian defects leading to amenorrhoea are correctable by gonado-tropin induction followed by IUI or IVF. Except in pituitary adenoma leading to hyperprolactinaemia, all space-occupying lesions of hypothalamus and pituitary are life threatening, and therefore, require more attention towards other manifestations rather than primary amenorrhoea. PCOS is a rare cause of primary amenorrhoea and when present can be treated for restoration of menstruation and reproductive function. Ovarian tumours leading to primary amenorrhoea are usually malignant and malignancy demands more attention than menstruation and reproduction. Similarly, primary ovarian failure can sometimes be treated with IVF and egg donation.

iv. **Thyroid and adrenocortical abnormalities:** Unless they are very gross or severe they do not present with primary amenorrhoea. Under such circumstances (severe CAH and cretinism), restoration of menstrual and reproductive function are not the primary objectives of treatment. However, in modest varieties of CAH, pregnancies have been recorded following control of adrenal hyper-activity with corticosteroids. Gender abnormality correction and rehabilitation in childhood and adolescence are the primary objectives of management.

v. **Endometrial unresponsiveness and uterine synechiae:** There are the difficult areas to treat in primary amenorrhoea although pregnancies have been reported following synechiotomy but results in general are not very satisfactory. If ovarian function is normal, surrogacy is the only treatment which may be rewarding.

REFERENCES

1. Wendy J Schillings, Howard D McClamrock. Primary amenorrhoea. Berek and Novak's Gynecology 2007; 14: 1035–1065.

2. Kiningham RB, Apgar BS, Schwenk TL. Evaluation of amenorrhea. *Am Fam Physician.* 1996; 53: 1185–94.

3. Pletcher JR, Slap GB. Menstrual disorders. *Pediatr Clin North Am.* 1999; 46: 505–18.

4. Reindollar RH, Byrd JR, McDonough PG. Delayed sexual development: A study of 252 patients. *Am J Obstet Gynecol.* 1981; 140: 371–80.

5. Saenger P. Turner's syndrome. N Engl J Med 1996; 335: 1749.

6. Massarano AA, Adams JA, Preece MA, Brook CG. Ovarian ultrasound appearances in Turner syndrome. J Pediatr 1989; 114: 568.

7. Wyss D, DeLozier CD, Daniell J, Engel E. Structural anomalies of the X chromosome: Personal observation and review of non-mosaic cases. Clin Genet 1982; 21: 145.

8. Portuondo JA, Neyro JL, Benito JA, et al. Familial 46XX gonadal dysgenesis. Int J Fertil 1987; 32: 56.

9. Blagowidow N, Page DC, Huff D, Mennuti MT. Ullrich-Turner syndrome in an XY female fetus with deletion of the sex-determining portion of the Y chromosome. Am J Med Genet 1989; 34: 159.

10. Krasna IH, Lee ML, Smilow P, et al. Risk of malignancy in bilateral streak gonads: The role of the Y chromosome. J Pediatr Surg 1992; 27: 1376.

11. Bradshaw Karen D Schorge, John O Schaffer, Joseph, Lisa M. Halvorson, Hoffman, Barbara G. Chapter on Amenorrhea: *Williams' Gynecology.* McGraw-Hill Professional 2008.

12. T Morgan. Turner syndrome: Diagnosis and management. Am Fam Physician 2007; 76; 405–10.

13. M.E. Rubio-Gozalbo, C.S. Gubbels, J.A. Bakker, PPCA. Menheere, WKWH. Wodzig, and JA. Land. Gonadal function in male and female patients with classic galactosemia. Human Reproduction update, 2010; 16, No. 2; 177–188.

14. Hoek A, Schoemaker J, Drexhage HA. Premature ovarian failure and ovarian autoimmunity. Endocr Rev. 1997; 18(1): 107–34.

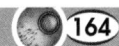
15. Nelson LM AJ, Flack MR. Premature ovarian failure. In: Adashi EY RJ, Rosenwaks Z, ed. Philadelphia: Lippincott-Raven; 1996. p. 1393–410.

16. Morris JM, Mahesh VB. Further observations on the syndrome, "Testicular Feminization Syndrome". Am J Obst Gynecol 1963; 15: 731–45.

17. Viner RM, Test Y, Willams DM, Patterson MN. Androgen Insensitivity Syndrome: a survey of diagnostic procedures. Arch Dis Child 1997; 77: 305–09.

18. Adachi M, Takayang R, Tomura A. Androgen Insensitivity Syndrome: as a possible coactivator Disease. N Engl J Med 2001; 344 (9): 696.

19. Manual M, Katayama KP, Jones HW, JR. The age of occurrence of gonadal tumors in intersex patients with a Y chromosome. Am J Obstet Gynec 1976; 124: 293.

20. Rutgers JL, Scully RE. The Androgen Insensitivity Syndrome: A clinicopathologic study. Int J Gynecol Path 1991; 10: 126.

21. Simpson JL. Genetics of sexual differentiation: Pediatric and Adolescent Gynecology, Ravan Press, New York: 1992: 1–37.

22. Griffin JE. Androgen Resistance: The clinical and molecular spectrum. N Engl J Med 1992; 326: 611.

23. Mecklenburg, Robert S, Loriaux, D. Lynn, Thompson, Ronald H, Andersen, Arnold E, Lipsett, Mortimer B. Hypothalamic Dysfunction in Patients With Anorexia Nervosa. Medicine: March 1974, Volume 53, Issue 2, 147.

24. Liuzzi A, Chiodine PG, Botalla 1, et al. J: "Decreased plasma growth hormone(GH) levels in acromegalics following CB 154 (2-Br-alpha-ergocryptine) administrating;" Clin. Endocrinol. Metab. 1972; 35: 941–43.

25. Barkan AL. Endocrine Metab. Clin. North Am 18:277–310, 1989. Shenker Y; Grekin RJ, et al: Acromegaly diagnosis and therapy; Clin. Endocrinol Metab. 1989; 69: 557–562.

26. Tay CCK, Glasier A, Mcneilly AS. Twenty-four hours secretory profiles of gonadotropins and prolactin in breast feeding women, Hum. Reprod 1992, 7: 951.

27. Green JS, Paffrey PS, Harnett JD, et al. Cardinal manifestations of 'Lawrance-Moon-Biedl' syndrome; N Eng. J. Med. 1989; 321: 1002.

28. Jeffcoate, WJ, Lawrance BM, Edward CRW, Besser GM. Endocrine function in Prader Willi Syndrome; Clin. Endocrin. (Oxford) 1980; 12: 81.

29. Jenkins JS, Gilbert C. Hypothalamic pituitary function in patients with craniopharyngiomas: J. Clin Endocrin. Metab. 1976; 43: 394–99.

30. Kitay JI. Altschule MD. The pineal gland Cambridge, MA. Harvard University Press, 1954.

31. Wurtman RJ, Kammer HN. Eng. Melatonin Synthesis by an ectopic pinealoma: J. Med. 1966; 274: 1233–37.

32. Lichter AS; Wara WM, Sheline GF, et al. Treatment of Craniopharyngeomas; Int. J. Radiat. Oncol. Bio. Phys. 1977; 2:675–683.

33. Walters W, Wilder RM, Kepler EJ. The suprarenal cortical syndrome with presentation of ten cases: Ann Surg. 1934; 100: 670–88.

34. Meador CK, Liddle GW, Island DP, et al. Causes of Cushing's syndrome in patients with tumours arising from non-endocrine tissue; J. Clin. Endocrinol. Metab. 1962; 22: 693–703.

35. Krieger, DT, Amorosa L, Linick F. Cyprohrptadine—induced remission of Cushing's disease; N. Eng. J. Med. 1975; 293: 893–96.

36. Jeffcoate WJ, Rees LH, Tomlin S, et al. Metyrapone in long term management of Cushing's disease; Br. Med. J. 1977; 2:215–17.

37. Poretsky L, Garber J, Kleenfield J: Primary amenorrhoea and pseudoprolactinoma in a patient with primary hypothroidism; Am. J: Med. 1986; 81: 180.

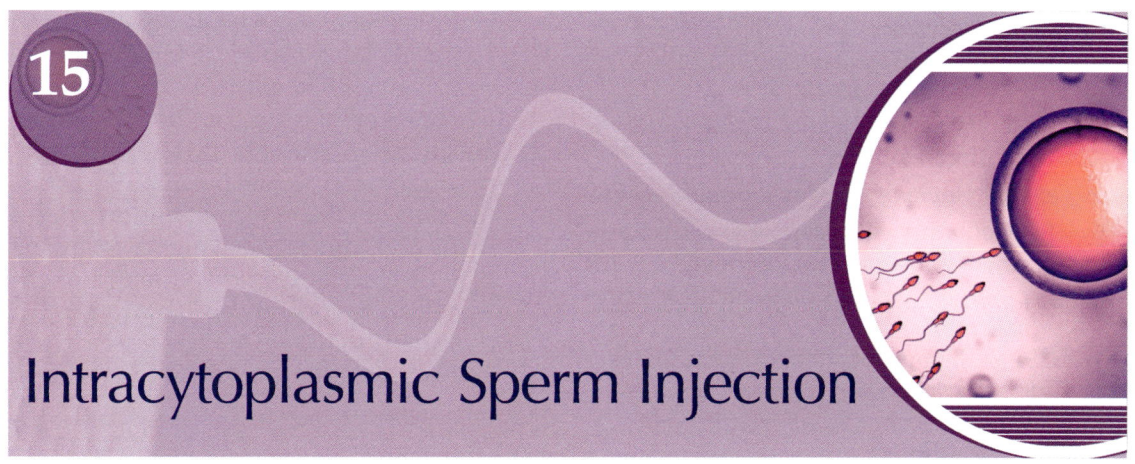

Intracytoplasmic Sperm Injection

INTRODUCTION

Intracytoplasmic sperm injection (ICSI) is a procedure of assisted fertilisation and considered to be an unique treatment for male infertility. Initially, the procedure of gamete micromanipulation for assisted reproduction was introduced for repeated fertilisation failure. The technology was sporadically used to overcome the barrier of zona pellucida because it is possible that the zona becomes hard for sperm penetration due to its prolonged exposure to culture media. The injection of sperm into ooplasm as a successful method of assisted fertilisation was established only by chance. ICSI has now become a very popular method of achieving pregnancy primarily in medically or surgically untreatable azoospermic husband and in addition, in many other complex infertility situations like unexplained infertility, repeated fertilisation failure, etc. The practice started with semi invasive procedure of zona hatching or drilling and subsequently the technology has gone up to the level of intracytoplasmic injection of spermatozoa. So the definition of intracytoplasmic sperm injection (ICSI) is one of the procedures of micromanipulation of oocytes and spermatozoa.

GRADUAL EVOLUTION OF ICSI

As already stated, in cases of repeated fertilisation failure, partial zona dissection was performed, and was followed by insemination as in ordinary IVF procedure. Idea was to overcome the barrier formed by zona pellucida.

When this technique also failed to achieve successful fertilisation the next step which evolved was subzonal insemination (SUZI). The procedure consists of injection of several motile sperms into the perivitelline space.[1] Injection of sperms into cytoplasm crossing not only zona, but also oolemma was a more invasive procedure and was first used in rabbit.[2] The first human pregnancy and birth by ICSI was reported by Palermo (1992) from Brussels, Belgium.[3]

INDICATIONS OF ICSI

Indications of ICSI have now widely been expanded. In some indications, the sperms are collected from testes, while in others the sperm collection is done from ejaculated semen.[4–6] Accordingly indications may be classified depending on the method of collection of spermatozoa.

A. ICSI with ejaculated spermatozoa
Following are the indications:

   a. Oligospermia (< 5,00,000) with normal motility and morphology

   b. Asthenozoospermia (even in Kartagener's syndrome—100% immotile spermatozoa), provided HOST (hypo-osmotic swelling test) is satisfactory.

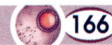

c. Teratozoospermia (when at least 4% sperms have normal morphology—Kruger's 'strict criteria')

d. Repeated fertilisation failure in conventional IVF

e. High level of ASA in seminal plasma

f. Ejaculatory disorders, e.g. retrograde ejaculation (sperm recovered from postmasturbated or postcoital urine sample)

B. ICSI with sperm collected from testes

This may be either from epididymis or interstitial tissue or seminiferous tubules:

i. With epididymal spermatozoa:

   a. Congenital absence of vas deferens

   b. Obstruction of ejaculatory duct

   c. Absence of seminal vesicles

ii. With testicular spermatozoa

   a. Azoospermia due to testicular failure (maturation arrest—germ cells aplasia)

   b. All indications of epididymal sperm

   c. Necrozoospermia

For testicular sperm aspiration especially in germ cell aplasia (Sertoli-cell–only syndrome), multiple biopsies of the testes may be necessary.

PARTIAL LIMITATIONS OF ICSI

a. Globozoospermia—even with globozoospermia pregnancy has been reported, but the chances of fertilisation are less. Though acrosomal reaction is not essential in ICSI fertilisation, failure is still quite common in this situation. This may be due to genetic defect in globozoospermic sperms.

b. Totally immotile or probably non-vital; chances of fertilisation are less even if 'HOST' is positive. Fertilisation rate is poor.

c. Germ cell aplasia (Sertoli-cell–only syndrome)—even in these individuals sperm may be available after multiple biopsy.

d. 3% cancellation rate is associated with absence of cumulus-corona-oocyte complex or metaphase-II oocytes or no sperm in TESE testicular failure in non-obstructive azoospermia.

e. Chromosomal abnormalities are more frequent in individuals with oligo- or oligoasthenozoospermia. So transmission of chromosomal abnormalities in the offspring is much higher following ICSI. ROSNI or round spermatid nuclei injection is preferable than aged or dysfunctional sperm, but miscarriage rate is more following ROSNI.

REQUIREMENTS FOR ICSI

Essential requirements and their functions are summarised below:

i. Inverted microscope fitted with 37°C heated plate (TOKAI) and Hoffman modulator which provides 3D configuration of the gametes (Fig. 15.1).

ii. *Bilateral micromanipulators:*

Functions of micromanipulators: They allow 3-dimensional manipulations (through coarse and fine movements) of the holding pipette on the left and an injection pipette on the right side respectively. Holding pipette is used to fix and injection pipette is used to release the sperm after injection. Injection pipette aspirates some amount of ooplasm before injecting the spermatozoa. Injectors can be either air filled or filled with mineral oil. A micrometer controls the plunger. The whole setup is placed on vibration-proof table to avoid interference by the motion. Some centres prepare their own microtools, but it

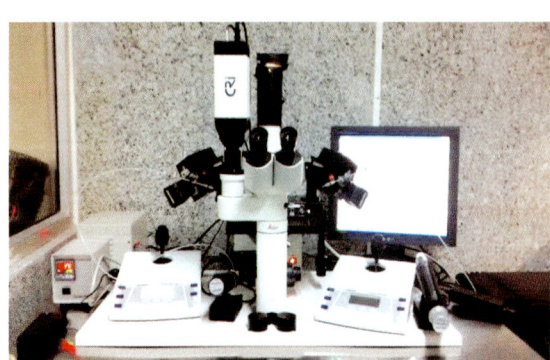

Fig. 15.1: ICSI setup

demands extra effort, time and specialised equipment.

iii. Injecting and holding pipette

iv. Requirements for oocyte and sperm preparation:

- Hyaluronidase, PVP, sperm washing media (pure sperm/all grad 100%), fertilisation media and mineral oil (Fig. 15.2).

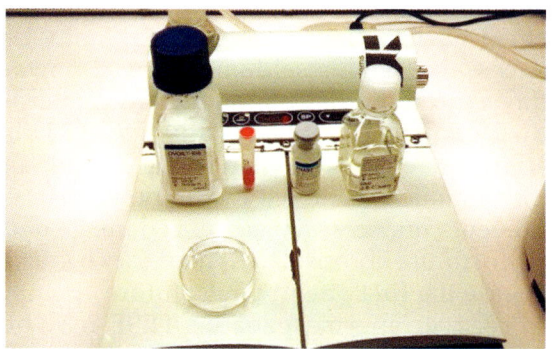

Fig. 15.2: Components for gamete preparation

Normal cellular morphology of sperm and normal ultrastructure of oocyte are essential for healthy fertilisation.

STEPS OF ICSI

Important and vital steps are summarised below:

a. Gamete collection

   i. Oocyte retrieval (same as in conventional IVF)

   ii. Sperm recovery/retrieval

b. Gamete preparation

   i. Oocyte preparation

   ii. Sperm preparation

c. ICSI dish preparation

d. Injection

GAMETE HANDLING PRIOR TO ICSI

Identification of M-II oocyte and oocyte preparation: The first step is denudation.

a. Oocyte denudation: Except for immature oocyte, denudation can be performed between 0 and 4 hours. It does not make any difference in fertilisation rate. The denudation should be performed by combination of enzymatic and mechanical procedures. Enzyme used is hyaluronidase. The concentration and duration of exposure of the oocyte to the enzyme are crucial for success of fertilisation. Unless this limitation is followed, it may lead to parthenogenetic activation of the oocyte. Usually 80 IU/ml hyaluronidase is used for oocyte denudation and oocytes are exposed for 40 seconds in hyaluronidase.

After denudation has been completed the oocyte should be examined under microscope for the following parameters: (i) Zona integrity, (ii) oocyte cytoplasm granularity, (iii) germinal vesicles (nucleus) and (iv) presence of first polar body in the perivitelline space. Absence of germinal vesicles and the presence of first polar body, with 'sun-burst' appearance of cumulus cell around zona indicate the classical characteristics of mature oocyte.

Following retrieval, 95% of cumulus-corona complex contains an intact oocyte (Fig. 15.3a). 5% represents empty zona, cracked zona or morphologically abnormal oocyte. Approximately 4% oocytes are at metaphase I stage with breakdown of GV, but not with extrusion of first polar body. 10% of intact oocytes are at GV stage. 86% are in metaphase II stage with presence of first polar body. ICSI is performed on metaphase II oocytes (Fig. 15.3b), oocyte quality may be assessed with polscopic evaluation of meiotic spindle (Fig. 15.4).

However, metaphase I oocytes may also achieve meiosis after a few hours of incubation

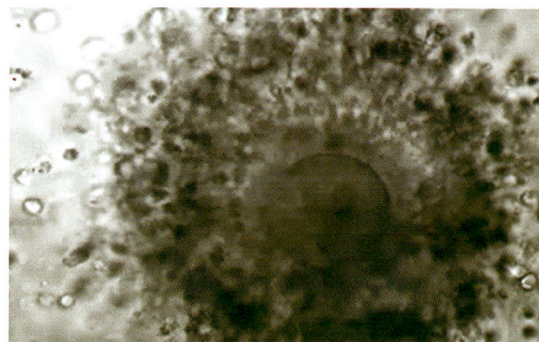

Fig. 15.3a: Mature oocyte before denudation

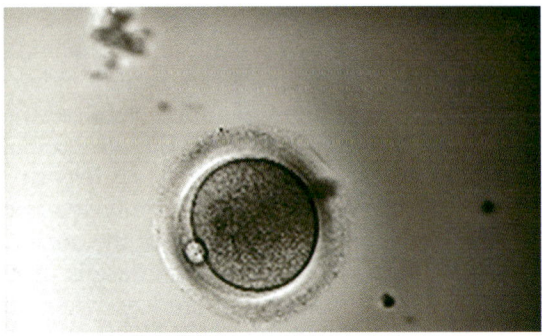

Fig. 15.3b: Metaphase-II oocyte

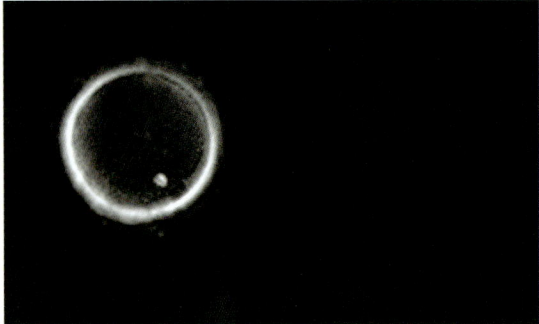

Fig. 15.4: Metaphase-II oocyte with MS under polscope

and may be available for ICSI on the day of OPU.[7] Mature metaphase I oocyte can also be directly subjected to ICSI but fertilisation rate (53%) is much less than what is achieved following injection of metaphase II oocytes. Denuded oocytes are kept in the incubator till the time of microinjection.

Sperm Aspiration/Extraction and Preparation

Sperm retrieval for ICSI procedure is performed in four different ways: (i) PESA—percutaneous epididymal sperm aspiration,[8–10] (ii) TESE or TESA—testicular sperm extraction or testicular sperm aspiration,[11] (iii) microdissection TESE—similar to TESE but using an operative microscope to identify the seminiferous tubules and avoiding vascular damage and (iv) testicular biopsy—seldom performed nowadays.

Procedures 1 and 2 can be performed under local xylocaine infiltration of the scrotal skin. But microsurgical dissection and testicular biopsy requires general anaesthesia. For PESA, the distended epididymis is identified

and using a butterfly needle (Fig. 15.5) (used for pediatric IV infusion) the epididymal fluid is aspirated and immediately examined under microscope to examine the presence of spermatozoa. For TESE, testicular sperm extraction needles are used which are larger than injection pipette (outer diameter 8–10 μm instead of 6–7 μm). Sometimes with a wide bore needle (as used in FNAC) the entire seminiferous tubule can be aspirated (Figs 15.6a and b). If the above two methods fail, surgical biopsy (multiple biopsy) may be necessary. This is seldom essential nowadays. On the other hand, currently microdissection TESE is being advocated. This allows exact identification of the location of the seminiferous tubule and at the same time prevents unnecessary vascular damage and risk of future fibrosis. This is necessary because in case the first attempt fails, future attempt to recover spermatozoa by TESE may be difficult.

Testicular tissues thus obtained are minced in small volume of media into small pieces with two needles or sterile microscopic slides on the heated stage of a microscope. Mincing is to be continued till no single seminiferous tubule (Fig. 15.7) remains intact. Homogenised solution is to be checked under the inverted microscope to confirm the presence of spermatozoa. This determines if further attempt of aspiration is necessary or not.

If the sample is not mixed with other cells (RBC, round cell, etc.) (Fig. 15.8) and adult spermatozoa are less in number (less than 10,000) simple washing is preferable. Sperm preparation is to be done by centrifugation of

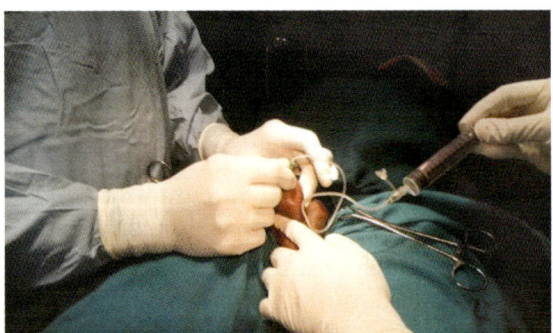

Fig. 15.5: Butterfly needle with tubing used for PESA

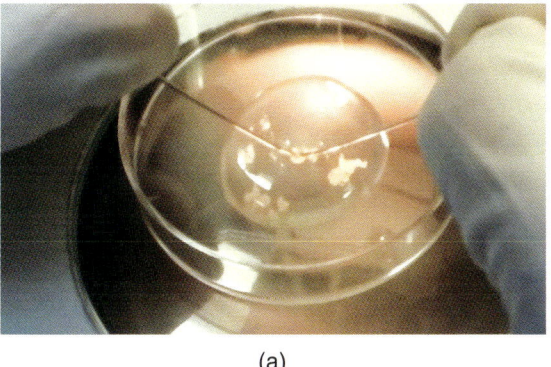

(a)

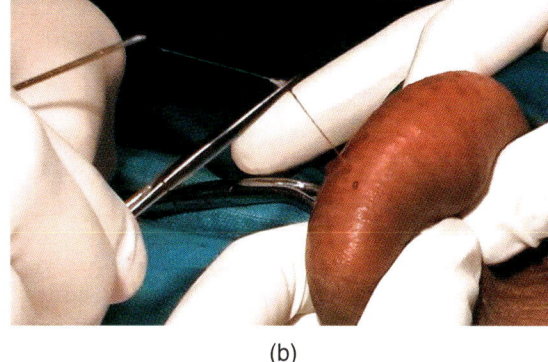

(b)

Figs 15.6a and b: TESE wide bored needle used for extraction of seminiferous tubules

the homogenised solution at 300 g for 5 minutes. The pellet should be suspended in 0.2–0.5 ml of fertilisation media and incubated for at least ½ hour before injection.

If the sample is mixed with blood cells and other cells (Fig. 15.9) sperm preparation by density gradient technique is mandatory.

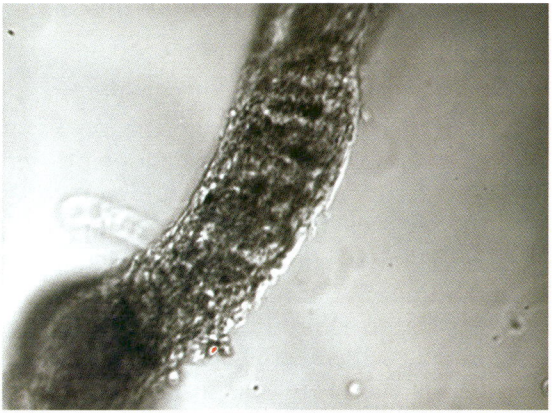

Fig. 15.7: Seminiferous tubule

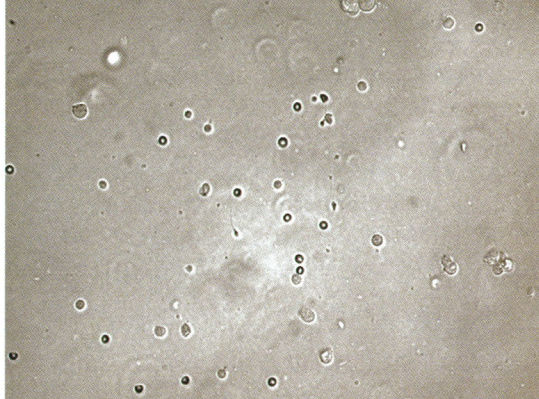

Fig. 15.8: Mature spermatozoa in clear TESA sample (after mincing)

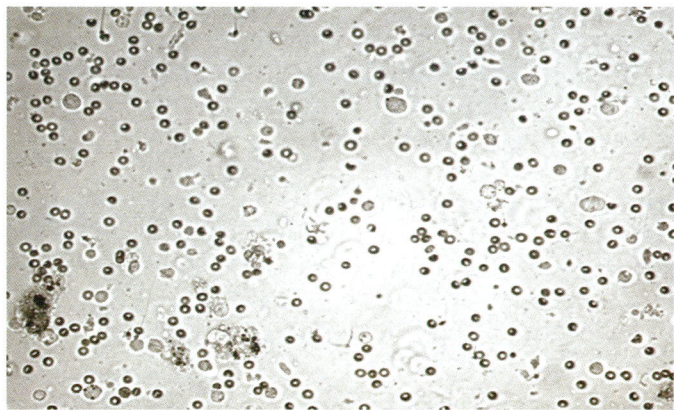

Fig. 15.9: TESA sample containing spermatozoa mixed with other cells (after mincing)

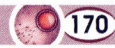

If no sperm cells are found in the first examination under microscope, tissue pieces can be treated with— (a) red blood cell lysis buffer—which dissolves RBCs or (b) an enzymatic collagen digestion medium—which dissolves the collagen tissues around spermatozoa. These procedures help and facilitate search for sperm cells.[12]

If only a few sperm cells are aspirated through fine needle aspiration, further sample processing is not necessary. Collecting single motile sperm with microneedle is necessary prior to ICSI.

Sperm Preparation Method

In ICSI procedure, density gradient centrifugation (using saline coated silica particle colloid solution) is always used. This procedure enhances the number of motile and morphologically normal sperm cells.[13]

Exception is extreme degree of oligozoospermic sample—because density gradient method of semen preparation results in insufficient yield of sperm cells for ICSI. In these cases, simple washing is advocated to reduce loss of sperm cell. In such poor recovery, immediate injection of washed spermatozoa into the oocyte is advocated, otherwise there is a risk of sperm to be damaged by ROS, produced by abnormal sperm cells, or leukocyte as they have not been filtrated by density gradient.

ICSI Dish Preparation (Fig. 15.10)

a. The procedure is carried out in plastic microinjection dish containing microdroplets of medium covered with mineral oil.

b. A fraction of sperm suspension is added to the periphery of the central PVP droplet. Viscous character of PVP is an advantage which slows down sperm motility and allows better control of fluid in the injection needle and prevents sperm cell from sticking to the pipettes.

c. The denuded oocytes are placed in the peripheral medium droplets.

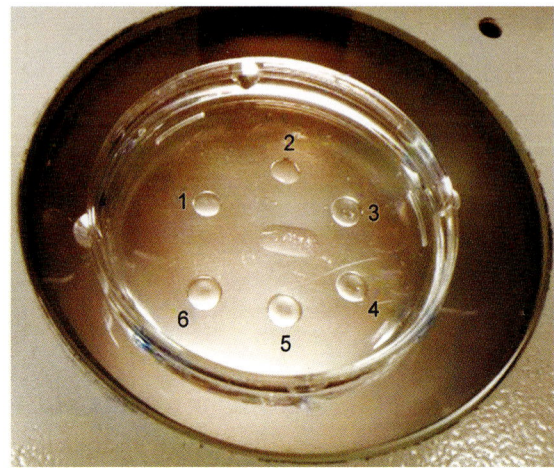

Fig. 15.10: ICSI dish with droplets (central droplet containing spermatozoa—peripheral droplets contain denuded oocyte)

The Dish Should be Incubated Till Injection

Intracytoplasmic injection procedure (Fig. 15.11):

The following steps are to be followed:

i. ICSI dish is brought from the incubator and placed on the heated stage of inverted microscope. The next step is alignment of the pipettes (Fig. 15.12).

ii. Selection and immobilisation of the spermatozoa: A single viable sperm is aspirated (Fig. 15.13) in the injection pipette which is filled with PVP. Sperm cell is then released in perpendicular position from the injection pipette—to facilitate sperm immobilisation. Sperm tail is rubbed against the petridish preferably

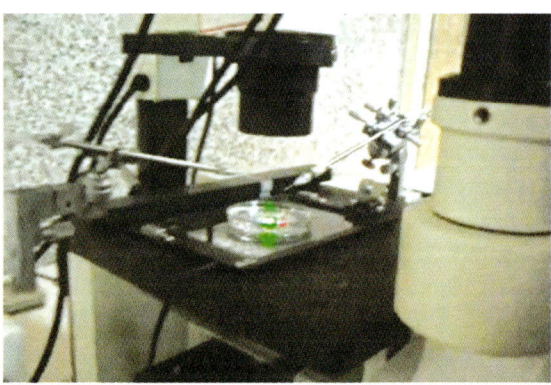

Fig. 15.11: ICSI Procedure

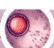

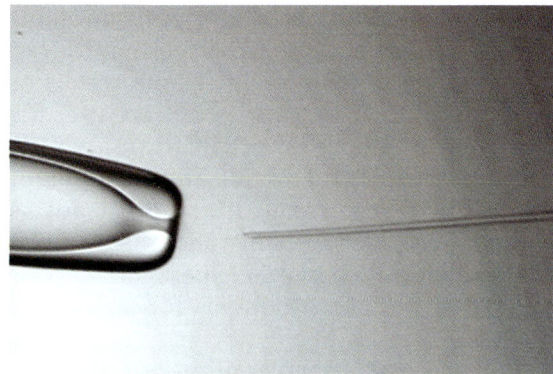

Fig. 15.12: Alignment (holding and injection) pipettes

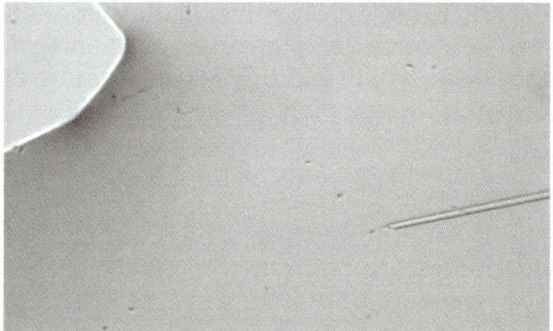

Fig. 15.13: Aspiration of spermatozoa

below the mid-piece. Immobilisation by rubbing the tail is important for oocyte activation.[14-16] This occurs through release of sperm cytosolic factors by the ruptured sperm membrane.

Advancing technology for identification of abnormal sperms has been introduced using higher magnification.

Sperm with big vacuole (> 0.8 μ) or more than one small vacuole in the nucleus which is usually associated with abnormal DNA should not be selected during injection—this procedure is possible under high magnification (6,000–8,000) and the procedure is known as intra-cytoplasmic morphologically selected sperm injection (IMSI). Fertilisation and pregnancy rate could be improved by IMSI.[17]

iii. Holding of the oocyte (Fig.15.14)—the oocyte is to be held with holding forceps in left hand in such a way that the first

polar body is at 6 or 12 o' clock position, to prevent injury to the meiotic spindle. In a good quality oocyte, meiotic spindle and first polar body lie very close to each other. So injection at 3 o' clock position should not injure the meiotic spindle in good quality oocyte.

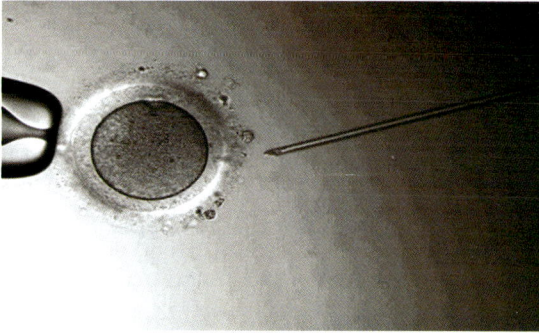

Fig. 15.14: Holding oocyte—PBI at 12 o' clock

iv. Injecting pipette should be brought very close to the 3 o'clock position, thereby proper puncture of the oolemma become easy by gentle pushing of the injecting pipette.

v. The next step is aspiration of the ooplasm to activate the oocyte and procedure also helps to ensure the entry of the injection needle through the oolemma.

vi. Disposal of aspirated ooplasm

vii. Injection of the sperm along with minimal volume of media (Fig. 15.15)

viii. Withdrawal of the injecting pipette

ix. Withdrawal of suction from holding pipette to release the injected oocyte.

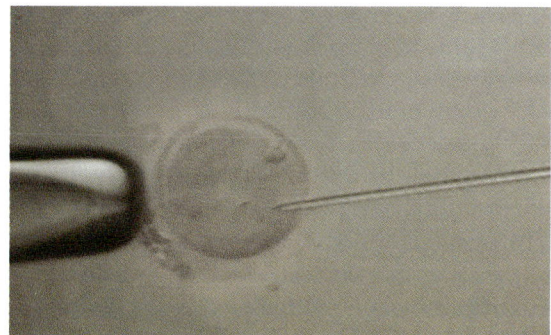

Fig. 15.15: Sperm in the ooplasm after injection

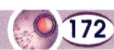

After the procedure all the injected oocytes should be washed in oocyte washing media and dipped in fertilisation or cleavage media layered with liquid paraffin in multiwell dish. Within 16 to 18 hours of injection, fertilisation is to be evaluated by pronuclear scoring on day 1. Rest of the procedure is similar to that in IVF.

Abnormal Fertilisation Following ICSI

This may happen following immature spermatid injection, round spermatid injection or secondary spermatocyte injection. These procedures may lead to incomplete chromatin condensation of sperm head, functional inferiority of cytoplasmic components, inferior quality of centriole; and these poor oocyte-activating factors may ultimately lead to subnormal fertilisation.

Other causes of abnormal or subnormal fertilisation in ICSI are—(a) incomplete calcium oscillation or waves (inefficient oocyte activation)—may lead to incomplete 2nd meiotic division resulting in aneuploidy, (b) defective microtubule organising centres (MTOC)—which may be responsible for defective mitotic and meiotic spindle and formation and (c) microtubules are essential for pronuclear apposition. Oocyte MTOC disappears after fertilisation. Sperm MTOC exists at the centriolar region. If sperm centriole is also defective, microtubules cannot form and pronuclear apposition is not possible. The procedure ends with abnormal fertilisation.

Summary

ICSI is a method of assisted fertilisation through micromanipulation of both male and female gametes. The procedure of injecting a single sperm into oocyte cytoplasm was discovered accidentally while attempting to overcome barrier of fertilisation (in conventional IVF) induced by culture medium exposed zona pellucida by injecting a few motile sperm into the subzonal space. This 'surprise' discovery not only helped in overcoming the problem of repeated fertilisation failure but also was accepted as a 'breakthrough' treatment of male infertility. ICSI is

now possible not only with sperms available in the ejaculate but also from sperm retrieved from testicular tissue—either epididymis or from seminiferous tubules of azoospermic husband. For oocyte fertilisation a single sperm is essential hence the number of sperms retrieved is not that significant as compared to sperm vitality and morphology. Morphologically abnormal sperms with poor vitality carry poor prognosis for successful fertilisation in ICSI.

For successful fertilisation, out of many steps in ICSI 4 are critical and vital. These are: (a) Denudation and identification of M-II oocyte, (b) selection and immobilisation of available sperm cells, (c) correct positioning of the oocyte before injection and (d) rupture of oolemma by aspirating ooplasm in the injecting needle prior to release of sperm.

Abnormal or subnormal fertilisation following ICSI may be a consequence of poor quality sperm which has been injected or inferior quality of oocyte response which has been generated following sperm injection. Poor quality sperms include immature spermatid injection or secondary spermatocyte injection. Defective oocyte response may lead to incomplete 2nd meiotic division or defective microtubule organising centre (MTOC) development which helps in pronuclear apposition. MTOC develops from sperm centriolar region. So defective MTOC formation again indicates sperm centriolar defect.

REFERENCES

1. Ng SC, Bongso A, Ratnam SS, et al. Pregnancy after transfer of sperm under zona. Lancet 1988; 2(8614): 790

2. Iritani A. Micromanipulation of gametes for *in vitro* assisted fertilisation. Mol Reprod Dev 1991; 28(2): 199–207.

3. Palermo G, Joris H, Devroey P, et al. Pregnancies after intracytoplasmic Injection of single spermatozoon into an oocyte. Lancet 1992; 340 (8810): 17–18

4. Palermo GD, Cohen J, Alikani M, Adler A, Rosenwaks Z. Intracytoplasmic sperm injection: A novel treatment for all forms of male factor infertility. Fertil Steril 1995; 63: 1231–40

5. Palermo GD, Cohen J, Rosenwaks Z. Intra-cytoplasmic sperm injection: a powerful tool to overcome fertilisation failure. Fertil Steril 1996; 65: 899–908.

6. Palermo GD, Schlegel PN, Hariprashad JJ, et al. Fertilisation and pregnancy outcome with intracytoplasmic sperm injection for azoospermic men. Hum Reprod 1999; 14: 741–8.

7. De Vos A, Van de Velde H, Joris H, Van Steirteghem A. *In vitro* matured metaphase-I oocytes have a lower fertilisation rate but similar embryo quality as mature metaphase-II oocytes after intracytoplasmic sperm injection. Hum Reprod 1999; 14: 1859–63.

8. Schlegel PN, Berkeley AS, Goldstein M, et al. Epididymal micropuncture with *in vitro* fertilisation and oocyte micromanipulation for the treatment of unreconstructable obstructive azoospermia. Fertil Steril 1994; 61: 895–901.

9. Schlegel PN, Cohen J, Goldstein M, et al. Cystic fibrosis gene mutations do not affect sperm function during *in vitro* fertilisation with micromanipulation for men with bilateral congenital absence of vas deferens. Fertil Steril 1995; 64: 421–6.

10. Tsirigotis M, Pelekanos M, Yazdani N, et al. Simplified sperm retrieval and intracytoplasmic sperm injection in patients with azoospermia. Br J Urol 1995; 76: 765–8.

11. Friedler S, Raziel A, Strassburger D, et al. Testicular sperm retrieval by percutaneous fine needle sperm aspiration compared with testicular sperm extraction by open biopsy in men with non-obstructive azoospermia. Hum Reprod 1997; 12: 1488–93.

12. Ramasamy R, Reifsnyder JE, Bryson C, et al. Role of tissue digestion and extensive sperm search after microdissection testicular sperm extraction. Fertil Steril 2011; 96: 299–302

13. Claassens OE, Menkveld R, Harrison KL. Evaluation of three substitutes for Percoll in sperm isolation by density gradient centrifugation. Hum Reprod 1998; 13: 3139–43.

14. Dozortsev D, Rybouchkin A, De Sutter P, Qian C, Dhont M. Human oocyte activation following intracytoplasmic injection: The role of the sperm cell. Hum Reprod 1995; 10: 403–7.

15. Fishel S, Lisi F, Rinaldi L, et al. Systematic examination of immobilizing spermatozoa before intracytoplasmic sperm injection in the human. Hum Reprod 1995; 10: 497–500

16. Palermo G, Joris H, Derde MP, et al. Sperm characteristics and outcome of human assisted fertilisation by subzonal inseminastion and intracytoplasmic sperm injection. Fertil Steril 1993; 59: 826–35.

17. Berkovitz A, Eltes F, Yaari S, et al. The morphological normalcy of the sperm nucleus and pregnancy rate of intracytoplasmic injection with morphologically selected sperm. um ReprodHHum Reprod 2005; 20: 185–90.

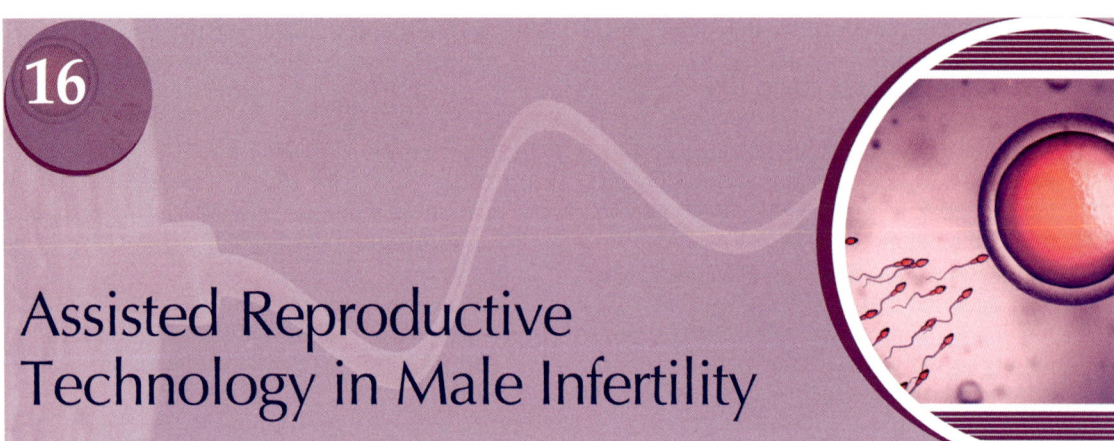

16

Assisted Reproductive Technology in Male Infertility

INTRODUCTION

Male reproductive dysfunction is the sole or contributory cause in half of couples presenting for treatment of infertility. Systematic clinical and laboratory evaluation of the male, and the application of cost-effective management strategies tailored to the individual patient's need are vital components of fertility practice.[1, 2]

Since medical and surgical procedures in male infertility are not very rewarding,[3, 4] assisted reproductive techniques (ART) have become popular adjunctive treatments for alleviating male factor problems. With our current knowledge of treatment of male infertility, the practical dictum has been—"We treat the gametes and not the individual". This is because in male infertility, gamete manipulation followed by ART is more rewarding than treating the person with hormones, antioxidants, vitamins or surgical correction. Gamete micro-manipulation technology has enabled the reproductive biologist to circumvent inefficient steps in the fertilisation process. Instead of simply facilitating sperm-egg interaction *in vivo*, sperm-egg interaction is enhanced by manipulation of the gametes *in vitro*.

With this background, this chapter is discussed under following headings:

- Choice of ART in male infertility
- Advancement of knowledge of ART in male infertility

- Three important steps of ART (IVF/ICSI) in male infertility
  - Selection of normal efficient sperm
    - Prior to ART
    - During semen preparation
    - During ICSI
  - Sperm extraction
    - In obstructive azoospermia, diagnosis and extraction
    - In non-obstructive azoospermia, diagnosis and extraction
  - Sperm protection against damage by ROS
- Conclusion.

CHOICE OF ART IN MALE INFERTILITY

Defining when and which technique to choose remains an important issue. Although good prospective evidence is lacking, often the choice of ART is made according to the semen parameters like total motile count before and/or after sperm preparation.

Three types of ART are possible for treatment of male infertility, namely IUI, conventional IVF and IVF with ICSI. IUI can be suggested as a first line approach when at least 0.8×10^6 motile sperms can be recovered after preparation.[5] IUI being a cost-effective alternative, it is to be proposed before more invasive and expensive treatment options like conventional IVF or IVF with ICSI.[6, 7] Although there are no studies available in the literature demonstrating increased live-birth rates after IUI in male factor infertility, six randomised controlled trials (RCTs) showed a significant increase in pregnancy rates after IUI, compared to timed intercourse in case of male factor infertility.[8]

While IVF was introduced in the late 1970s as a treatment for tubal infertility, it quickly became apparent that it was also an excellent therapeutic option for male subfertility.[9] When no conception has occurred after 3–4 IUI cycles in couples with moderate male factor subfertility with at least one million motile sperms after semen preparation IVF is proposed.

The prevalence of complete fertilisation failure after conventional IVF is reported to be as high as 50%.[10, 11] The causes of total fertilisation failure during standard IVF are related to either oocyte, sperm or laboratory factors; this is also true for ICSI cycles in which complete fertilisation failure occurs in less than 3% of started cycles.[12]

The cut-off values in non-azoospermic and acceptable TMC values used to decide between conventional IVF and ICSI are generally experience-based. TMC (in the native semen sample or after sperm preparation) and sperm morphology (strict criteria) have been used as criteria for determining, if conventional IVF treatment can be recommended to the couple. In this regard, Kastrop, et al.[13] proposed a minimum motile count of at least one million spermatozoa in the native semen sample. Other authors use the motile progressive count after sperm preparation as their criterion, with suggested lower limits of one million[14] to 0.5 million progressive motile spermatozoa[15] or even 0.2 million motile progressive spermatozoa.[16] When morphology is used as a gauge, 5% normal forms is the cut-off value, below which poor fertilisation after conventional IVF is anticipated.[17] Occasionally, a combination of morphology and motile count is analysed. Plachot, et al.[18] proposed that at least 0.5 million normal, progressively motile sperm per millilitre must be present in the ejaculate in order to recommend conventional IVF.

Though there is no good clinical evidence available, there are well-accepted, absolute indications for ICSI: Use of surgically retrieved testicular and epididymal sperm, use of immotile, but viable, ejaculate spermatozoa (e.g. flagellar dyskinesia and immotile cilia syndromes) and use of round-headed spermatozoa (globozoospermia). Presence of significant levels of antisperm antibodies is an indication for ICSI,[19, 20] despite a recent meta-analysis concluding that there is no benefit of ICSI over IVF in cases of antisperm antibody-mediated male factor infertility.[21]

For cryopreserved sperm from cancer patients, ICSI should be the method of choice when assisted reproduction is indicated.[22–25] Based on retrospective case series, it may be prudent that for most of these patients, there may be limited numbers of spermatozoa available due to poor quality of cryopreserved sperm and the post-thaw sperm damage that may occur.

ICSI preceded by PESA or TESE is the only treatment for the azoospermic males.

However, if affordable, IVF/ICSI are superior in all types of male infertility—whether related or unrelated to sperm abnormalities. This means that IVF and ICSI are more rewarding in infertile male, either with azoospermia, oligozoospermia, asthenozoospermia, OTA syndrome as well as in erectile, ejaculatory dysfunction, immune incompatibility, oxidative stress, etc.

ADVANCEMENT OF KNOWLEDGE OF ART IN MALE INFERTILITY

During last 20 years our knowledge in ART, especially with regard to male infertility has significantly advanced in four specific areas.

The four specific areas are:

a. Successful fertilisation does not require epididymal transit of sperm.

b. ICSI requires a single sperm—may be non-motile, but should be viable.

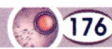

c. Even in Sertoli-cell–only syndrome, microscopic foci of spermatogenesis exist in either testis.

d. With the help of operating microscope—selection and extraction of seminiferous tubules which contain active spermatozoa is possible even in men with Sertoli-cell–only syndrome.

THREE IMPORTANT STEPS OF IVF/ICSI

   i. Sperm selection

  ii. Sperm extraction for ICSI

 iii. Sperm protection against ROS.

Sperm Selection

Even in *in vivo* pregnancies—millions of sperms are deposited in vagina—the competent sperms reach the fallopian tube and the most efficient one fertilises the oocyte—hence there is a need for efficient sperm selection.

At coitus, human sperms are deposited into the anterior vagina, where to avoid vaginal acid and immuno responses, they quickly contact cervical mucus and enter the cervix. Cervical mucus filters sperm with poor morphology and motility and as such only a minority of ejaculated sperms actually enter the cervix. In the uterus, muscular contractions may enhance passage of sperm through the uterine cavity. A few thousand of sperms swim through the uterotubal junctions to reach the fallopian tubes (uterine tubes, oviducts) where sperms are stored in a reservoir, or at least maintained in a fertile state, by interacting with endosalpingeal (oviductal) epithelium. As the time of ovulation approaches, sperms become capacitated, and hyperactivated, which enables them to proceed towards the tubal ampulla. Sperm may be guided to the oocyte by a combination of thermotaxis and chemotaxis. Motility hyperactivation assists sperm in penetrating mucus in the tubes and the cumulus oophorus and zona pellucida of the oocyte, so that they may finally fuse with the oocyte plasma membrane known as oolemma. Knowledge of the biology of sperm transport can help in improving techniques like artificial insemination and IVF.

In IVF/ICSI, inefficient sperms are discarded during sperm processing (density gradient)—morphologically normal sperms are screened and are used for insemination or injection.

In IVF following insemination, still there is a scope and need for natural selection of the most efficient sperms—because fertilisation is not assisted.

But in ICSI, there is no scope for natural sperm selection—because fertilisation occurs by 'assisted-sperm injection'. Hence in ICSI sperms to be injected—should be carefully selected.

How to Select Normal Efficient Sperm?

Sperm selection is performed at three stages of the ICSI procedure. For non-azoospermic subjects sperm assessment is done prior to actual ICSI procedure and also at the time of semen preparation. In azoospermic husbands, sperm selection is carried out during sperm preparation (when adequate number of sperms has been retrieved) or during actual ICSI procedure (when limited number of sperms are available for injection).

The details have already been discussed in some other chapters related to male infertility, but a brief description with relevant photographs, are being presented below for recapitulation.

Sperm Assessment Prior to ART

Conventionally three tests are performed:

a. Tests for absence of motility—hypo-osmotic swelling test (HOST): If more than 60% sperms exhibit coiling and swelling of mid-piece and tail, the test is positive (immotile but viable) (Fig. 16.1).

b. Tests for acrosome integrity—intact acrosome is essential for acrosome reaction at the time of fertilisation. Depletion or absence of acrosome is ascertained by various biochemical and polscopic evaluations (during IVF/ICSI). Details have been described in some other chapters of this book.

c. Tests for nuclear DNA fragmentation—a few common tests are: TUNEL assay—

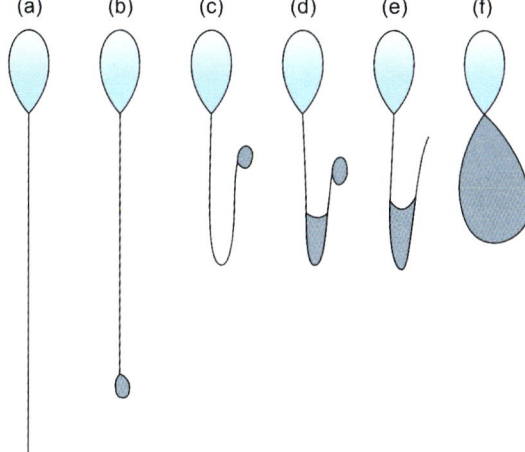

(a)   (b)   (c)   (d)   (e)   (f)

Figs 16.1a to f: Hypo-osmotic swelling test (HOST)

analysed by fluorescence activated cell sorting; COMET assay, after biochemical treatment looks like "comet under fluorescence microscope"; halo-sperm test—the test is performed by commercially available kit (Fig. 16.2).

Complete asthenozoospermia, i.e. 100% immotile spermatozoa in the ejaculate, is reported at a frequency of one out of 5,000 men. It is extremely important to determine the underlying etiology, e.g. primary ciliary dyskinesia (spermatozoa are immotile but viable) or necrozoospermia (spermatozoa are non-viable as may occur in near-complete occlusion of the vas or ejaculatory ducts). In the former category, electron microscopy is the gold standard to diagnose specific sperm defects.[26] Correction should be carried out when possible (e.g. transurethral resection of the ejaculatory ducts in partial ejaculatory duct obstruction). Injection of uncharacterised

immotile sperm makes fertilisation after ICSI unpredictable and decreases both fertilisation and pregnancy rates.[27, 28]

When no motile spermatozoa are found in the ejaculate, the patient should produce a second ejaculate. In most patients, the second semen sample often contains a few motile spermatozoa for use with ICSI. In patients with absolute asthenozoospermia, even after extensive processing of the semen specimen, different strategies can be applied to improve ICSI outcome. Immotile but vital spermatozoa may be selected by a hypo-osmotic swelling test. Since the hypo-osmotic swelling test depends, in part, on the sperm tail membrane, it is not very useful when there are anatomical sperm tail deficiencies, functional sperm tail and flagellar defects.[29] Apart from the hypo-osmotic swelling test, additional corrective measures can be tried such as exposure of the sperm to pentoxifylline, application of laser-assisted immotile sperm selection or the use of a birefringence polscope.[29]

If only dead sperms are present in repeated ejaculates (necrozoospermia), viable spermatozoa may be recovered from a testicular biopsy, and lead to normal fertilisation and pregnancies after ICSI.[30]

Globozoospermia is the morphological end result of disturbed spermiogenesis, and recently, genetic etiologies have been described.[31, 32] Various case reports have detailed the birth of ICSI-conceived offspring using round-headed acrosome-less spermatozoa, but in consecutive case series, the results after ICSI are poor and unpredictable, even when artificial oocyte activation with calcium ionophore is applied.[33]

Apart from globozoospermia and structural abnormalities involving the mid-piece or

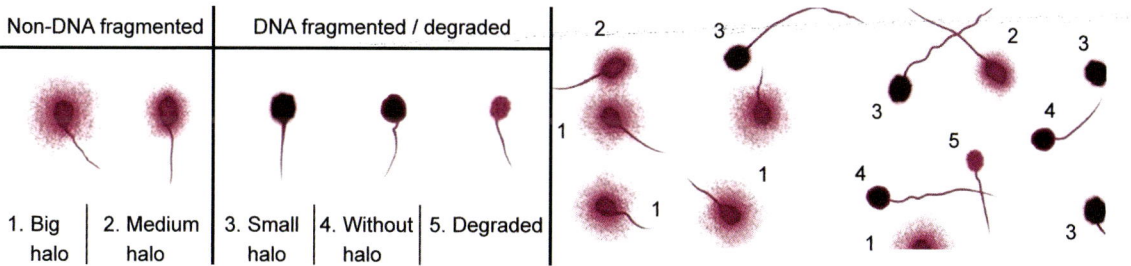

Non-DNA fragmented		DNA fragmented / degraded		
1. Big halo	2. Medium halo	3. Small halo	4. Without halo	5. Degraded

Fig. 16.2: Halo-sperm test

sperm tail, as mentioned above, the impact of teratozoospermia on the outcome after ICSI remains limited. A meta-analysis of studies focusing on teratozoospermia concluded that no decrease in the probability of conception is observed after ICSI using sperm from men with isolated teratozoospermia.[34] However, when only embryos resulting from ICSI using morphologically abnormal spermatozoa are transferred implantation rates are lower.[35]

Loss of DNA integrity may also have an impact on ICSI outcome.[36]

Sperm Selection during Sperm Preparation

Conventional: Density gradient technique is used which removes immature sperms, debris, leukocytes, etc. Otherwise they generate reactive oxygen species.

Special method: Annexin V MACS separation—this is a special method which is used to separate apoptotic from non-apoptotic sperms. Apart from ROS, apoptosis of sperms occurs due to hyperactivity of a plasma membrane enzyme called phosphotidyl serine (PS). This can be detected by ANNEXIN-V microbeads which can be used during sperm preparation.

Sperm Selection during ICSI

This has also been detailed in chapter of ICSI, however, brief description with similar photographs are detailed below:

Unfortunately, there are no real-time methods available to discard spermatozoa with ultrastructural tail deficiencies, DNA damage or chromosomal instability. Yet novel methods to improve selection of spermatozoa for ICSI have been introduced.

PICSI

A technique that depends on binding of spermatozoa to solid state hyaluronan has been introduced in an effort to select mature spermatozoa with lower levels of chromosomal instability for the use in conjunction with ICSI.[37] Intact sperm contains hyaluronic acid receptor on the sperm membrane. Since the bound mature spermatozoa have to be 'harvested' from a petridish coated with solid state hyaluronan; this selection method has been named 'PICSI'. Unfortunately, to date, no data from RCTs are available in order to evaluate the benefit from this novel method.

IMSI: MSOME (Motile Sperm Organelle Morphology Examination)

In the technique of intracytoplasmic morphologically selected sperm injection, spermatozoa are selected by high-power magnification (about × 6000). Based on the few studies available in the literature, a recent albeit premature, meta-analysis concluded that intracytoplasmic morphologically selected sperm injection may significantly improve implantation and pregnancy rates while also reducing miscarriage rates after ICSI.[38]

Are these Tests Indicated in all Cases of Male Infertility Undergoing ICSI?

No; except in repeated fertilisation failure. In addition, the tests may be helpful in all cases with apparent chromosomal/genetic defect; for example, Klinefelter syndrome, XX male, undescended testis, post-chemotherapy azoospermia. However, genetic counseling is mandatory in all cases of male infertility undergoing IVF and ICSI.

Sperm Extraction

Sperm extraction is necessary in azoospermia followed by ICSI. Azoospermia may be of two types—obstructive azoospermia (OA) and non-obstructive azoospermia (NOA). In obstructive azoospermia, obstruction may exist in five different areas of seminal pathway, namely—(a) Rete testis, (b) epididymis (c) vas-deferens, (d) seminal vesicle, and (e) ejaculatory duct. Occasionally vas deferens and seminal vesicle may be absent.

Diagnosis is not difficult except in rete testis obstruction. The salient diagnostic parameters of OA (except rete testis obstruction) are:

a. Epididymis is distended.
b. Serum FSH is normal.
c. Fructose in seminal plasma is absent in ejaculatory duct and seminal vesicle obstruction.
d. Azoospermia in semen analysis.

Sperm extraction in obstructive azoospermia (OA) is not difficult as epididymis is almost always distended. Microsurgical epididymal sperm aspiration (MESA) involves the aspiration of sperm-containing fluid from individual epididymal tubules and the use of the sperm to fertilise oocytes *in vitro*. Use of this technique, first employed in the treatment of men with congenital vasal agenesis, has since been extended to include the treatment of men with other forms of vasal and epididymal obstruction. Another approach to epididymal sperm harvesting is the use of percutaneous epididymal sperm aspiration (PESA).[39] This procedure is somewhat less invasive than MESA, but the yield of motile sperm is lower than that achieved with MESA.

Details of the procedure have been described in Chapter on ICSI.

Genetic defect may coexist. Hence counselling is essential—vertical transmission in male child is a risk factor.

The etiology of non-obstructive azoospermia (NOA): May be genetic—as in Klinefelter's syndrome or in 46XX males. The acquired causes are—undescended testis, systemic chemotherapy and excessive scrotal thermal exposure. The clinical diagnostic parameters include—finding of small testis and flat empty epididymis. Diagnosis is confirmed by low serum FSH level and testicular biopsy reveals evidences of hypospermatogenesis, maturation arrest and Sertoli-cell–only syndrome.

The actual procedures of sperm extraction are as follows:
a. TESE with testicular biopsy under local or general anaesthesia—not commonly performed nowadays.
b. Fine needle or wide bore aspiration biopsy—commonly performed and currently used with 23–19 gauge needle. This not only allows aspiration of testicular tissue but also of seminiferous tubules.
c. Under special situations and in some cases of Sertoli-cell–only syndrome 'micro-dissection TESE' may be useful. This is usually difficult, but a more rewarding technique.

Advantages of micro-dissection TESE over conventional techniques:
- Selective extractions of tubules containing active spermatozoa
- Microscopic vessels can be avoided or cauterised avoiding haematoma or devascularisation
- Avoids unnecessary trauma to already compromised testis.

Disadvantages
- Time consuming
- Surgeon has to be especially trained.

Cumulative delivery rates in couples where testicular sperm is used are low. In obstructive azoospermia of the male partner, the cumulative chance for a delivery after 3 cycles is reported to be 35%, but without drop-out, this figure would be expected to be around 50%.[40] Men suffering from NOA undergoing TESE are to be counseled that not only are the sperm recovery rates limited but also the fertilisation, implantation and conception rates are decreased compared to men with normal spermatogenesis.[41]

Since the introduction of ICSI by Gianpiero Palermo in 1991, there has been much controversy concerning its safety, mainly because of concerns about potential damage to the cytoskeleton and meiotic spindle from the process itself, deleterious modifications that may occur in genomic imprinting and transmission of genetic risks.[42, 43] According to different cohort studies, the prevalence of major congenital malformations after ICSI is comparable to the major congenital malformation rate as reported for conventional IVF and, reassuringly, even large-population studies.[44–46]

However, the mean sex chromosome aneuploidy rate after ICSI (0.8%) is significantly higher than in the general population (0.2%).[47] Neither obstetric outcome of ICSI pregnancies nor child development of ICSI offspring is different from conventional IVF and they are not influenced by sperm origin or quality.[48, 49]

When epididymal sperm is used for ICSI, stillbirths or congenital malformations are not

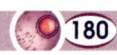

more prevalent in comparison to IVF and ICSI using ejaculated sperm, while cognitive development is also similar.[50, 51] While aneuploidy screening on embryos obtained after ICSI for NOA showed increased aneuploidy and mosaicism,[52] and karyotypes of miscarriages occurring after TESE–ICSI showed higher aneuploidy rates than expected.[53] A few publications focusing on the outcome of children born after ICSI using testicular sperm concludes that no significant differences exist between ICSI using ejaculated spermatozoa or ICSI using testicular spermatozoa in terms of birth weight, perinatal mortality and major malformation rate.[50, 51, 54–57]

Both IVF and ICSI parents should be informed about the uncertainties concerning the long-term issues of these techniques with regard to their future offspring. In addition, patients need genetic testing prior to ICSI, not only for pure diagnostic reasons but also to prevent the transmission of genetic traits associated with their infertility problem.

Sperm Protection Against Damage by Reactive Oxygen Species (ROS)

Aerobic metabolism generates reactive oxygen species—hydroxyl radicals, superoxide anion, hydrogen peroxide and nitric oxide. They are small and highly reactive due to unpaired valence shell electrons that are capable of initiating an uncontrolled cascade of chain reactions.

ROS may block or retard early embryonic development by affecting key cellular organelles required for rapid cell division. The ROS may cause aggregation of cytoskeleton components, condensation of the endoplasmic reticulum, loss of membrane fluidity and embryo fragmentation.[58, 59] Free radicals have many pathological effects including DNA damage. Balance between ROS in the culture media and the ability of embryo to neutralise them may affect *in vitro* embryo development.

Sperms are vulnerable to damage by ROS attack because:

- Sperm head plasma membrane is made up of polyunsaturated fatty acid (PUFA), which is an unstable fatty acid.

- Premature fusion and disintegration of membranes lead to exocytosis of acrosin before sperm head reaches zona pellucida.
- During maturation of spermatozoa, extrusion of cytoplasm allows more place for nuclear DNA—resulting in loss of repair and defence mechanism.
- In ICSI (PESA-ICSI)—presence of abnormal and immature sperms enhances ROS production.

But there are compensatory mechanisms also in seminal plasma. The compensatory plasma antioxidants are superoxide dismutase (SOD), catalase and glutathione. However, these defense mechanisms are disrupted during sperm preparation for IVF or ICSI. For example, high speed centrifugation adds more damage to sperm membrane. Sperm freezing and thawing increase ROS concentration.

Strategies to reduce ROS damage to sperm in ART treatment are discussed below.

The following procedures are practiced to reduce ROS damage:

a. Antioxidant use *in vivo*—treating individuals with antioxidants for three months before ART—results are not very encouraging.
b. Antioxidant use *in vitro*—adding anti-oxidants (vitamin E, vitamin C and CoQ, etc.) to culture media, results are controversial.
c. Adding human serum albumin to culture media—this is believed to be more pro-tective against oxidative stress (OS).

The current conventional practice for reducing OS and to enhance sperm motility for mild to moderate asthenospermic sample is to add either pentoxyfylline (PTX) or platelet activating factor. Undoubtedly the procedure enhances sperm motility *in vitro* but their functional potential for increasing pregnancy rate is still doubtful.

Summary

ART though expensive, is a rewarding treatment for male infertility. IUI has a limited scope with acceptable sperm count and motility in postwash sample. Even in dubious cases of non-obstructive azoospermia, sperm retrieval is possible with advancing technology of microdissection TESE enhancing success rate in fertilisation and pregnancy outcome. Appropriate steps are to be taken for sperm protection against ROS damage in ART procedure.

In all cases of male infertility, genetic counseling is mandatory prior to ICSI procedure.

REFERENCES

1. Baker HW. Clinical Management of Male Infertility in Male Reproduction, Chap. 7, de Groot L, McLachlan R, editors. South Dartmouth MA; MD Text Com. Inc. 2008.

2. Krausz C. Male infertility: pathogenesis and clinical diagnosis. Best Pract Res Clin Endocrinol Metab 2011; 25: 271–85.

3. O' Donovan PA, Vandekerckhove P, Lilford RJ, Hughes E. Treatment of male infertility: Is it effective? Review and meta-analyses of published randomized controlled trials. Hum Reprod 1993; 8: 1209–22.

4. Kamischke A, Nieschlag E. Analysis of medical treatment of male infertility. Hum Reprod. 1999; 14 Suppl 1: 1–23.

5. van Weert JM, Repping S, van Voorhis BJ, van der Veen F, Bossuyt PM, et al. Performance of the postwash total motile sperm count as a predictor of pregnancy at the time of intrauterine insemination: A meta-analysis. Fertil Steril. 2004; 82: 612–20.

6. Goverde AJ, McDonnell J, Vermeiden JP, Schats R, Rutten FF, et al. Intrauterine insemination or *in vitro* fertilisation in idiopathic subfertility and male subfertility: A randomised trial and cost-effectiveness analysis. Lancet 2000; 355: 13–8.

7. Karande VC, Korn A, Morris R, Rao R, Balin M, et al. Prospective randomized trial comparing the outcome and cost of *in vitro* fertilisation with that of a traditional treatment algorithm as first-line therapy for couples with infertility. Fertil Steril 1999; 71: 468–75.

8. Cohlen BJ. Should we continue performing intrauterine inseminations in the year 2004. Gynecol Obstet Invest 2004; 59: 3–13.

9. Brzechffa P, Buyalos R. Female and male partner AE and menotrophin requirements influence pregnancy rates with human menopausal gonadotrophin therapy in combination with intrauterine insemination. Hum Reprod 1997; 12: 29–33.

10. Molloy D, Harrison K, Breen T, Hennessey J. The predictive value of idiopathic failure to fertilise on the first *in vitro* fertilisation attempt. Fertil Steril 1991; 56: 285–9.

11. Coates TE, Check JH, Choe J, Nowroozi K, Lurie D, et al. An evaluation of couples with failure of fertilisation *in vitro*. Hum Reprod 1992; 7: 978–81.

12. Liu J, Nagy ZP, Joris H, Tournaye H, Camus M, et al. Analysis of 76 total-fertilisation-failure cycles out of 2732 intracytoplasmic sperm injection cycles. Hum Reprod 1995; 10: 2630–6.

13. Kastrop PM, Weima SM, van Kooij RJ, te Velde ER. Comparison between intracytoplasmic sperm injection and *in vitro* fertilisation (IVF) with high insemination concentration after total fertilisation failure in a previous IVF attempt. Hum Reprod 1999; 14: 65–9.

14. Fisch B, Kaplan-Kraicer R, Amit S, Zukerman Z, Ovadia J, et al. The relationship between sperm parameters and fertilizing capacity *in vitro*: a predictive role for swim up migration. J *In vitro* Fert Embryo Transf 1990; 7: 38–43.

15. Verheyen G, Tournaye H, Staessen C, de Vos A, Vandervorst M, et al. Controlled comparison of conventional *in vitro* fertilisation and intracytoplasmic sperm injection in patients with asthenozoospermia. Hum Reprod 1999; 14: 2313–9.

16. Payne D, Flaherty SP, Jeffrey R, Warnes GM, Matthews CD. Successful treatment of severe male factor infertility in 100 consecutive cycles using intracytoplasmic sperm injection. Hum Reprod 1994; 9: 2051–7.

17. Grow DR, Oehninger S, Seltman HJ, Toner JP, Swanson RJ, et al. Sperm morphology as diagnosed by strict criteria: Probing the impact of teratozoospermia on fertilisation rate and pregnancy outcome in a large *in vitro* fertilisation population. Fertil Steril. 1994; 62: 559–67.

18. Plachot M, Belaisch-Allart J, Mayenga JM, Chouraqui A, Tesquier L, et al. Outcome of conventional IVF and ICSI on sibling oocytes in mild male factor infertility. Hum Reprod 2002; 17: 362–9.

19. Nagy ZP, Verheyen G, Liu J, Joris H, Janssenswillen C, et al. Results of 55 intracytoplasmic sperm injection cycles in the treatment of male-

immunological infertility. Hum Reprod 1995; 10: 1775–80.

20. Lahteenmaki A, Reima I, Hovatta O. Treatment of severe male immunological infertility by intracytoplasmic sperm injection. Hum Reprod 1995; 10: 2824–8.

21. Zini A, Fahmy N, Belzile E, Ciampi A, Al-Hathal N, et al. Antisperm antibodies are not associated with pregnancy rates after IVF and ICSI: Systematic review and meta-analysis. Hum Reprod 2011; 26: 1288–95.

22. Kelleher S, Wishart SM, Liu PY, Turner L, di Pierro I, et al. Long-term outcomes of elective human sperm cryostorage; Hum Reprod. Volume 16, Issue 12, pp. 2632–2639.

23. Tournaye H, Goossens E, Verheyen G, Frederickx V, de Block G, et al. Preserving the reproductive potential of men and boys with cancer: Current concepts and future prospects. Hum Reprod Update 2004; 10: 525–32.

24. Hourvitz A, Goldschlag DE, Davis OK, Gosden LV, Palermo GD, et al. Intracytoplasmic sperm injection (ICSI) using cryopreserved sperm from men with malignant neoplasm yields high pregnancy rates. Fertil Steril 2008; 90: 557–63.

25. Dohle G. Male infertility in cancer patients: Review of the literature. Int J Urol 2010; 17: 327–31.

26. Mobberley MA. Electron microscopy in the investigation of asthenozoospermia. Br J Biomed Sci. 2010; 67: 92–100.

27. Tournaye H. Clinical aspects of ICSI with immotile sperm. In: Hamamah S, Olivennes F, Mieusset R, Frydman R, editors. Male Sterility and Motility Disorders. New York; Springer-Verlag; 1999: pp. 135–40.

28. Mitchell V, Rives N, Albert M, Peers MC, Selva J, et al. Outcome of ICSI with ejaculated spermatozoa in a series of men with distinct ultrastructuralflagellar abnormalities. Hum Reprod 2006; 21: 2065–74.

29. Ortega C, Verheyen G, Raick D, Camus M, Devroey P, et al. Absolute asthenozoospermia and ICSI: What are the options? Hum Reprod Update 2011; 17: 684–92.

30. Tournaye H, Liu J, Nagy Z, Verheyen G, van Steirteghem A, et al. The use of testicular sperm for intracytoplasmic sperm injection in patients with necrozoospermia. Fertil Steril 1996; 66: 331–4.

31. Dam AH, Koscinski I, Kremer JA, Moutou C, Jaeger AS, et al. Homozygous mutation in

SPATA16 is associated with male infertility in human globozoospermia. Am J Hum Genet 2007; 81: 813–20.

32. Liu G, Shi QW, Lu GX. A newly discovered mutation in PICK1 in a human with globozoospermia. Asian J Androl 2010; 12: 556–60.

33. Tournaye H. Sperm parameters, globozoospermia, necrozoospermia and ICSI outcome. In: Filicori M, editor. Treatment of Infertility: The New Frontiers. Princeton NJ; Communications Media for Education; 1998: pp. 259–68.

34. Hotaling JM, Smith JF, Rosen M, Muller CH, Walsh TJ. The relationship between isolated teratozoospermia and clinical pregnancy after *in vitro* fertilisation with or without intracytoplasmic sperm injection: A systematic review and meta-analysis. Fertil Steril 2010; 95:1141–5.

35. de Vos A, van de Velde H, Joris H, Verheyen G, Devroey P, et al. Influence of individual sperm morphology on fertilisation, embryo morphology, and pregnancy outcome of intracytoplasmic sperm injection. Fertil Steril 2003; 79: 42–8.

36. Zini A, Jamal W, Cowan L, Al-Hathal N. Is sperm DNA damage associated with IVF embryo quality? A systematic review. J Assist Reprod Genet 2011; 28: 391–7.

37. Huszar G, Jakab A, Sakkas D, Ozenci CC, Cayli S, et al. Fertility testing and ICSI sperm selection by hyaluronic acid binding: Clinical and genetic aspects. Reprod biomed online 2007; 14: 650–63.

38. Tournaye H. Update on surgical sperm recovery—the European view. Hum Fertil (Camb) 2010; 13: 242–6.

39. Temple-Smith PD, Southwick GJ, Yates CA, et al. Human pregnancy by in vitro fertilisation (IVF) using sperm aspirated from the epididymis. J *In vitro* Fert Embryo Transf 1985; 2:119–122.

40. Osmanagaoglu K, Tournaye H, Kolibianakis E, Camus M, van Steirteghem A, et al. Cumulative delivery rates after ICSI in women aged >37 years. Hum Reprod 2002; 17: 940–4.

41. Vernaeve V, Tournaye H, Osmanagaoglu K, Verheyen G, van Steirteghem A, et al. Intracytoplasmic sperm injection with testicular spermatozoa is less successful in men with nonobstructiveazoospermia than in men with obstructive azoospermia. Fertil Steril 2003; 79: 529–33.

42. Osmanagaoglu K, Vernaeve V, Kolibianakis E, Tournaye H, Camus M, et al. Cumulative

delivery rates after ICSI treatment cycles with freshly retrieved testicular sperm: A 7-year follow-up study. Hum Reprod 2003; 18: 1836–40.

43. Tournaye H. Intracytoplasmic sperm injection: a time bomb? In: De Jonge C, Barratt C, editors. Assisted Reproductive Technology: Accomplishments and Horizons. Cambridge; Cambridge University Press; 2002. pp. 397–406.

44. Nikolettos N, Asimakopoulos B, Papastefanou IS. Intracytoplasmic sperm injection—an assisted reproduction technique that should make us cautious about imprinting deregulation. J SocGynecol Investig 2006; 13: 317–28.

45. Ponjaert-Kristoffersen I, Bonduelle M, Barnes J, Nekkebroeck J, Loft A, et al. International collaborative study of intracytoplasmic sperm injection-conceived, *in vitro* fertilisation-conceived, and naturally conceived 5-year-old child outcomes: Cognitive and motor assessments. Pediatrics 2005; 115: e 283–9.

46. Bonduelle M, Ponjaert I, Steirteghem AV, Derde MP, Devroey P, et al. Developmental outcome at 2 years of age for children born after ICSI compared with children born after IVF. Hum Reprod 2003; 18: 342–50.

47. Bonduelle M, Liebaers I, Deketelaere V, Derde MP, Camus M, et al. Neonatal data on a cohort of 2889 infants born after ICSI (1991–1999) and of 2995 infants born after IVF (1983–1999) Hum Reprod 2002; 17: 671–94.

48. Bonduelle M, Wilikens A, Buysse A, van Assche E, Devroey P, et al. A follow-up study of children born after intracytoplasmic sperm injection (ICSI) with epididymal and testicular spermatozoa and after replacement of cryopreserved embryos obtained after ICSI. Hum Reprod 1998; 13 Suppl 1: 196–207

49. Wennerholm UB, Bergh C, Hamberger L, Westlander G, Wikland M, et al. Obstetric outcome of pregnancies following ICSI, classified according to sperm origin and quality. Hum Reprod 2000; 15: 1189–94.

50. Wennerholm UB, Bonduelle M, Sutcliffe A, Bergh C, Niklasson A, et al. Paternal sperm concentration and growth and cognitive development in children born with a gestational age more than 32 weeks after assisted reproductive therapy. Hum Reprod 2006; 21: 1514–20.

51. Belva F, de Schrijver F, Tournaye H, Liebaers I, Devroey P, et al. Neonatal outcome of 724 children born after ICSI using non-ejaculated sperm. Hum Reprod 2011; 26: 1752–8.

52. Woldringh GH, Horvers M, Janssen AJ, Reuser JJ, de Groot SA, et al. Follow-up of children born after ICSI with epididymal spermatozoa. Hum Reprod 2011; 26: 1759–67.

53. Silber S, Escudero T, Lenahan K, Abdelhadi I, Kilani Z, et al. Chromosomal abnormalities in embryos derived from testicular sperm extraction. FertilSteril 2003; 79: 30–8.

54. Bettio D, Venci A, Levi Setti P. Chromosomal abnormalities in miscarriages after different assisted reproduction procedures. Placenta 2008; 29 Suppl B: 126–8.

55. Palermo G, Schlegel PN, Hariprashad JJ, Ergün B, Mielnik A, et al. Fertilisation and pregnancy outcome with intracytoplasmic sperm injection for azoospermic men. Hum Reprod 1999; 14: 741–8.

56. Ludwig M, Katalinic A. Malformation rate in fetuses and children conceived after ICSI: results of a prospective cohort study. Reprod biomed online 2002; 5: 171–8.

57. Vernaeve V, Bonduelle M, Tournaye H, Camus M, van Steirteghem A, et al. Pregnancy outcome and neonatal data of children born after ICSI using testicular sperm in obstructive and non-obstructive azoospermia. Hum Reprod 2003; 18: 2093–7.

58. Agarwal A, Gupta S, Sharma RK. Role of oxidative stress in female reproduction. Reprod Biol Endocrinol 2005; 3:28.

59. Gupta S, Agarwal A, Banerjee J, Alvarez JG. The role of oxidative stress in spontaneous abortion and recurrent pregnancy loss: A systematic review. Obstet Gynecol Sur 2007; 62: 335–47.

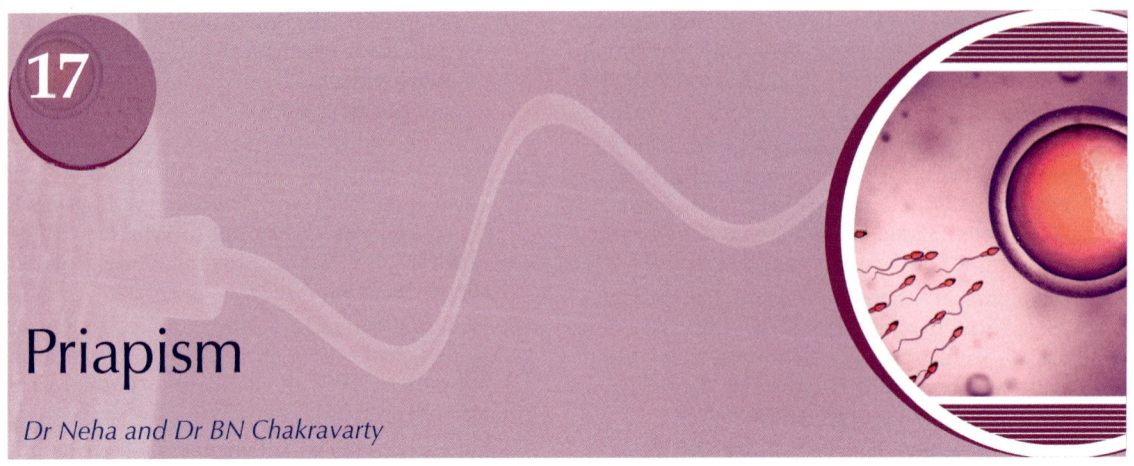

Priapism

Dr Neha and Dr BN Chakravarty

Priapism is a condition in which an erect penis fails to return to flaccid state within four hours in absence of physical and psychological stimulation. The condition develops when blood in the penis becomes trapped and is unable to drain. The term "Priapism" is derived from the word PRIAPUS, the Greek God of fertility and lust, who has been depicted with large phallus.[1]

Typically, only the corpora cavernosa are affected; rarely spongiosum and glans penis.[2] If the condition is not treated immediately, it can lead to scarring and permanent erectile dysfunction. It is a medical emergency, especially ischaemic priapism and early treatment is important for full functional restoration.

The incidence is 1.5 in 100,000 persons per year[3] and is particularly common in those with sickle cell disease. It can occur in all age groups. Priapism has a bimodal peak incidence and is most common between ages 5 years and 10 years in boys and ages 20 years and 50 years in men.[4] Common association amongst adults is the use of medication specially with intracavernosal injection accounting for about 25% of adult cases.[5] The common association in children is sickle cell disease.

TYPES

1. Ischaemic (veno-occlusive, low flow or anoxic) priapism constitutes 80–90% cases.

It is a nonsexual, persistent erection, resulting from blood not adequately draining from the penis to the body due to impaired relaxation instead of paralysis of cavernosal smooth muscles.[6–8] Consequently, blood gets trapped in the erection chambers and corpus cavernosa. It is a type of compartment syndrome.[9] A variety of etiologic factors may contribute to the failure of the detumescence mechanism in this condition. Dysfunction of nitric oxide pathway can result in priapism in some group of patients, especially those with sickle cell disease.[10] Ischaemic priapism is an emergency and a painful condition. Due to stagnation of blood, over a period of time—hypoxia, hypercarbia and acidosis sets in the penile tissue. The corpora cavernosa becomes rigid and penile tissue becomes oedematous. As a result of these changes, structural damage to erectile tissues at microscopic level can occur as early as four to six hours of onset of erection. Irreversible damage with necrosis of endothelial cells and cavernosal smooth muscles can occur, if the condition persists for 24 to 48 hours, followed by fibroblastic proliferation and fibrosis of erectile tissues. Thus the duration of priapism is strongly correlated with erectile dysfunction in future.

Resolution of ischaemic priapism results in penis returning to a flaccid, non-painful state. Using colour Doppler ultrasonography and by measuring the oxygen and CO_2 content and the pH of the blood in cavernosa, resolution of priapism can be verified.

2. Non-ischaemic (arterial, high flow or congenital) priapism constitutes 10–20% of cases. It is a nonsexual and persistent erection caused by unregulated cavernous arterial inflow and usually less painful. It mostly results from a fistula between the cavernosal artery and corpus cavernosum occurring as a congenital defect. The defect also may be secondary to trauma in the perineal region, which prevents blood in the penis from circulating normally, with increased flow and accumulation of blood in cavernosa. The onset of posttraumatic non-ischaemic priapism can occur up to 72 hours after injury. Congenital arterial malformation may also be a cause of non-ischaemic priapism. Typically the penis is neither fully rigid nor painful. This condition is not an emergency. In 62% cases, this type of priapism resolves spontaneously.[11] On resolution of nonischaemic priapism, the penis becomes completely flaccid.

3. Stuttering (intermittent or recurrent) priapism is a type of ischaemic priapism, in which unwanted, unstimulated painful erections occur repeatedly with intervening periods of detumescence. It most commonly occurs in individuals with sickle cell disease. Initially the duration of erection is short, but with time, these episodes of erection become prolonged and more frequent, finally leading to full-blown ischaemic priapism. Dysfunction of nitric oxide pathway and phosphodiesterase type 5 in erectile tissues has been implicated in the pathogenesis.

Etiology

It is a poorly understood phenomenon and involves vascular and neurological factors.

It can be associated with:

a. Congenital arterial malformations involving penile arteries

b. *Haematological condition*: Sickle cell disease and sickle cell trait, leukaemia, thalassaemia

c. *Neurological disorders*: Spinal cord trauma, spinal cord lesions

d. *Iatrogenic complication of intracavernosal injection of prostaglandin E1*: It occurs in almost 5% of cases.

e. *Medications*: A common cause of priapism is the use and/or misuse of medications. Drugs that may cause priapism are antihypertensives, anticoagulants and antidepressants.

f. Glucose-6-phosphate dehydrogenase deficiency is associated with priapism. The enzyme deficiency leads to decreased levels of NADPH (nicotinamide adenine dinucleotide phosphate hydrogenase), which is a cofactor involved in formation of NO.

g. In extreme cases of rabies

h. Illicit drug use, such as marijuana and cocaine

i. In rare cases, priapism may be related to cancers that can affect the penis and prevent the outflow of blood.

Clinical Features and Diagnosis

The diagnosis is self-evident. Persistent erection in absence of sexual excitement, leads to diagnosis. Using colour Doppler ultrasonography and/or cavernosal blood gas analysis, ischaemic and non-ischaemic varieties can be distinguished.

Complications of Priapism

- Clotting of blood retained in the penis (thrombosis).
- Damage to the blood vessels of the penis resulting in impaired erectile function or impotence.
- Ischaemia of penis
- In serious cases, ischaemia may lead to gangrene which could necessitate penis removal (amputation).

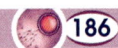

Management

History and Clinical Examination

The diagnosis of priapism is self-evident. One's main aim should be to differentiate ischaemic from nonischaemic priapism, as ischaemic condition is an emergency. Patient's history, clinical examination and laboratory/radiologic assessment helps in reaching diagnosis and consequently determining treatment.

The Important Points in History

- Duration of erection and any history of prior similar episode and treatment taken
- Associated pain
- History of any haematological condition especially, sickle cell disease.
- Medication history, use of antihypertensives; anticoagulants; antidepressants and other psychoactive drugs; alcohol, marijuana, cocaine and other illegal substances. History of intracavernosal injection of prostaglandin E1.
- History of perineal or pelvic injury.

The genitalia, perineum and abdomen should be carefully examined. Examination of penis, in cases of priapism, reveals engorgement of corpora cavernosa, but corpus spongiosum and glans penis remain flaccid in most cases in contrast to normal erection. Abdominal, pelvic and perineal examination may reveal evidence of trauma or malignancy.

The Laboratory and Radiologic Tests

- **Complete blood count with haemoglobin electrophoresis:** These tests can be helpful to diagnose haemoglobinopathies, like sickle cell disease, thalassaemia.
- **Psychoactive medication screening and urine toxicology:** These tests can be done, if priapism is suspected due to misuse or side effect of drugs.
- **Cavernosal blood gas analysis:** Due to stagnation of blood, in case of ischaemic priapism, over a period of time hypoxia, hypercarbia and acidosis sets in. In case of nonischaemic variety, blood gas analysis is normal.

- **Colour Doppler ultrasonography:** By using colour Doppler ultrasonography, ischaemic type can be differentiated from nonischaemic variety. In ischaemic variety there is minimal or absent blood flow in contrast to normal or high blood flow observed in nonischaemic type.[12]
- Penile arteriography

Using colour Doppler ultrasonography and/or cavernosal blood gas analysis ischaemic and nonischaemic varieties can be distinguished.

Treatment

The goal of the treatment is to achieve detumescence and preserve erectile function.

Treatment depends on the cause, in sickle cell anemia, the first step in management is blood exchange transfusion. The treatment options in other cases are as follows:

- **Ice packs:** Ice applied to the penis and perineum may reduce swelling.
- **Oral analgesics:** If the patient is complaining of pain, oral analgesics can be used.
- **Drugs:** α-agonist agents like pseudoephedrine are used which exert a constriction effect on smooth muscles of corpora cavernosa, that in turn facilitates venous outflow.
- Intracavernous injection of sympathomimetic drugs, which induce contraction of cavernosal smooth muscles thus promoting venous drainage. During this treatment drugs known as α-agonists are injected into the penis. Phenylephrine is the drug of choice. Oral α-agonists have also been used for the acute treatment of priapism.
- **Aspiration:** After numbing the penis, aspiration of blood from cavernosa is done with heparinised needle to reduce pressure and swelling.
- **Surgical shunt:** A shunt is a passageway that is surgically created between corpus cavernosum and the corpus spongiosum, glans penis or one of the penile veins to

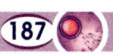

divert the blood flow and allow circulation to return to normal.

- Arteriography with embolisation of the fistulous connection can be done.

- **Surgical ligation:** Used in cases where an artery has been ruptured. Ligation of the fistula or ruptured artery that is causing the priapism in order to restore normal blood flow is also recommended.

Summary

Priapism is a state of prolonged penile erection in absence of sexual or psychological stimulation. Priapism occurs because blood is trapped in the erectile cavernous tissues of penis and is unable to drain.

There are three clinical types; low flow or ischaemic, high flow or non-ischaemic, stuttering or intermittent. Low flow or ischaemic priapism constitutes 80–90% cases of clinically presented priapism.

Basically, priapism occurs due to vascular or neurological defect. Haematological disorders like sickle cell trait, leukaemia, thalassaemia may be associated with priapism. Similarly, spinal cord trauma or lesions may be associated with priapism.

Complications include subsequent erectile dysfunction and in extreme cases gangrene of the penis. Priapism is an emergency condition. The principle of management consists of prevention of complications. In early cases local application of ice or use of drugs like α-agonist agents may help. But for intractable cases, intracavernous injection of α-agonist agents, surgical ligation of artery, surgical shunt or aspiration of blood from corpus cavernosa may be required.

REFERENCES

1. Papadopoulos, I; Kelâmi, A. Priapus and priapism. From mythology to medicine. Urology 1988; 32:385.
2. Lewis, JH; Javidan, J; Keoleian, CM; Shetty, SD. Management of partial segmental priapism. Urology 2001; 57:169.
3. El and, IA; van der Lei, J; Stricker, BH; Sturkenboom, MJ. Incidence of priapism in the general population. Urology 2001; 57:970.
4. Cherian, J; Rao, AR; Thwaini, A, et al. Medical and surgical management of priapism. Postgrad Med J 2006; 82:89.
5. Burnett, AL; Bivalacqua, TJ. Priapism: current principles and practice. Urol Clin North Am 2007; 34:631.
6. Broderick, GA; Gordon, D; Hypolite, J; Levin, RM. Anoxia and corporal smooth muscle dysfunction: a model for ischemic priapism. J Urol 1994; 151:259.
7. Kim, NN; Kim, JJ; Hypolite, J, et al. Altered contractility of rabbit penile corpus cavernosum smooth muscle by hypoxia. J Urol 1996; 155:772.
8. Moon, DG; Lee, DS; Kim, JJ. Altered contractile response of penis under hypoxia with metabolic acidosis. Int J Impot Res 1999; 11:265.
9. Pryor, J; Akkus, E; Alter, G, et al. Priapism. J Sex Med 2004; 1:116.
10. Burnett, AL. Nitric oxide in the penis—science and therapeutic implications from erectile dysfunction to priapism. J Sex Med 2006; 3: 578.
11. Montague, DK; Jarow, J; Broderick, GA, et al. American Urological Association guideline on the management of priapism. J Urol 2003; 170:1318.
12. Metawea, B; El-Nashar, AR; Gad-Allah, A, et al. Intracavernous papaverine/phentolamine induced priapism can be accurately predicted with color Doppler ultrasonography. Urology 2005; 66: 858.

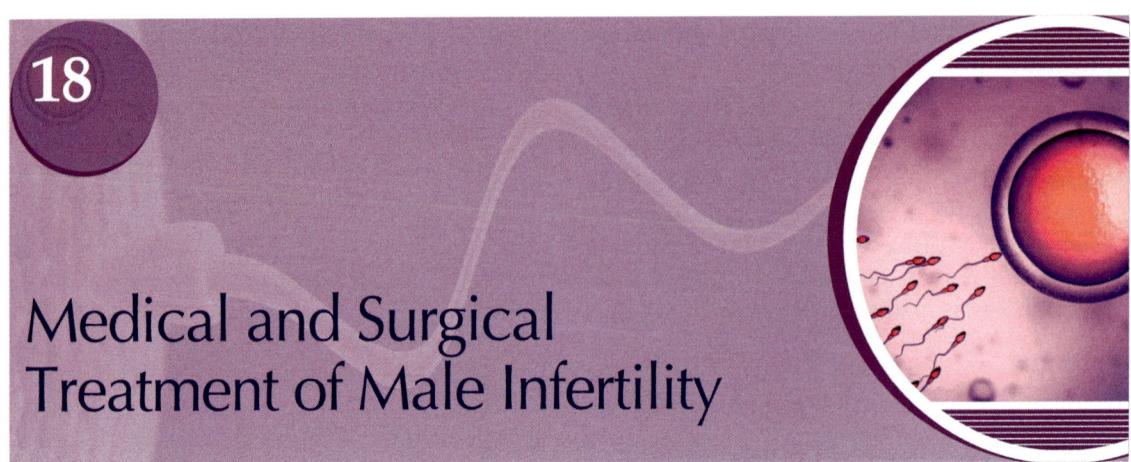

18

Medical and Surgical Treatment of Male Infertility

Medical management of male infertility is not very rewarding. Though there are sporadic reports of improvement of semen parameters with medical therapy, the overall experience of uniform benefit is far from satisfactory. However, the alternative treatment of assisted reproductive technology is very expensive and may not be affordable by all patients. Moreover, a few types of male reproductive abnormalities though limited, may exhibit favourable improvement with medical therapy.

This limited group includes oligo- and rarely a few selected cases of oligoasthenospermia, due to endocrine abnormalities, semen or seminal tract infection or inflammation including these affecting testis or scrotal skin. Some cases of erectile and ejaculatory dysfunction may also be treated by medical therapy. These are examples where a specific medical therapy is rationally indicated.

Apart from directed therapy, the place of empiric medical treatment in male infertility cannot be totally ignored. Empiric treatment is based on theoretical concept or practical experience without proven efficacy. The word 'Emperic' is derived from Greek word 'Empeirikós' which means a doctor relying on experience only. It is difficult to predict who will respond to empiric medical treatment (hormonal, antioxidants, nutraceuticals), and who will not respond, but their correct choice and judicious application may be valuable

in conjunction with assisted reproductive technology. A few relevant circumstances are discussed in this chapter. Initially the place of specific medical therapy is discussed and subsequently role and rationality of empiric treatment is outlined.

ENDOCRINE DYSFUNCTION

Deficiency or excess of some of the hormones related to sperm development or maturation may be responsible for oligospermia or mild oligoasthenospermia. Endocrine substitution or regulation may help to improve semen parameters. The following are some of the examples:

A. Role of Gonadotropins

Both follicle-stimulating hormone (FSH) and luteinizing hormone (LH) are essential for spermatogenesis. LH acts on Leydig cells to produce androgen and FSH acts on Sertoli cells to generate androgen-binding globulin (ABG), a protein—which carries androgen into the lumen of seminiferous tubules for development and maturation of spermatozoa.

While FSH exerts a synergistic action with LH for initiating spermatogenesis, the ongoing role of FSH after initiation is controversial.[1]

It is surprising that germ cells do not have androgen receptors but androgens produced by Leydig cell act on germ cell through androgen binding-globulin generated by Sertoli cell.

It has been suggested that both hypo- and hyper-androgenism may adversely affect sperm production and maturation. In one variety which is more common—hypogonadotropism leads to hypoandrogenism (both serum and testicular). In this variety, pituitary is primarily at fault. While in the other, primary hyperandrogenism (mostly iatrogenic), through suppression of anterior pituitary leads to hypogonadotropism which in turn results in reduced intratesticular testosterone production. In the second variety, hyperandrogenism develops in consequence of administration of exogenous androgens or use of anabolic steroids mostly used for stimulating spermatogenesis in oligospermic subjects. Elevated serum level of androgen suppresses pituitary gonadotropin which in turn, reduces intratesticular testosterone production. In this variety, pituitary suppression is secondary to hyperandrogenism. In both varieties, the objective of treatment is replacement with exogenous gonadotropin therapy.

In the following paragraphs, the treatment of both the groups is outlined under separate headings:

a. Management of hypoandrogenic hypogonadotropic oligospermia: It has already been stated that hypogonadotropism results in androgen deficiency which leads to reduced sperm production and maturation. The basic etiology of this variety may be either congenital or acquired. One of the rare congenital causes is Kallmann's syndrome which is manifested by anosmia and oligo- or azoospermia. Other features of Kallmann's syndrome which may or may not exist are—cleft palate and cryptorchidism. Oligo- or azoospermia in Kallmann's syndrome is due to failure of hypothalamic gonadotropin-releasing hormone (GnRH) secretion. This leads to deficient secretion of FSH and LH. Acquired causes of hypogonadotropism leading to oligo- or azoospermia may be due to tumour or trauma. Medical treatment consists of substitution of gonadotropin therapy.

Classic regimen of HMG and hCG in oligospermia due to hypogonadotropic hypogonadism:

i. hCG injection (1500–2000 IU) SC/IM—three times a week for 3 to 6 months. hCG is a surrogate for LH. Therefore, the objective of use of hCG is to increase intratesticular testosterone level. If sperm count does not improve then hCG regimen is followed by.

ii. HMG injection (75–150 IU) SC/IM—three times a week for 3 to 6 months. Treatment response may be observed between six months and one year following commencement of therapy. Miyagawa Y, et al. reported, in a retrospective study, promising result following combination regimen of intramuscular injection of hCG (3000 IU) twice a week and HMG (75 IU) 3 times a week for a period of 3–6 months.[2]

However, currently with alternate option of IVF-ET very few patients will opt for medical therapy. This is because with medical treatment, the duration of therapy is longer and final outcome in terms of achieving pregnancy is more uncertain than in ART.

Clomiphene citrate has also been used for mild grades of hypogonadotropic hypoandrogenic oligospermia. The mechanism of action and the dose used are as follows:

Clomiphene binds to hypothalamic and pituitary oestrogen receptor sites, thereby blocking oestrogenic central feedback inhibition mechanism of gonadotropin secretion. This allows pituitary to release elevated level of gonadotropin—thereby increasing intratesticular testosterone production. Whitten and coworkers specifically evaluated effect of clomiphene citrate in men with hypogonadotropic hypogonadism.[3] They reported favourable response of these individuals with 50 mg of clomiphene citrate three times per day for 3–4 months. However, it must be noted that the use of clomiphene citrate

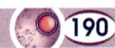

in this setting is currently considered to be an 'off-label' usage.

b. Management of hyperandrogenic hypogonadotropic oligospermia:

This rare variety of oligospermia is observed in some men taking exogenous testosterone or following use of illicit anabolic steroid supplementation. Hormone estimation reveals low FSH and LH and excess serum androgen level. Low level of serum FSH and LH leads to decreased intratesticular testosterone level resulting in partial or complete suppression of testicular sperm production.

Though research is currently ongoing with androgen as the major component of the medical male hormonal contraceptive agents, exogenous androgen should be withheld in men actively trying to achieve pregnancy. This also refers to hypogonadotropic oligospermic men being treated with androgens.

Treatment for hyperandrogenic hypogonadotropic men with excess androgens consists of avoiding use of exogenous androgen or anabolic steroids. If patients still have hypogonadism with persistent oligo- or azoospermia after cessation of androgen therapy, attempt to increase intratesticular testosterone with hCG with or without HMG may be beneficial.[4]

B. Role of Thyroid Hormone

Thyroid hormones are essential in organ development and routine metabolism. Hypothyroidism is a known cause of diminished libido and erectile dysfunction (Griboff, 1962). Hypothyroidism leads to oligospermia as well. Treatment with thyroxine helps in achieving improved sperm count and motility.

Similarly, hyperthyroidism (Graves' disease) also has a negative impact on spermatogenesis. This is because patients with hyperthyroidism have lower bioavailable testosterone, higher sex hormone-binding globulin, higher LH level compared to control. These patients also have remarkably abnormal semen parameters. The same author also stressed that deficits including semen abnormalities were normalised once euthyroid state is achieved.

C. Oestrogen Excess

Oestrogen excess in men may cause hypogonadotropic oligospermia. The normal ratio of testosterone to oestradiol in men should be > 10:1. The common clinical situation in men, where such abnormal ratio is observed, is obesity. In adipose tissues, testosterone is converted to oestradiol by aromatase enzyme. With increasing incidence of obesity increasing number of men are presenting with abnormal testosterone to oestradiol ratio. Liver failure is another cause of oestrogen excess. Excess oestrogen by negative 'feedback' mechanism inhibits pituitary gonadotropin secretion and thereby inhibits intratesticular testosterone production. It has been suggested[5] that oestrogen excess in combination with androgen deficiency results in deficient spermatogenesis.

Aromatase inhibitor by reducing oestradiol and increasing androgen level may be effective in improving spermatogenesis in oestrogen excess induced oligospermic individuals. The drug is available either in the steroidal (testolactone) or in non-steroidal (anastrozole) formulation. Significant improvement has been reported following daily use of 1 mg dose of non-steroidal aromatase inhibitor-anastrozole for a period of three months due to increase in the testosterone to oestradiol ratio.

D. Prolactin Excess

Hyperprolactinaemia may have a significant impact on male infertility. Excess prolactin leads to inhibition of hypothalamic secretion of GnRH which in turn results in diminished secretion of pituitary FSH and LH leading to diminished synthesis of intratesticular testosterone and impaired spermatogenesis.

Low level of testosterone is responsible for diminished libido, erectile dysfunction and abnormal semen parameters. Hence the overall effect of hyperprolactinaemia leads to diminished male reproductive potential.

Hyperprolactinaemia is more commonly associated with hypothyroidism. In addition, hyperprolactinaemia may also be due to stress, liver disease, use of certain medication (like phenothiazines and antidepressants) and prolactin-secreting tumours (prolactinoma). Hyperprolactinaemia in men is often asymptomatic or sometimes they may present with symptom of galactorrhoea. When routine testing of serum reveals evidence of hypothyroidism, testing for excess serum prolactin should also be performed. Diminished libido and erectile dysfunction also indicate possibility of hyperprolactinaemia.

In case of elevated serum prolactin (> 50 ng/ml), pituitary gland imaging is indicated. If adenoma is detected, this should be classified either as micro-(< 10 mm) or macro-(> 10 mm) adenomas. Microadenomas are always treated medically whereas selected cases (neurological or ophthalmological symptom producing) macroadenomas require surgical intervention.

Treatment of hyperprolactinaemia with or without prolactinoma primarily consists of use of dopamine agonists. The commonly used drugs are either bromocriptine or cabergoline.

Regarding efficacy, cabergoline appears to be more effective than bromocriptine specially when prolactinoma has been detected on CT scan or MRI. Resistance to the drug is less compared to bromocriptine. Patients resistant to bromocriptine respond well to cabergoline. Cabergoline appears to be the first choice specially when prolactinoma is present.

In symptom producing prolactinomas (visual disturbances, persistent headache) transphenoidal surgical excision or radiotherapy may be necessary. With treatment either medical or surgical, it is expected that there may be reversal of GnRH inhibition of pituitary. But it is essential that patients' serum gonadotropin level should be assessed in the postoperative period because patient may require gonadotropin therapy, even after resolution of hyperprolactinaemia.

INFECTION OR INFLAMMATION

Infection and inflammation have significant impact on semen parameters. Evidence of infection is ascertained by finding of leukocytes in seminal plasma under the microscope or by presence of bacteria revealed by semen culture. Identification of leukocytes under microscope should be done with caution as immature germ cells also look like leukocytes or round cells. Similarly, collection of semen for bacterial culture should also be done very carefully. Before collection, penis and external urethral meatus should be properly cleaned with antimicrobial soap. Because pathogens present in these areas are—*Ureaplasma urealyticum*, *Escherichia coli*, enterococci, *Proteus mirabilis* and *Micoplasma hominis*. They have not been found very significant for adversely affecting semen parameters. So presence of these pathogens does not indicate active medical treatment.[6]

On the other hand, organisms such as Chlamydia, *Neisseria gonorrhoea*, *Treponema pallidum*, *Mycobacterium tuberculosis*, *Haemophilus ducreyi*, herpes simplex virus (HPV) and *Trichomonas vaginalis* may have deleterious effect on sperm function.[7, 8] Therefore, treatment of sperm infection with these organisms appears to be beneficial. Apart from bacteria, presence of leukocytes itself may require active management. Because presence of more than 6–8 leukocytes per high power field (hpf) may induce sperm damage through production of reactive oxygen species (ROS).[9] Presence of leukocytospermia with or without active bacterial infection indicates antimicrobial therapy. In infection or inflammation the four major pharmacological approaches are:

a. Antimicrobial therapy to treat clinical or subclinical infection
b. Anti-inflammatory medication (such as CoX2 inhibitor)
c. Antioxidant therapy to minimise oxidative stress
d. Antihistaminics to stabilise mast cells.

TESTICULAR/SCROTAL FACTOR

Testicular hyperthermia is associated with decreased semen quality mainly low density of sperms. It was reported that testicular hypothermia device (THD) which provides scrotal skin evaporative cooling demonstrated an improvement in sperm density. Scrotal

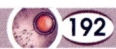

dermatitis (wash leather scrotum) may be responsible for male infertility due to its hyperthermic effect. Antibiotics and anti-inflammatory agents may improve the condition.

Sexual Dysfunction

Medical treatment is also available for various sexual dysfunctions—the commonest ones are erectile and ejaculatory dysfunctions. They have been elaborately discussed in subsequent chapters of this book.

Other Medical Therapies

While medical treatment may improve male fertility potential in certain situations discussed above, in contrast, a large number of drugs and substances can also adversely affect male reproductive capability. It is important to know these agents as substitution or cessation of these substances may improve male fertility potential. The names of these drugs and substances which have detrimental effect on male fertility potential are listed in Table 18.1.

Table 18.1: Possible adverse impact of drugs on male fertility potential	
Alcohol	Gentamicin
Allopurinol	Heroin
α-adrenergic blockers	Lithium
Anabolic steroids	Marijuana
Antipsychotics	Methadone
β-blockers	Monoamine oxidase inhibitors
Erythromycin	Nitrofurantoin
Calcium channel blockers	Phenothiazines
Chemotherapy	Spironolactone
Cimetidine	Sulphasalazine
Cocaine	Tetracycline
Colchicines	Thiazide diuretics
Cyclosporine	Tobacco
Dilantin	Tricyclic antidepressants

EMPIRIC THERAPY

Besides specific directed therapy outlined above, often empiric therapy is used to treat men with idiopathic infertility or infertility with oligospermic and oligoasthenospermic semen samples.

The drugs which may be used are low dose androgens (low dose testosterone—mesterolone), antioestrogen (clomiphene), gonadotropin, antiprostaglandins, pentoxifylline and nutraceuticals. Besides low dose testosterone, gonadotropin and nutraceuticals, other drugs are not commonly used in clinical practice.

Low dose testosterone

Previously, high dose testosterone therapy (testosterone enanthate 200 to 500 mgm intra-muscularly every 2 weeks) was administered to suppress spermatogenesis temporarily with the idea that after discontinuation, the rate of sperm production is higher compared to presuppression level through a rebound phenomenon. Theoretically sound, but practically the protocol did not work satisfactorily.[10, 11] Currently low dose testosterone (mesterolone) is used to augment intratesticular testosterone to improve spermatogenesis in borderline hypogonadotropic or even normogonadotropic oligospermic individuals. The reasons for empiric use of low dose testosterone is that sometimes with idiopathic male infertility with normal level of FSH and LH, Leydig cell function may be sub-normal resulting in deficient intratesticular testosterone production with reduced spermatogenesis. Use of gonadotropin (FSH, hCG) is the alternate option. But because of cost, low dose testosterone as the substitution is the preferred choice.

Antioestrogens

Clomiphene citrate and tamoxifen are antioestrogens which exert their action by competing with oestrogen for oestrogen receptors at the hypothalamic pituitary level. They inhibit the inhibitory effect of oestrogen at the hypothalamic and pituitary areas thereby increasing pituitary gonadotropin secretion.

Increased level of gonadotropin results in elevated intratesticular testosterone which hopefully stimulates improved spermatogenesis. Elevated oestradiol (low SHBG as in obesity and hypothyroidism, etc), also has a negative impact on Leydig cell, and therefore, antioestrogenic effect of clomiphene citrate may improve testicular function by this mechanism also.

Therefore, men with mild oligospermia, low normal serum gonadotropin and elevated oestradiol level are more likely to respond to clomiphene or tamoxifen therapy. Association of asthenospermia or abnormal morphology or high elevated gonadotropin are contraindications for use of clomiphene treatment.

Recently clomiphene has been used to improve intratesticular spermatogenesis even in hypogonadotropic azoospermic men for the purpose of successful sperm retrieval in ICSI. Following 3 to 9 months of clomiphene therapy nearly 100% sperm retrieval has been reported by Hussain and colleagues.[12] The recommended dose of clomiphene citrate is 25 mg daily with 5 days rest a month or 25 mg on alternate days which may reduce pituitary receptor downregulation with consequent increase in gonadotropin to help further improve sperm count.[13] Dose should be adjusted not only to increase testosterone level but also to maintain the level of testosterone within normal range.

Testolactone is another antioestrogen which also improves testicular function by decreasing conversion of testosterone to E2 through aromatase inhibition. Increase of intratesticular testosterone stimulates spermatogenesis. Though uncontrolled studies recorded encouraging results with clomiphene and tamoxifen treatment, report of World Health Organisation showed no effect with these drugs.[14]

Similarly, testolactone used in a dose of 1 gm daily for 6–12 months has shown some promise in uncontrolled studies but in placebo controlled crossover report very little importance was recorded.[15, 16]

Gonadotropin

Empiric treatment of idiopathic male infertility with gonadotropin (hCG, HMG and rFSH) is very controversial.[17, 18] But many uncontrolled studies have published encouraging results which have stimulated interest in continued investigation with exogenous gonadotropin.

Also development of rFSH has prompted recommendation of FSH treatment in some special situations of idiopathic male infertility.[19]

Situations in which empiric use of gonadotropin in idiopathic male infertility has been useful are:

a. Patients have normal plasma levels of FSH and inhibin B with hypospermatogenesis detected in seminiferous tubules but without maturation disturbances.[20, 21]

b. In infertile men who have significant number of apoptotic or immature sperms, FSH has the potential to improve sperm microorganelles.[22, 23]

c. In idiopathic oligospermia, use of FSH for the husband before attempting IVF/ICSI has produced better quality embryo and resulted in improved pregnancy rates.[24, 25]

SURGICAL MANAGEMENT OF MALE INFERTILITY

Apart from sperm retrieval techniques in ART (ICSI), there are two common surgical approaches for the treatment of male infertility. These are:

a. Repair of varicocele and

b. Management of vasal or vaso-epididymal obstruction.

On rare occasions, repair of congenital defect like hypospadiass or transurethral excision of müllerian cyst at the point of entry of ejaculatory duct into prostatic urethra may be rewarding.

Repair of Varicocele

Though several studies have reported favourably in support of varicocele repair, controversy still exists about its utility in the surgical management of male infertility.

Varicocele has been reported to be associated with 35 to 40% in men with primary infertility and 75 to 80% of men with secondary infertility. However, this is found only in 15% of general population.[26, 27] The cause of subfertility in varicocele is attributed to venous dilatation.[28] Stasis of blood increases intratesticular temperature which reduces testicular function. It causes testicular

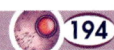

damage, decreases testosterone production by interfering with Leydig cell function leading to decreased sperm production.

Several studies have demonstrated improved semen parameters, testosterone production and pregnancy outcomes following varicocele repair. *Repair of large (Gr. II and Gr. III) varicocele in younger men may have greater beneficial effect on sperm parameters and androgen production than in older men.*[29, 30]

Surgical Repair of Vasal or Epididymal Obstruction

VAS obstruction is more common after vasectomy or secondary to some injuries like childhood hernia repair, orchidopexy or following hydrocele operation.[31] Obstruction following infection (gonococcal, chlamydial) causes permanent damage to vasal epithelial lining with fibrosis of muscular layer, and therefore, surgical canalisation rarely helps.

Microsurgical vasovasostomy has significantly improved results compared to those with older techniques.[32, 33] Patency and pregnancy rates vary directly with the period of obstruction. Results of surgery following obstruction for less than 3 years resulted in patency rate of 97% and pregnancy rate of 96%.[34] Results are better following microsurgical procedures with use of multilayered repair as against single layer repair which was practised in older technique. Multilayer technique ensures watertight anastomosis which prevents formation of sperm granulomas. Watertight anastomosis is important because there is no constituent of vasal fluid which helps in sealing the anastomosis site internally.

VASOEPIDIDYMOSTOMY

It is a technically challenging microsurgical procedure. If epididymal obstruction is present, vasoepididymostomy may be required proximal to obstruction to restore continuity of sperm transport. In these situations, the decision is made during the surgery and is based on microscopic examination of the proximal vasal fluid (for sperm) and the duration of obstruction.[35, 36]

Five basic principles to remember during microsurgical reconstructive surgery are:
  i. Adequate mobilisation of vas deferens before anastomosis.
  ii. Maintenance of blood supply to vas deferens with its adventitial covering
  iii. Tension-free anastomosis
  iv. Meticulous placement of sutures
  v. Adequate haemostasis to prevent postoperative haematoma.

Summary

In certain situations of male infertility medical treatment may have a positive role. The situations include a group of abnormalities-such as endocrine dysfunction, infection, inflammation, ejaculatory and erectile problems. Even if duration of therapy is prolonged, and outcome more often unpredictable yet medical therapy is acceptable by some couples because this is less expensive than alternative therapy of assisted reproductive technology. Though controversial, empiric use of clomiphene, tamoxifen, testolactone, FSH and antioxidants has been rewarding.

Clomiphene and tamoxifen have been used in selected cases of hypogonadotropic hypoandrogenic oligospermic individuals. They act by inhibiting the inhibitory effect of oestrogen at the hypothalamic and pituitary level, thereby increasing secretion of pituitary gonadotropin. Gonadotropin increases the level of intratesticular testosterone which stimulates spermatogenesis in idiopathic or hypogonadotropic oligospermic men.

Testolactone also improves testicular function by decreasing conversion of testosterone to E2 through aromatase inhibition. Also empiric use of gonadotropin may be helpful in idiopathic oligospermia who have normal FSH, but have testicular tubular hypospermatogenesis or those attempting IVF and ICSI. Though not yet well established, role of antioxidants in oligoasthenospermic male infertility is quite promising in future.

Surgical correction of testicular defect is indicated in congenital defects like correction of hypospadias, excision of ejaculatory duct

cyst, or correction of acquired lesion like varicocele or reversal of obstruction at the region of vas deferens or epididymis. With advent of ART these regimens are becoming less popular but when performed with judicious selection of drugs or with judicious application of selected techniques in properly selected cases the result may be encouraging.

REFERENCES

1. Plant TM, Marshall GR. The functional significance of FSH in spermatogenesis and the control of its secretion in male primates. Endocr Rev 2001; 22: 764 –786.

2. Miyagawa Y, Tsujimura A, Matsumiya K, et al. Outcome of gonadotropin therapy for male hypogonadotropic hypogonadism at university affiliated male infertility centres: A 30-year retrospective study. J Urol 2005; 173: 2072–2075.

3. Whitten SJ, Nangia AK, Kolettis PN. Select patients with hypogonadotropic hypogonadism may respond to treatment with clomiphene citrate. Fertil Steril 2006; 86: 1664–1668.

4. Menon DK. Successful treatment of anabolic steroid-induced azoospermia with human chorionic gonadotropin and human menopausal gonadotropin. Fertil Steril 1003; 79 (Suppl 3): 1659–1661.

5. Jones TM, Fang VS, Landau RL, Rosenfield R. Direct inhibition of Leydig cell function by estradiol. J Clin Endocrinol Metab 1978; 47: 1368–1373.

6. Chan PT, Schlegel PN. Inflammatory condition of the male excurrent ductal system. Part I. J Androl 2002a; 23: 453–460—Chan PT, Schlegel PN. Inflammatory conditions of the male excurrent ductal system. Part II. Androl 2002b; 23: 461–469.

7. Hosseinzadeh S, Brewis IA, Pacey AA, Moore HD, Eley A. Coincubation of human spermatozoa with Chlamydia trachomatis *in vitro* causes increased tyrosine phosphorylation of sperm proteins. Infect Immun 2000; 68: 4872–4876.

8. Kohn FM, Erdmann I, Oeda T, et Mulla KF, Schiefer HG, Schill WB. Influence of urogenital infections on sperm functions. Andrologia 1998; 30 (Suppl 1): 73–80.

9. Sharma RK. Agarwal A. Role of reactive oxygen species in male infertility. Urology 1996; 48: 835–850.

10. Gerris J, Comhaire F, Hellemans P, et al. Placebo controlled trial of high-dose mesterolone treatment of idiopathic male infertility. Fertile Steril 55: 603, 1991.

11. Comhaire FH. Treatment of idiopathic testicular failure with high dose testosterone undecanoate: A double-blind pilot study. Fertil Steril 54, 689, 1990.

12. Hussein A, et al. Clomiphene administration for cases of nonobstructive azoospermia: A multicenter study. J Androl 2005; 26(6): 787–91; (discussion: 792–3).

13. Homonnai ZT, et al. Clomiphene citrate treatment in oligozoospermia: Comparison between two regimens of low-dose treatment. Fertil Steril 1988; 50(5): 801–4.

14. World Health Organization: A double blind trial of clomiphene citrate for the treatment of idiopathic male infertility. Int J Androl 15: 299, 1992.

15. Vigersky RA, Glass AR. Effect of delta-1-testolactone on the pituitary-testicular ais in oligospermic men. J clin Endocrinol Metab 52: 897, 1981.

16. Clark RV, Sherins RJ. Clinical Trial of testolactone for treatment of idiopathic male infertility. J Androl 10: 240, 1989.

17. Kamischke A, et al. Recombinant human follicle stimulating hormone for treatment of male idiopathic infertility: a randomized, double blind, placebo-controlled. Clinical trial. Hum Reprod 1998; 13(3): 596–603.

18. Knuth UA, et al. Treatment of severe Oligospermia with human chronic gonadotropin/human menopausal gonadotropin: a placebo-controlled, double blind trial. J Clin Endocrinol Metabl 1987; 65.

19. Merino G, et al. Sperm characteristics and hormonal profile before and after treatment with follicle stimulating hormone in fertile patients. Arch Androl 1996; 37(3): 197–200.

20. Foresta C, et al. Use of recombinant human follicle stimulating hormone in the treatment of male factor infertility. Fertil Steril 2002; 77(2): 238–44.

21. Foresta C, et al. FSH in the treatment of oligozoospermia. Mol. Cell Endocrinol 2000; 161 (1–2): 89–97.

22. Baccetti B, et al. The effect of follicle stimulating hormone therapy on human sperm structure (Notulae seminologicae 11). Hum Reprod 1997; 12(9): 1955–68.

23. Ben-Rafael Z, et al. Follicle-stimulating hormone treatment for men with idiopathic oligoteratoasthenozoospermia before *in vitro*

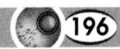

fertilisation: The impact on sperm microstructure and fertilisation potential. Fertil Steril 2000; 73(1): 24–30.

24. Caroppo E, et al. Recombinant human follicle-stimulating hormone as a pretreatment for idiopathic oligoasthenoteratozoospermic patients undergoing intracytoplasmic sperm injection. Fertil Steril 2003; 80(6): 1398–403.

25. Ashkenazi J, et al. The role of purified follicle stimulating hormone therapy in the male partner before intracytoplasmic sperm injection. Fertil Steril 1999; 72(4): 670.

26. Goelick JI, Goldstein M. Loss of fertility in men with Varicocele. Fertil Steril 1993; 59(3): 613–6.

27. Kim ED, et al. Varicocele repair improves semen parameters in azoospermic men with spermatogenic failure. J Urol 1999; 162(3 Pt l): 737–40.

28. Dubin L, Amelar RD. etiologic factors in 1294 consecutive cases of male infertility. Fertil Steril 1971; 22(8): 469–74.

29. Hadziselimovic F, et al. Testicular and vascular changes in children and adults with Varicocele.

J Urol 1989; 142 (2 Pt 2): 583–5 [discussion: 603–5].

30. Scherr D, Goldstein M, Comparison of bilateral versus unilateral varicocelectomy in men with palpable bilateral varicoceles. J Urol 1999; 162(1): 85–8.

31. Sheynkin YR et al. Microsurgical repair of iatrogenic injury to vas deferens. J Urol 1998; 159(1): 139–41.

32. Silber SJ. Microscopic vasectomy reversal. Fertil Steril 1977; 28(11): 1191–202.

33. Owen ER. Microsurgical vasovasostomy: a reliable vasectomy reversal. AUST N Z J SURG 1977; 47(3): 305–9.

34. Belker AM, et al. Results of 1,469 microsurgical vasectomy reversals by the Vasovasostomy Study Group. J Urol 1991; 145(3): 505–11

35. Chawla a, et al. Should all urologists performing vasectomy reversals be able to perform vasoepididymostomies if required? J Urol 2004; 172(3): 1048–50

36. Thomas AJ. Infertility. New York: Lippincott Williams and Wilkins; 2004, p. 829–30.

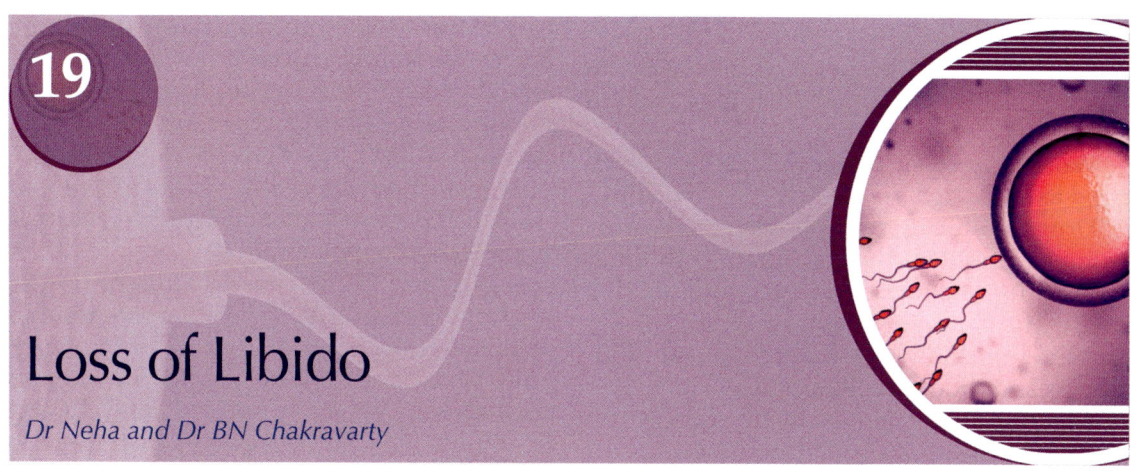

Loss of Libido

Dr Neha and Dr BN Chakravarty

Loss of libido refers to a condition when a patient presents with decrease or loss of sexual desire and/or sexual drive.

Since it is a condition which occurs naturally with ageing and might be affected by various physical or psychological conditions and also by mental state of patient, defining loss of libido is not easy. Also due to the social stigma at times many patients do not seek medical advice due to which quantification of the problem prevalent in society is difficult.

ASSESSMENT OF PATIENT

History of patient often leads to some outstanding facts about the patient and their psychological as well as sexual conditions. The sexual drive normally decreases with age,[1] but the degree is variable. Qualitative aspects of sexual activity may change and improve with age.[2] As with other medical conditions, attempt should be made to find out what the patient actually means when he complains of loss of libido. Detailed history of onset and progress needs to be elicited. History of any comorbidity, e.g. chronic disease, hypertension, diabetes, cancer or drugs which are known to affect metabolic or hormonal levels in body is important. Sexual trauma, dyspareunia or incompatibility with particular partner is enquired. Excessive physical or psychological stress, work stress, family issues or financial issues may affect the hormonal balance and lead to decrease of sexual activity. Alcohol or drug dependence decreases sexual activity. Fear of getting pregnant in young working ladies or general attitude to shy away from commitment might be another aspect which the clinician must not miss. Mental condition like depression and depressive phase of bipolar disorders are associated with decreased libido. Hence mental status of patient should be thoroughly evaluated.

Physical examination—local examination is important to rule out any cause of dyspareunia. Systemic examination may reveal some systemic diseases like hypertension or prostatomegaly in men which might be associated with loss of libido. However, apart from such specific conditions physical examination is not very helpful.

Investigations

Diagnosis is usually made by history. Investigation helps to rule out diabetes, hypothyroidism, decreased sex hormones—oestrogen, testosterone, FSH, LH or hyper-prolactinaemia. Deranged liver functions, high cholesterol, poor diabetic control are associated with loss of libido and hence specific tests for same are useful.

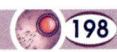

MANAGEMENT

Counseling forms a major role in management. Psychologist as well as sex therapist need to be involved.

Work related or financial related issues need to be tackled.

Drugs related to loss of libido can be overcome by intelligent substitution with other medication. Examples of antihypertensive medication or antidepressive or cancer medications leading to loss of libido are well-known and should be modified.

Alcohol abuse needs to be tackled by counseling and appropriate medications.

Thyroid disorders and diabetes should be controlled with help of endocrinologist.

Since there is no specific cause associated with loss of libido and at times there are multiple associated factors, no specific guidelines and algorithm for treatment can be outlined. More often multidisciplinary approach needs to be adopted.

Role of hormone treatment in augmenting libido is controversial. It seems that androgens have an important role in improving libido in both men and women, but the use of testosterone for increasing libido is controversial both in men and women.[3] Lack of androgens and excess of prolactin have important roles in regulating libido.[4]

In women, use of 17β-oestradiol is less effective than tibolone in raising libido.[5] Addition of growth hormone along with dihydroepiandrosterone (DHEA) may improve well-being and libido in both sexes but more in women than in men.[6]

Summary

Loss of sexual desire or sexual drive is known as loss of libido. Apart from age, chronic illness, mental or sexual trauma, psychosocial or financial stress, or partner incompatibility may be some of the important causes of deficient libido. Use of drugs, specially antihypertensives, anticancer, antipsychotics or excessive alcohol may be other contributory factors for the problem of loss of libido.

Management consists of counseling about relationship rehabilitation with partner, lifestyle modification or substitution of drug in case a specific drug is the cause of loss of libido. Androgens may have a positive role in both men and women. Use of growth hormone, in both sexes and 17β-oestradiol in women approaching menopause have doubtful efficacy. Sildenafil may be effective in case there is simultaneous erectile dysfunction.

REFERENCES

1. Araujo AB, Mohr BA, Mc Kinlay JB. Changes in sexual functionbin middle-aged and older men: Longitudinal data from the Massachusetts Male aging study; J Am Geriatr Soc. 2004 Sep; 52(9): 1502–9.

2. Hurd Clarke L. Older women and sexuality: Experiences in marital relationships across the life course. Can J Aging. 2006 Summer; 25(2): 129–40.

3. Margo K, Winn R. Testosterone treatments: Why, when, and how?; Am Fam Physician. 2006 May 1; 73(9): 1591–8.

4. Corona G, Petrone L, Mannucci E, et al. The important couple: Low desire.; Int J Androl. 2005 Dec; 28 Suppl 2; 46–52.

5. Somunkiran A, Erel CT, Demirci F, et al. The effect of tibolone versus 17 beta-estradiol on climacteric symptoms in women with surgical menopause: Arandomized, cross-over study; Maturitas. 2006 Jul 8.

6. Brooke AM, kalingag LA, Miraki-Moud F, et al. Dehydroepiandrosterone (DHEA) improves psychological well-being in male and female hypopituitary patients on maintenance growth hormone replacement. J Clin Endocrinol Metab. 2006 Jul 18.

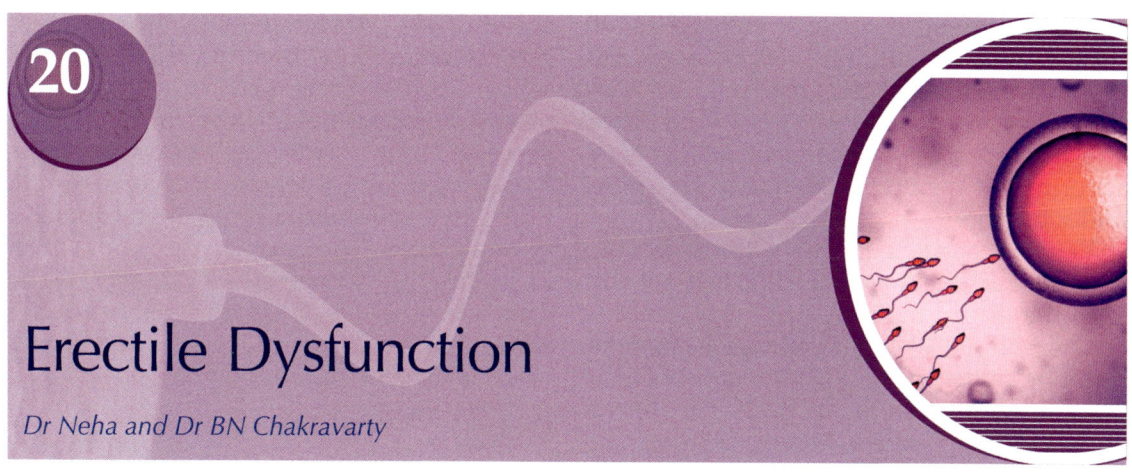

Erectile Dysfunction

Dr Neha and Dr BN Chakravarty

The NIH consensus conference in 1993 defined erectile failure as "the inability of a male to attain and maintain an erection of the penis that is sufficient to permit satisfactory intercourse".[1] Erectile failure or dysfunction is also sometimes called impotency.

The incidence of erectile failure increases with age, with an incidence of around 5% in age group of 40 years, increasing to around 25–30% in 50 years and above. It can be due to psychological or organic causes, organic being more common. It can result in low self-esteem, performance anxiety, depression, stress and infertility. Currently with change of lifestyle, modern professional and social stress, erectile dysfunction is becoming an increasingly common problem for male infertility.

ANATOMY AND PHYSIOLOGY OF ERECTION

Erection is a complex phenomenon which requires adequate and healthy vascular tissue in penis, intact nervous system, adequate amount of circulating testosterone and psychological impulses from brain.

There are three erectile components in the penis, two corpora cavernosa and one corpus spongiosum. The two corposa cavernosa are present in the shaft of the penis side by side and attached to each other by dense fibrous septum and in the depression formed by this septum lies corpus spongiosum ventrally. A

dense layer of fibrous tissue binds and contains three erectile components and there is a fascia, known as Buck's fascia which holds these components together (Fig. 20.1).

These erectile tissues have cavernous spaces which are lined by smooth muscles. In flaccid state, these muscles are contracted and cavernous space collapses, while during

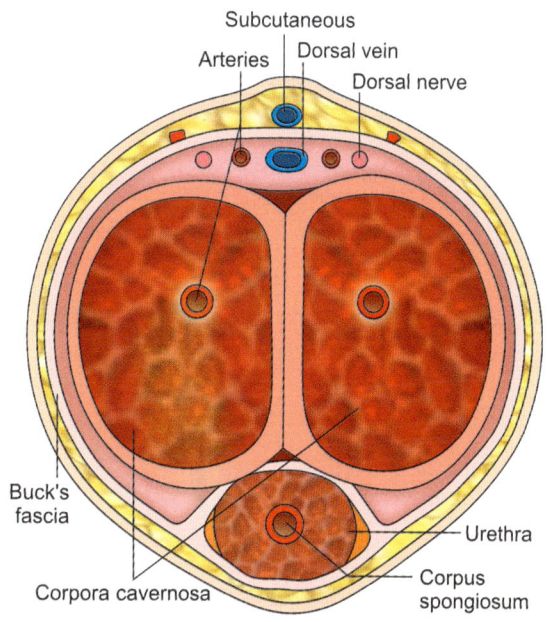

Fig. 20.1: Erection occurs when erectile tissues are filled with blood supplied by arteries and remain trapped within cavernous spaces because of temporary obstruction of venous drainage

erection, these spaces greatly enlarge due to relaxation of smooth muscles. The arterial blood flow into these spaces markedly increases and the penis becomes engorged with blood and this puts the non-distensible fibrous coverings of the erectile tissue in the penis under tension.

Venous channels draining these erectile tissues leave them in a tangential manner and with the increasing pressure in the erectile components, their venous drainage is impaired resulting in distension and elongation of the tissues and thus the penis itself. Due to the non-distensible fibrous coverings of the erectile tissues, the arterial blood pressure increases considerably in these tissues leading to expansion and distension of the erectile tissues which in turn straightens and hardens the penis (Figs 20.2 and 20.3).

Erection Mostly a Vascular Phenomenon

The neurological drive in erection involves both the parasympathetic and sympathetic

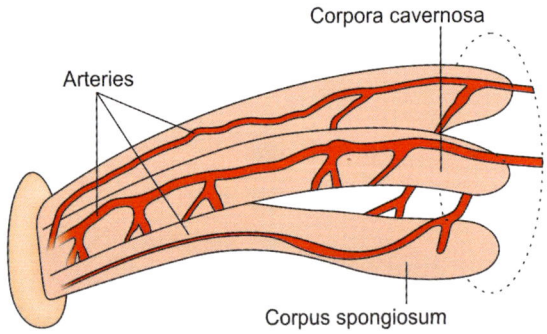

Fig. 20.2: Arteries entering into the cavernous spaces

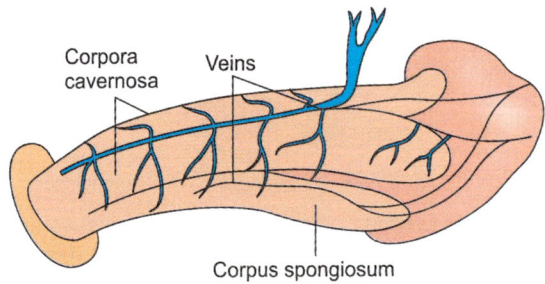

Fig. 20.3: Venous channels leave in a tangential manner

systems, but parasympathetic system plays the dominant role. Erection is initiated by sexual stimulation that can be visual, tactile or even olfactory and these impulses are processed in the medial pre-optic areas of the hypothalamus. The central nervous system thus plays an important role in erection and its separation from part of the spinal cord frequently leads to erectile dysfunction. The pudendal nerve is the main sensory supply from penis and section of this nerve may result in erection failure.

Etiology

Erectile dysfunction can be due to psychological, neurological, endocrine, vascular or muscular disorders.

Age: The incidence increases with age, around 5% affected at the age of 40 years, 50% at the age of 70 years.

Disorders of nervous system: Peripheral neuropathies, pudendal nerve injury, damage to spinal cord and spinal cord lesion like prolapsed intervertebral disc, spinal cord tumour, cauda equina, multiple sclerosis.

These disorders either damage the reflex arc involved in erection or dissociate the central nervous system from the spinal cord.

Vascular disorders: Arteriosclerosis is a condition in which arterial dimensions are compromised and it can result in decreased arterial flow to erectile tissues, hampering erection, when penile arteries are affected by arteriosclerosis. So patients with cardiovascular disease can have coexisting erectile dysfunction.[2] As much as 30% reduction in arterial supply can result in total erectile failure. The incidence of arteriosclerosis increases with age.

Penile artery damage due to any cause, can also result in similar problem and thus erectile dysfunction can be a complication of penile surgeries.

Cavernous smooth muscle dysfunction: Earlier known as idiopathic erectile failure, this is a condition in which the smooth muscle in the penis fails to relax which can be due to intrinsic muscle problem or inadequate formation of nitric oxide (NO).

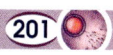

Secondary to surgery of prostate: Erectile dysfunction can occur after prostatic surgery. It can be seen in 10% of cases following transurethral resection of the prostate and in almost 30% cases after radical prostatectomy.

Endocrine causes: Low androgen secretion has variable effect. In some cases a small reduction in secretion can result in erectile failure while in others no problem occurs. Hyperprolactinaemia can result in erectile failure, as it reduces the LH levels and thus the circulating androgen levels.

Diabetes mellitus, especially type 1 is a common cause of erectile dysfunction in young men. Autonomic dysfunction is mostly the cause but it can also be due to associated hypertension and arteriosclerosis.

Drugs: β-blockers are the most common group of drugs causing erectile dysfunction. Other group of drugs are antihistaminics, antihyperlipidaemics, H_2 inhibitors like ranitidine and chemotherapeutic agents.

Recreational drugs like cannabis and narcotics can result in erectile failure. Chronic heavy alcohol consumption and smoking can result in erectile failure.

Chronic illness: Renal failure, hepatic failure, liver cirrhosis and depressive illness can cause erectile problem.

Psychogenic: Sympathetic outflow is increased in anxiety and can overcome the parasympathetic outflow needed for erection. In men with psychogenic erectile failure, the normal morning erection (stiffness) is perceived (elicited by leading question), and this distinguishes psychogenic from organic causes.

Management

Patient's history: A complete medical, surgical and sexual history from the patient is to be taken which include chronic illness, endocrinopathies, prostatic, penile, spinal surgeries, drug history and history of chronic smoking or alcohol abuse. Gradual onset of problem with associated loss of morning stiffness indicates organic cause.

Physical examination: A complete physical examination especially cardiovascular or neurological examination is important in cases of erectile dysfunction. The penis should also be carefully examined for sensation and any fibrous plaques caused by Peyronie's disease.

Investigations

Laboratory Investigations

- Blood count (TLC, DLC)
- Fasting and postprandial blood sugar
- Lipid profile
- Urine analysis
- Liver function test

Hormone levels: Total and free testosterone, SHBG, FSH, LH, TSH and serum prolactin levels.

Psychosocial evaluation: A psychological evaluation is important using a questionnaire and an interview. Sexual partner should also be evaluated to know expectations and perceptions during sexual intercourse.

Ultrasound examination of penis: USG of the penis is useful in evaluation of erectile failure, especially Doppler study of penile arteries for arteriosclerotic changes.

Pharmacocavernosography: It involves in determining the flow needed to maintain erection. Saline is infused in corpora cavernosa to cause erection. If the flow needed to generate erection is more than 120 ml/min and that to maintain erection is more than 20 ml/min, it indicates venous leak. Using contrast medium, site of leak can be determined.

Rigiscan: It is a device that has a snap gauge band that breaks when penile tumescence occurs and can be helpful in demonstrating nocturnal tumescence and erection that occurs on waking in the morning. This can be used to differentiate organic from psychogenic erectile failure.

Prevention and Treatment

Prevention

The risk of developing erectile dysfunction is increased in individuals with diabetes,

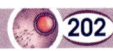

heart disease and hypertension, and optimal management of these conditions is helpful in preventing the onset of ED.[3-5] Lifestyle changes that improve vascular functions like avoiding smoking, having an ideal body weight and exercising regularly may help to prevent or reverse erectile dysfunction. However, only minimal data is there to support this supposition.[6, 7]

Treatment

Sexual counseling: Sexual counseling and sex therapy may be effective in a group of patients with minor sexual problems, especially when these are caused by sexual ignorance and psychological factors. Sex education, support, and reassurance may help to restore sexual function in some and in others, referral to a more specialised and intensive counseling may be necessary.[8]

Medical Treatment

Phosphodiesterase inhibitors: Oral phosphodiesterase type 5 inhibitors are the first line therapy, unless contraindicated. The drug blocks the action of phosphodiesterase enzyme and helps to build up cGMP with consequent enhancement of erection. They only enhance the natural response of sexual stimulation and cannot stimulate erection in absence of normal stimuli. Almost 70 to 80% patients respond to this treatment, e.g. sildenafil, tadalafil and vardenafil. Side effects consist of sudden fall in pressure especially when used along with nitrites or hypotensive therapy or α-blockers. Other reactions consist of facial flushing and mild headache.

These drugs potentiate the hypotensive effects of drugs like organic nitrates and nitrites, e.g. amyl nitrite.[9, 10] So their concomitant use is contraindicated.

Oral Testosterone in Medical Treatment after Phosphodiesterase Inhibitor

Oral testosterone may be helpful in some men with low level of endogenous serum or intratesticular testosterone. Prolonged use, however, may be ineffective and may damage the liver. Testosterone therapy is not recommended in individuals with normal serum testosterone levels.

In Central Africa and the United States, **Yohimbe bark (active component–Yohimbine) is widely used in numerous dietary supplements to correct erectile dysfunction.**

Intracavernous injection of vasoactive agents: It can be used in those who fail to respond to oral treatment. Alprostadil (prostaglandin E1), papaverine, and phentolamine are the most commonly used vasoactive drugs and PGE1 is the most popular agent. PGE1 is injected in the corpora cavernosa. The patients have to be trained regarding the use, doses and complications of these agents. The usual dose required is 10 to 20 µm and it takes 2 to 3 minutes for erection to start and in almost 10 to 15 minutes full erection is achieved. The drug is to be injected using an insulin syringe at right angle to the shaft. Other drugs previously used and now discarded are papaverine hydrochloride, phentolamine, alprostadil, etc.

Complications: Priapism, haematoma formation and bruising, infection, fibrous tissue formation within erectile tissue.

Topical and urethral agents: Medicated urethral system for erection (MUSE). In this procedure; alprostadil, a synthetic vasodilator similar to PGE1 is used in a liposomal form as a topical agent applied inside the urethra. In 3% of patients, hypotension can occur after first dose,[11] so initially it should be used under supervision of healthcare personnel.

Alprostadil, organic nitrates, minoxidil, papaverine and yohimbine have been tested via topical administration to the glans penis or penile shaft, with limited benefit.

Vacuum constriction devices: In a selected group of patients with erectile dysfunction, vacuum constriction devices are a low cost and effective treatment option. Devices with vacuum limiters to avoid injury to the penis by preventing establishment of extremely high negative pressure, is advised.

Penile prostheses: Various penile prostheses are available that can be inserted in the erectile tissue of the penis. It can be malleable or non-inflatable and inflatable. These are used in cases who are refractory to medical treatment. Inflatable prostheses are mostly used nowadays. These provide closer to normal flaccidity and erection of penis. Penile prostheses should not be used in presence of cutaneous, systemic or urinary tract infection. These prostheses can be implanted under general, spinal, or epidural anaesthesia, but it can be performed under local anaesthesia also.[12, 13]

Disadvantage: Once penile prostheses are inserted, erectile tissue is effectively destroyed and its function can never be regained.

Complications: Perforation of urethra, tunical perforation, glandular perforation, infection, erosion and malfunction of inflatable device.

Surgical

Penile arterial reconstructive surgery: Microvascular surgery involving bypassing any arteriosclerotic obstruction to blood flow in penile arteries. Careful selection of patient for surgery gives good result with the advantage of providing natural and non-pharmacologically induced erection for many years. Ultrasonography and Doppler studies can be helpful in determining the site and extent of damage prior to surgery.

Penile venous reconstructive surgery: These are useful in cases where erectile failure is the result of venous leak. Venogenic erectile dysfunction can be diagnosed by pharmaco-cavernosography. The site of venous leak is identified and these can be ligated.

Summary

Erectile dysfunction may be organic or psychogenic in origin. Though more commonly due to organic defect, erectile failure simply due to apprehension and anxiety is also frequently observed nowadays.

Apart from age, (disorder starts at 50 years, reaches a peak after 70 years) neurological and vascular lesions are common causes of erectile dysfunction. Lesions of spinal cord like tumour, disc prolapse, multiple sclerosis, surgery on spinal cord are common causes of erectile failure. Similarly, arteriosclerosis, diabetic vasculopathy are the significant vascular causes.

There are three erectile components containing cavernous spaces in the penis lined by smooth muscles. The erectile components are covered by non-distensible fibrous covering. When erectile tissues are filled up with blood and remain trapped because of temporary obstruction of venous drainage, penile erection occurs.

Apart from local erectile tissues, central nervous system through sexual stimulation plays an important role in the mechanism of erectile function.

Besides history, blood biochemistry, significant hormone assessment and in some cases imaging of the penile blood flow are the meaningful investigations. Before treatment starts functional erectile dysfunction should be differentiated from organic lesions. Use of some drugs such as antihistaminics, anti-hypertensives, H_2 inhibitors such as ranitidine or recreational drugs like cannabis, narcotics can result in erectile failure. Rarely chronic illness (e.g. renal or hepatic failure) may also cause erectile dysfunction.

Medical treatment, unless contraindicated, with sidenefil, tadenafil or vardenafil are the currently used drugs which provides satisfactory results. Contraindications consist of heart disease, hypertension and use of nitrites. In exceptional cases venous or arterial surgery has been attempted. Intra-cavernosal injection of prostaglandin or topical use of urethral agents (MUSE) are rarely used in current treatment of erectile dysfunction.

REFERENCES

1. Impotence. NIH Consens Statement, 10: 1, 1992.

2. Feldman HA, Goldstein I, Hatzichristou DG, Krane RJ, McKinlay JB. Impotence and its medical and psychosocial correlates: Results of the Massachusetts Male Aging Study. J Urol, 151: 54, 1994.

3. Johannes CB, Araujo AB, Feldman HA, Derby CA, Kleinman, KP and McKinlay, JB: A incidence of erectile dysfunction in men 40 to 69 years old: Longitudinal results from the

Massachusetts male aging study. J Urol, 163: 460, 2000.

4. Bacon CG, Mittleman MA, Kawachi I, Giovannucci E, Glasser DB, Rimm EB. Sexual function in men older than 50 years of age: Results from the health professionals' follow-up study. Ann Intern Med, 139: 161, 2003.

5. U.S. Department of Health and Human Services. Physical Activity and Health: A Report of the Surgeon General. Atlanta, GA: U.S. Department of Health and Human Services, Centers for Disease Control and Prevention, National Center for Chronic Disease Prevention and Health Promotion, 1996.

6. Esposito K, Giugliano F, Di Palo C, Giugliano G, Marfella R, D' Andrea, F, et al. Effect of lifestyle changes on erectile dysfunction in obese men: A randomized controlled trial. JAMA, 291: 2978, 2004.

7. Derby CA, Mohr BA, Goldstein I, Feldman HA, Johannes, CB, McKinlay JB. Modifiable risk factors and erectile dysfunction: Can lifestyle change modify risk? Urology, 56: 302, 2000.

8. World Health Organization. A Second International Consultation on Erectile and Sexual Dysfunction. Paris: June 2003.

9. Kloner RA, Mullin SH, Shook T, Matthews R, Mayeda, G, Burstein S et al. Erectile dysfunction in the cardiac patient: How common and should we treat? J Urol, 170: S46, 2003.

10. Kloner RA, Hutter AM, Emmick JT, Mitchell, MI, Denne J, Jackson G. Time course of the interaction between tadalafil and nitrates. J Am Cardiol, 42: 1855, 2003

11. Padma-Nathan H, Hellstrom WJ, Kaiser, FE, Labasky RF, Lue TF, Nolten WE et al. Treatment of men with erectile dysfunction with transurethral alprostadil. Medicated Urethral System for Erection (MUSE) Study Group. N Engl J Med. 336: 1, 1997.

12. Dos Reis JM, Glina S, Da Silva MF, Furlan V. Penile prosthesis surgery with the patient under local regional anesthesia. J Urol, 150: 1179, 1993.

13. Kaufman JJ. Penile prosthetic surgery under local anesthesia. J Urol, 28: 1190, 1982.

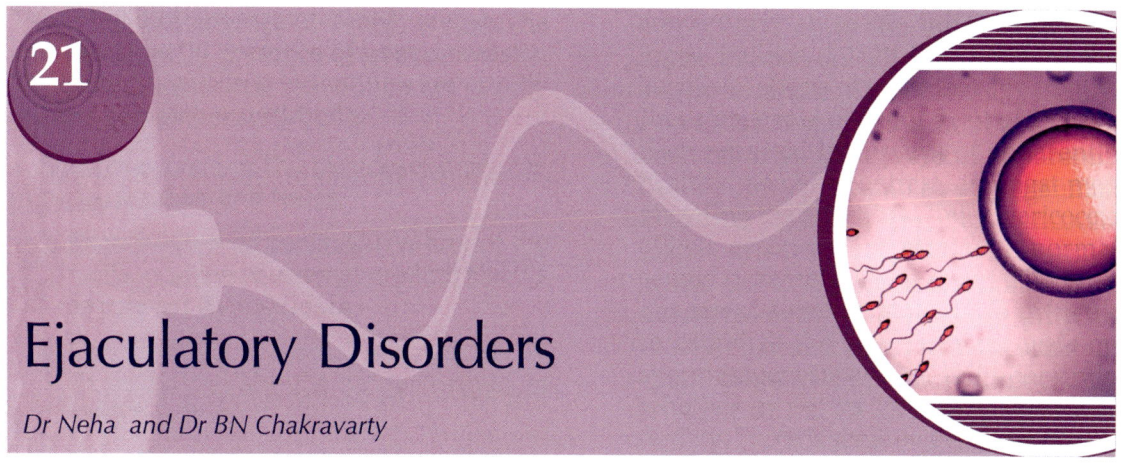

21

Ejaculatory Disorders

Dr Neha and Dr BN Chakravarty

Ejaculation is the process of forcilble ejection of seminal fluid through urethral meatus and is accompanied by orgasm, but it is a distinct entity from orgasm. Ejaculatory disorders are the most common type of male sexual disorders.[1] Ejaculatory disorders can be of following types:

- Retrograde ejaculation
- Premature ejaculation
- Ejaculatory failure

All ejaculatory disorders can result in infertility.

ANATOMY AND PHYSIOLOGY OF EJACULATION

Ejaculation involves two distinct phenomena: emission and expulsion.

Emission: The process of emission is a sympathetic phenomenon, controlled by sympathetic nervous system, originating in the thoracolumbar spine (T10-L2). It involves closure of bladder neck muscle, to prevent retrograde flow of ejaculate in the bladder. Seminal fluid originating in seminiferous tubules and epididymis receives additional contribution from vas deferens, seminal vesicles, prostate, Cowper's glands and is finally deposited into prostatic urethra.

Expulsion: Expulsion involves the coordinated rhythmic action of the bladder neck, urethra, bulbospongiosus, pelvic striated muscle and external urethral sphincter to propel semen through the urethra and out of the meatus. Somatic nervous system mediates the process and involves relaxation of external urethral meatus with simultaneous clonic contractions of prostate, bulbocavernosus muscle, ischiocavernosus, levator ani, and transverse perineal muscles, propelling the seminal fluid out of the urethra.

RETROGRADE EJACULATION

Retrograde ejaculation is a phenomenon in which, due to incomplete closure of bladder neck, the seminal fluid is passed into the bladder instead of expulsion outside the urethra. Instead of semen, small amount of secretion from urethra and bulbourethral glands are passed through urethra.

Etiology of Retrograde Ejaculation

Drugs

Various drugs have been implicated in causing retrograde ejaculation. Common examples are: α-receptor antagonists for lower urinary tract symptoms; a common α-receptor blocker 'tamsulosin' used for benign hypertrophy of prostate can also cause retrograde ejaculation. In addition, other agents like sympatholytics for hypertension, antidepressants, and antipsychotics, may also be responsible for retrograde ejaculation by affecting the contractility of bladder neck muscles.

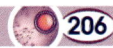

Diabetic Complication

Diabetes, especially long-standing uncontrolled, is a common cause of autonomic neuropathy and can result in ejaculatory disorders in 5–30% of men due to affection of few sympathetic and parasympathic nerve fibres.

Neurological Disorders

Various neurological disorders like spinal cord injury, prolapsed intervertebral disc, multiple sclerosis, motor neuron disease can result in retrograde ejaculation.

Urethral Obstructive Lesions

In case of severe urethral obstruction or urethral strictures, the pressure generated for ejaculation may overcome bladder neck closure pressure and leads to retrograde ejaculation.

Surgical Damage of Bladder Neck Integrity

Retrograde ejaculation can occur as a post-operative complication secondary to damage of bladder neck muscle or damage to sympathetic nerve fibres. Transurethral prostectomy, urethrotomy, surgery for posterior urethral valves, para-aortic lymphadenectomy, retroperitoneal surgeries, colorectal surgery, and spine surgery are the common surgical procedures adversely affecting bladder neck muscles or their nerve supply. Development of nerve-sparing retroperitoneal lymph node dissection (RPLND) techniques are less damaging to patients' ejaculatory function.

Idiopathic

In some men despite a complete investigation, no cause can be identified for retrograde ejaculation. This may be a variety of 'functional' retrograde ejaculation. Functional retrograde ejaculation can be easily differentiated from organic lesions by simple interrogation—if the patient gets nocturnal emission the possibility of organic lesion can be safely ruled out.

Diagnosis

A little or no semen is discharged from the urethra during the male sexual climax (during ejaculation). This is a significant cause of male infertility. In addition, urine passed after intercourse or masturbation is usually cloudy in nature. This is because of mixture of seminal fluid with urine.

Investigation

Investigation consists of examination of urine sample after intercourse or masturbation. This will reveal presence of sperm, either living or dead.

Treatment

Prophylactic

- If possible, withdrawal of drugs like α-blockers which may be responsible for retrograde ejaculation.
- Development of nerve sparing surgery performed around prostate or during retroperitoneal lymph node dissection.

Drugs

Drugs used to treat retrograde ejaculation include sympathomimetics like α-adrenergic agonist (e.g. imipramine 25 mg b.d. and phenylpropalamine 50 to 75 mg b.d.) which are detailed in Table 21.1.

Table 21.1: Drugs used to treat retrograde ejaculation

Agent	Drug class	Dosage (mg)	Frequency (per day)
Ephedrine sulfate	α- and β-adrenergic agonists	25	2x
Imipramine hydrochloride	Tricyclic antidepressant	25	3x
Pseudoephedrine hydrochloride	α- and β-beta adrenergic agonists	120	2x

(Ohl et al. 2008)

Surgical Treatment

Bladder neck tightening surgeries like Young-Dees-Leadbetter surgery can be performed when retrograde ejaculation occurs as postoperative complication due to injury to bladder neck.[2]

Bladder Sperm Retrieval

Cases that do not respond to medical treatment and in whom infertility is a concern, bladder sperm retrieval can be performed. Bladder is evacuated and then around 100 ml of buffer media is introduced and the person is asked to perform masturbation. The ejaculated sperm deposited in the bladder can be catheterised to retrieve sperms.

Another method and which is commonly practised, is to ask the patient to restrict fluid intake for 3 to 4 hours and to take alkaline agent by mouth like sodium bicarbonate to increase the pH level of urine. The objective is to minimise the detrimental effect of acidic urine on sperms. Ejaculation is induced by masturbation and sample retrieved by bladder catheterisation.

PREMATURE EJACULATION

Premature ejaculation (PE) is a condition in which a man experiences orgasm and ejaculation occurs quickly after initiation of sexual activity and with minimal penile stimulation. Premature ejaculation (PE) is characterised by a lack of voluntary control over ejaculation. There is no uniform cut-off definition for "premature", but a consensus of experts at the International Society for Sexual Medicine, endorsed a definition which states: "Ejaculation which always or nearly always occurs prior to or within about one minute".[3] The International Classification of Diseases (ICD-10) applies a cut-off of 15 seconds from the beginning of sexual intercourse.[4]

PE is also known as *early ejaculation, rapid ejaculation, rapid climax and premature climax.*

Etiology

Several theories have been suggested for premature ejaculations like:
- *Early conditioning*
- *Performance anxiety*
- Passive aggressiveness
- Infrequent sex

But there is little evidence to support any of these possibilities.[5]

Recent studies suggest that serotonin, a neural substance (neurohormone) produced by nerves, is significantly related to premature ejaculation (PE). Dysfunction of the actions of serotonin in the brain may result in PE. A few studies revealed that increased amount of serotonin in the brain delays ejaculation while low amount can produce a condition similar to PE.

Psychological factors are also commonly involved in premature ejaculation. Conditions like depression, stress, lack of confidence, performance anxiety, history of sexual repression can result in PE. PE can be result of strained relationship between partners and childhood sexual abuse.

PE may occur secondary to prostatitis[6] or as side effect of certain group of drugs.

Treatment

Medication

Antidepressant: Selective serotonin reuptake inhibitors can delay orgasm in men—so use of these drugs as 'off-label' medication may help to solve the problem of premature ejaculation. The drug can be taken daily about two to six hours before sexual activity.

Anaesthetic Cream

Anaesthetic creams are applied to the head of the penis about 20 to 30 minutes before intercourse to lessen the sensitivity and 'damp down' sexual sensation in the penis and thus may be helpful in premature ejaculation.

Psychiatric Therapy

It addresses the feelings of a man has about his sexuality and sexual relationship. It can be used along with medications and behavioural therapy. Psychological therapy can also help a man learn to be less anxious about his sexual performance and have greater sexual confidence.

Behavioural Therapy

In this therapy, a man makes use of exercises to develop tolerance to sexual stimulation and, as a result, delay ejaculation.

Squeeze Method

This was introduced by Masters and Johnson. In this procedure, the partner stimulates the man's penis till the point he is about to ejaculate. At the climax, the partner squeezes the head of the penis hard enough, the finger-grip abolishes the desire to climax, and the man partially loses his erection.[7–9] The goal of this technique is to let the man realise sensations leading up to orgasm, and then to voluntarily control and delay his orgasm.

Stop-start Method

In this method, the partner stimulates the man's penis till the point just before climax, after which they stop all stimulation till the urge to ejaculate subsides.[10–14] As the urge settles down, the partner is asked to begin stimulating his penis again. The procedure is repeated a few times, before the man finally ejaculates.

FAILURE OF EMISSION OR EJACULATION FAILURE (ASPERMIA)

It is a condition in which contraction of the ductal system which occurs during the emission phase of ejaculation does not occur resulting in failure of any ejection of secretion in the posterior urethra and sperms remain in the cauda epididymis and the ampullae of each vas deferens.

Etiology

Neurological disorders

Spinal cord injuries are the most commonly related to ejaculatory failure. Other neurological conditions that can lead to this type of defect are multiple sclerosis, Parkinson's disease, spina bifida, damage to the pelvic nerves.

Diabetes mellitus

It can lead to autonomic neuropathy and is a common cause of ejaculatory disorders.

Treatment

When failure of emission is the reason for infertility, the aim is to retrieve sperm which can be done in following ways.

Electroejaculation

Electroejaculation is the standard method for sperm retrieval in these men. Depending on the number of sperms retrieved, IUI or ICSI may be planned.

Vibratory stimulation

Vibrators applied to the glans penis can be an effective method for ejaculation and the sample can be used for insemination or cryopreserved for future use.

Surgical method of sperm collection like TESA or PESA

While intrauterine insemination is possible following collection of sperm by electro-ejaculators or vibrators—sperm retrieval with TESE (testicular sperm extraction) or PESA (percutaneous epididymal sperm aspiration) always requires the more expensive ICSI procedure for achieving pregnancy.

Summary

Ejaculation occurs in two phases—emission and expulsion. Following emission semen is deposited in the prostatic urethra. Expulsion involves propelling seminal fluid out of external urethral meatus. These two integrated mechanisms are controlled by coordinated thoracolumbar systemic nervous system and tightly regulated genitourinary ductal and pelvic flow muscular activity.

There are three types of ejaculatory disorders. Retrograde and premature ejaculations are relatively commoner than anejaculation or aspermia.

Failure of bladder neck to close at the time of emission or expulsion is primarily responsible for retrograde ejaculation. More often the defect is organic rather than functional. Organic defects consist of either vascular or neurological abnormalities. Use of α-receptor blocker as used in benign prostatic hypertrophy may lead to retrograde ejaculation. Sometimes bladder neck integrity is adversely affected following surgical intervention like prostatectomy or preaortic or para-aortic lyphadenectomy. Treatment consists of substitution, prevention or medical intervention. Substitution consists of procedures like change of drugs for α-receptor blocker as used in hypertensive disorders and prevention indicates nerve injury sparing surgery for surgeries performed for spinal cord lesions or on bladder and prostate. Medical intervention consists of use of sympathomimetics which may correct retrograde ejaculation. In intractable cases, harvesting of sperm from postcoital or postmasturbation sample of urine followed by ICSI is the accepted procedure of treatment.

Premature ejaculation (PE) is more often a psychiatric than an organic problem. However, recently serotonin, a neurohormone, has been involved in the mechanism of PE. Selective serotonin reuptake inhibitors can delay orgasm. So use of these drugs as 'off-label' therapy can help to cure PE.

Complete failure of ejaculation though not a very common problem in clinical practice, may sometimes be encountered in infertile men with neurological defects like multiple sclerosis, parkinsonism, spina bifida and following surgical damage to pelvic nerves. Diabetic neuropathy or vasculopathy may be amongst other causes.

For treatment of infertility, sperm collection is performed for either IUI or IVF/PESA following use of electroejaculator, vibrator or through TESE (testicular sperm extraction) or PESA (percutaneous epididymal sperm aspiration).

REFERENCES

1. Rosen RC. Prevalence and risk factors of sexual dysfunction in men and women. Curr Psychiatry Rep. 2000; 2:189–195.
2. Middleton RG, Urry RL. The Young-Dees operation for the correction of retrograde ejaculation. J Urol. 1986 Dec; 136(6): 1208–9.
3. Sharlip ID, Hellstrom WJ, Broderick GA. The ISSM definition of premature ejaculation: A contemporary, evidence-based definition. Journal of Urology, 179 (suppl), 340, abstract 988, 2008.
4. Althof SE. Treatment of rapid ejaculation: Psychotherapy, pharmacotherapy, and combined therapy (pp. 212–240). In S. R. Leiblum (Ed.), Principles and practice of sex therapy (4th ed.). NY: Guilford 2007.
5. Byers ES G Grenier. "Premature or Rapid Ejaculation: Heterosexual Couples' Perceptions of Men's Ejaculatory Behavior". Archives of Sexual Behavior, 2003, 32 (3): 261.
6. Althof SE et al. "International Society for Sexual Medicine's Guidelines for the Diagnosis and Treatment of Premature Ejaculation". Journal of Sexual Medicine, 2010. 7 (9): 2947.
7. Castleman, M Great Sex, Rodale, Inc., 2004: 137–138.
8. Masters W, V Johnson. Human Sexual Inadequacy, Little Brown and Company, 1970.
9. Belliveau F L Richter, Understanding Human Sexual Inadequacy, Hodder and Stoughton 1970.
10. Castleman M, Great Sex, Rodale, Inc., 2004: 136–137.
11. Kaplan, Helen S, PE: How to Overcome Premature Ejaculation, Brunner Mazel/New York Times, 1989: 48–58.
12. Metz M, B McCarthy, Coping with Premature Ejaculation, New Harbinger Publications, 2003: 123–128.
13. Silverberg, S. (1978, 2010), Lasting Longer: The Treatment Program for Premature Ejaculation, Physicians Medical Press, pp. 44–57.
14. Birch RW, A Short Book About Lasting Longer, PEC Publishing, 2007: 27–38.

Index

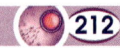